**Clinical Trials in Neurologic Practice**

Blue Books of Practical Neurology
*(Volumes 1–14 published as BIMR Neurology)*

1  **Clinical Neurophysiology**
Eric Stalberg and Robert R. Young

2  **Movement Disorders**
C. David Marsden and Stanley Fahn

3  **Cerebral Vascular Disease**
Michael J. G. Harrison and Mark L. Dyken

4  **Peripheral Nerve Disorders**
Arthur K. Asbury and R. W. Gilliatt

5  **The Epilepsies**
Roger J. Porter and Paolo I. Morselli

6  **Multiple Sclerosis**
W. Ian McDonald and Donald H. Silberberg

7  **Movement Disorders 2**
C. David Marsden and Stanley Fahn

8  **Infections of the Nervous System**
Peter G. E. Kennedy and Richard T. Johnson

9  **The Molecular Biology of Neurological Disease**
Roger N. Rosenberg and Anita E. Harding

10  **Pain Syndromes in Neurology**
Howard L. Fields

11  **Principles and Practice of Restorative Neurology**
Robert R. Young and Paul J. Delwaide

12  **Stroke: Populations, Cohorts, and Clinical Trials**
Jack P. Whisnant

13  **Movement Disorders 3**
C. David Marsden and Stanley Fahn

14  **Mitochondrial Disorders in Neurology**
A. H. V. Schapira and Salvatore DiMauro

15  **Peripheral Nervc Disorders 2**
Arthur K. Asbury and P. K. Thomas

16  **Contemporary Behavioral Neurology**
Michael R. Trimble and Jeffrey L. Cummings

17  **Headache**
Peter J. Goadsby and Stephen D. Silberstein

18  **The Epilepsies 2**
Roger J. Porter and David Chadwick

19  **The Dementias**
John H. Growdon and Martin N. Rossor

20  **Hospitalist Neurology**
Martin A. Samuels

21  **Neurologic Complications in Organ Transplant Recipients**
Eelco F. M. Wijdicks

22  **Critical Care Neurology**
David H. Miller and Eric C. Raps

23  **Neurology of Bladder, Bowel, and Sexual Dysfunction**
Clare J. Fowler

24  **Muscle Diseases**
Anthony H. V. Schapira and Robert C. Griggs

25  **Clinical Trials in Neurologic Practice**
José Biller and Julien Bogousslavsky

# Clinical Trials in Neurologic Practice

Edited by

**José Biller, M.D.**
Professor and Chairman, Department of Neurology, Indiana University School of Medicine, Indianapolis; Chief, Neurology Services, Department of Neurology, Indiana University Medical Center

*and*

**Julien Bogousslavsky, M.D.**
Professor and Chairman of Neurology, University of Lausanne, Switzerland; Chief of Neurology, University Hospital, Lausanne, Switzerland

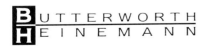

Boston    Oxford    Aukland    Johannesburg    Melbourne    New Delhi

Copyright © 2001 by Butterworth–Heinemann

 A member of the Reed Elsevier group

All rights reserved.

No part of this publication may be reproduced, stored in a retrieval system, or transmitted in any form or by any means, electronic, mechanical, photocopying, recording, or otherwise, without the prior written permission of the publisher.

Every effort has been made to ensure that the drug dosage schedules within this text are accurate and conform to standards accepted at time of publication. However, as treatment recommendations vary in the light of continuing research and clinical experience, the reader is advised to verify drug dosage schedules herein with information found on product information sheets. This is especially true in cases of new or infrequently used drugs.

Recognizing the importance of preserving what has been written, Butterworth–Heinemann prints its books on acid-free paper whenever possible.

 Butterworth–Heinemann supports the efforts of American Forests and the Global ReLeaf program in its campaign for the betterment of trees, forests, and our environment.

**Library of Congress Cataloging-in-Publication Data**
Clinical trials in neurologic practice / edited by José Biller, Julien Bogousslavsky.
 p. ; cm. — (Blue books of practical neurology ; 25)
 Includes bibliographical references and index.
 ISBN 0-7506-7140-8
 1. Nervous system—Diseases—Treatment. 2. Clinical trials. I. Biller, José. II. Bogousslavsky, Julien. III. Series
 [DNLM: 1. Nervous System Diseases—therapy. 2. Randomized Controlled Trials. WL 140 C6417 2001]
 RC346 .C557 2001
 616.8'046—dc21

00-056441

**British Library Cataloguing-in-Publication Data**
A catalogue record for this book is available from the British Library.

The publisher offers special discounts on bulk orders of this book.
For information, please contact:

Manager of Special Sales
Butterworth–Heinemann
225 Wildwood Avenue
Woburn, MA 01801-2041
Tel: 781-904-2500
Fax: 781-904-2620

For information on all Butterworth–Heinemann publications available, contact our World Wide Web home page at: http://www.bh.com

10 9 8 7 6 5 4 3 2 1

Printed in the United States of America

We dedicate this book to our families, and to Mark L. Dyken, M.D., and Franco Regli, M.D., mentors, colleagues, and friends.

# Contents

*Contributing Authors*                                                    ix
*Series Preface*                                                          xiii
*In Memory of C. David Marsden*                                            xv
*Preface*                                                                 xvii

1  Randomized Controlled Trials: Methodology, Outcomes,
     and Interpretation                          1
   *Linda S. Williams*

2  Clinical Trials in Stroke                                               27
   *John R. Marler*

3  Intracerebral Hemorrhage                                               49
   *Carlos S. Kase*

4  Aneurysmal Subarachnoid Hemorrhage Trials                              63
   *Luca Regli and Bernhard Walder*

5  Head Injuries                                                          77
   *Hugh J. L. Garton and Thomas G. Luerssen*

6  Clinical Trials in Spinal Cord Injury                                  99
   *Charles H. Tator and Michael G. Fehlings*

7  Clinical Trials in Epilepsy                                            121
   *Pierre Loiseau and Pierre Jallon*

8  Dementia                                                               147
   *Florence Pasquier and Jean-Marc Orgogozo*

9  Clinical Trials in Parkinson's Disease                                 173
   *Ergun Y. Uc, Andrea J. DeLeo, and Robert L. Rodnitzky*

10 Hyperkinetic Movement Disorders                                        201
   *Anna H. Hristova and William C. Koller*

viii  *Contents*

11  Multiple Sclerosis                                               221
    *Myriam Schluep and Julien Bogousslavsky*

12  Clinical Trials in Central Nervous System Infections             237
    *Cynthia M. Hingtgen and Karen L. Roos*

13  Peripheral Neuropathy Treatment Trials                           261
    *Christopher Klein, Michael Polydefkis, and Vinay Chaudhry*

14  Myasthenia Gravis: A Clinical Trials Perspective                 293
    *Robert M. Pascuzzi*

15  Clinical Trials in Muscle Disorders                              311
    *Renato Mantegazza, Carlo Antozzi, Ferdinando Cornelio,*
    *and Stefano Di Donato*

*Index*                                                              327

# Contributing Authors

*Carlo Antozzi, M.D.*
Neurologist, Neuromuscular Research Department, National Neurological Institute Carlo Besta, Milan, Italy

*José Biller, M.D.*
Professor and Chairman, Department of Neurology, Indiana University School of Medicine, Indianapolis; Chief, Neurology Services, Department of Neurology, Indiana University Medical Center

*Julien Bogousslavsky, M.D.*
Professor and Chairman of Neurology, University of Lausanne, Switzerland; Chief of Neurology, University Hospital, Lausanne, Switzerland

*Vinay Chaudhry, M.D., F.R.C.P. (U.K.)*
Associate Professor of Neurology, Johns Hopkins University School of Medicine and Johns Hopkins Hospital, Baltimore

*Ferdinando Cornelio, M.D.*
Director and Professor, Department of Neurology, National Neurological Institute Carlo Besta, Milan, Italy

*Andrea J. DeLeo, D.O.*
Fellow Associate, Department of Neurology, University of Iowa College of Medicine, Iowa City; Fellow in Movement Disorders, Department of Neurology, University of Iowa Hospitals and Clinics

*Stefano Di Donato, M.D.*
Department Head of Biochemistry and Genetics, National Neurological Institute Carlo Besta, Milan, Italy

*Michael G. Fehlings, M.D., Ph.D., F.R.C.S.C.*
Associate Professor of Surgery, University of Toronto Faculty of Medicine, Ontario; Staff Neurosurgeon, Department of Surgery, Toronto Western Hospital

x    *Contributing Authors*

*Hugh J. L. Garton, M.D., M.H.Sc.*
Lecturer, Department of Surgery, Division of Neurosurgery, University of Michigan, Ann Arbor; Attending Neurosurgeon, Department of Surgery, Division of Neurosurgery, University of Michigan Health Care System, Ann Arbor

*Cynthia M. Hingtgen, M.D., Ph.D.*
Assistant Professor, Department of Neurology, Indiana University School of Medicine, Indianapolis

*Anna H. Hristova, M.D.*
Fellow in Movement Disorders, Department of Neurology, University of Kansas Medical Center, Kansas City

*Pierre Jallon, M.D.*
Epilepsy Unit, Hospital Cantonal Universitaire, Geneva, Switzerland

*Carlos S. Kase, M.D.*
Professor of Neurology, Boston University School of Medicine; Attending Neurologist, Department of Neurology, Boston Medical Center

*Christopher Klein, M.D.*
Fellow in Clinical Neurophysiology, Department of Neurology, Johns Hopkins University School of Medicine and Johns Hopkins Hospital, Baltimore

*William C. Koller, M.D., Ph.D.*
Professor of Neurology, University of Miami School of Medicine

*Pierre Loiseau, M.D.*
Professor Emeritus of Neurology, University Hospital, Bordeaux, France

*Thomas G. Luerssen, M.D., F.A.C.S., F.A.A.P.*
Professor of Neurological Surgery, Indiana University School of Medicine, Indianapolis; Director of Pediatric Neurosurgery Service, James Whitcomb Riley Hospital for Children

*John R. Marler, M.D.*
Associate Director for Clinical Trials, National Institute of Neurological Disorders and Stroke, National Institutes of Health, Bethesda, Maryland

*Renato Mantegazza, M.D.*
Head of Neuroimmunology Laboratory, Department of Neuromuscular Diseases, National Neurological Institute Carlo Besta, Milan, Italy

*Jean-Marc Orgogozo, M.D.*
Professor of Neurology, University of Medicine, Bordeaux, France; Head of Neurology, CHU Pellegrin, Bordeaux, France

*Robert M. Pascuzzi, M.D.*
Professor and Vice Chairman, Department of Neurology and Co-Director of Resident Education, Indiana University School of Medicine, Indianapolis; Chief of Neurology, Wishard Health Services, Indianapolis

*Florence Pasquier, M.D., Ph.D.*
Professor of Neurology, Faculty of Medicine, Lille, France; Head of the Department of Neurology and Memory Center, University Hospital, Lille, France

*Michael Polydefkis, M.D.*
Fellow in Neurology, Johns Hopkins University School of Medicine and Johns Hopkins Hospital, Baltimore

*Luca Regli, M.D.*
Médecin Associé, M.E.R., Department of Neurosurgery, Centre Hospitalier Universitaire Vaudois, Lausanne, VD, Switzerland

*Robert L. Rodnitzky, M.D.*
Professor and Vice Chairman of Neurology, University of Iowa College of Medicine, Iowa City; Director of the Movement Disorders Clinic, University of Iowa Hospitals and Clinics

*Karen L. Roos, M.D.*
Professor, Department of Neurology, Indiana University School of Medicine, Indianapolis

*Myriam Schluep, M.D.*
Senior Resident in Neurology, Centre Hospitalier Universitaire Vaudois, Lausanne, Switzerland

*Charles H. Tator, M.D., M.A., Ph.D., F.R.C.S.C.*
Professor and Chairman of Neurosurgery, University of Toronto Faculty of Medicine, Ontario; Staff Neurosurgeon, Toronto Western Hospital

*Ergun Y. Uc, M.D.*
Assistant Professor of Neurology, University of Arkansas College of Medicine, University of Arkansas Medical Center, and Central Arkansas Veterans Health Care Systems, Little Rock

*Bernhard Walder, M.D.*
Research Fellow, Surgical Intensive Care Unit, University Hospitals of Geneva, Geneva, Switzerland

*Linda S. Williams, M.D.*
Assistant Professor, Department of Neurology, Indiana University School of Medicine and Roudebush VA Medical Center, Indianapolis

# Series Preface

The *Blue Books of Practical Neurology* series is the new name for the BIMR Neurology series, which was itself the successor of the *Modern Trends in Neurology* series. As before, the volumes are intended for use by physicians who grapple with the problems of neurologic disorders on a daily basis, be they neurologists, neurologists in training, or those in related fields such as neurosurgery, internal medicine, psychiatry, and rehabilitation medicine.

Our purpose is to produce monographs on topics in clinical neurology in which progress through research has brought about new concepts of patient management. The subject of each monograph is selected by the Series Editors using two criteria: first, that there has been significant advance in knowledge in that area and, second, that such advances have been incorporated into new ways of managing patients with the disorders in question. This has been the guiding spirit behind each volume, and we expect it to continue. In effect we emphasize research, both in the clinic and in the experimental laboratory, but principally to the extent that it changes our collective attitudes and practices in caring for those who are neurologically afflicted.

Arthur K. Asbury
Anthony H. V. Schapira
*Series Editors*

# In Memory of C. David Marsden

David Marsden was the first Series Editor for these monographs; he was asked by Butterworths in 1982 to take on this duty. Shortly thereafter, he recruited one of us (AKA) to join him. The principle that evolved for the Series was that each volume should feature practical aspects of neurology, with emphasis on those areas in which the fruits of research had improved and expanded the management of the neurologic disorders in question. This principle is the guiding spirit for the Blue Books of Practical Neurology and will remain so for as long as these volumes are published. It is one of the many legacies that David Marsden bequeathed to the fields of neurology and neuroscience and will serve as a living commemoration of this extraordinary man and his manifold accomplishments.

Arthur K. Asbury
Anthony H. V. Schapira
*Series Editors*

# Preface

The rapidly changing demographics of the world population create serious implications for society and its health care systems. Neurologic problems are common in general medical practice and often represent a heavy burden for patients and their families. The primary care physician will encounter these disorders with increasing frequency because of the change in demographics of the aging population ("the aging society") and the impact of managed care on health care delivery.

Since the early experiments on the treatment of scurvy in 1747, the controlled, randomized clinical trial has been increasingly recognized as the most reliable evidence of effectiveness and the best method of establishing the value of new and promising treatment approaches. There have been thousands of large randomized clinical trials relevant to neurologic disorders, and it would be exceedingly difficult for any one individual to keep track of all these trials. Randomized clinical trials are not only tools, they are also essential elements underlying high-quality medical care. To place the topic in context and to further facilitate and enhance the physician's ability to manage patients with neurologic disorders, this monograph, written by a distinguished group of trans-Atlantic experts, considers a selective list of highly prevalent neurologic disorders that demand not only the skilled competence of the neurologic practitioner but that also require familiarity of the primary care physician as well.

With this challenge in mind, Dr. Williams introduces this issue of the *Blue Books of Practical Neurology* by presenting a balanced and relevant review of clinical trial methodology and study design in Chapter 1.

Cerebrovascular disorders are a major health care problem. Stroke is the third leading cause of death in industrialized countries and the most common cause of disability. Each year there are, in the United States and European Union combined, approximately 1 million patients who have an acute stroke.[1] During the 1990s, investigators made great strides in preventing subsequent stroke in high-risk individuals. Likewise, the existence of a therapeutic window has formed the basis for the success of thrombolytic therapy in ischemic stroke if therapy is initiated within 3 hours. Drs. Marler, Kase, Regli, and Walder address these and other issues in an authoritative, comprehensive, and critical review in Chapters 2, 3, and 4.

xvii

xviii  *Preface*

Severe head injuries remain a leading cause of disability and death in young adults. Traumatic brain injury has an annual incidence ranging up to 430 per 100,000 population.[2] In the field of neurotrauma, the 1990s were characterized by great advances in our understanding of the pathophysiologic processes causing secondary brain and spinal cord damage. Current efforts in the management of spinal cord injury emphasize neuroprotective and regenerative approaches. Head and spinal cord injuries are discussed in Chapters 5 and 6 by Drs. Garton, Luerssen, Tator, and Fehlings, who provide full coverage on clinical trials in these areas.

Epilepsy affects approximately 1% of the world population at any one time. Epidemiologic studies have shown that the worldwide prevalence of epilepsy is 5–8 cases per 1,000. The pharmacologic treatment of epilepsy has made considerable progress in recent years, although 25–30% of patients will continue to have frequent epileptic seizures despite the use of antiepileptic drugs, or will experience unacceptable drug-related side effects.[3] Numerous novel antiepileptic drugs have been licensed around the world in the last few years. The exciting developments in randomized clinical trials in epilepsy are explored in Chapter 7 by Drs. Loiseau and Jallon, and practical considerations are offered on the rational use of monotherapy and polytherapy in the treatment of epilepsy.

Alzheimer's disease is the most common cause of dementia in the elderly, accounting for one-half to three-fourths of all cases. Vascular dementia, the second most common cause of dementia, may be preventable. Drs. Pasquier and Orgogozo provide a review of new cholinesterase inhibitors and other various therapeutic approaches in dementia in Chapter 8.

Extrapyramidal syndromes produce an array of motor symptoms that often burden already impaired patients. The identification of a marked decrease of dopamine content in the striatum of a patient with Parkinson's disease (PD) initiated a new era for the pharmacotherapy of PD. In addition, several other important biochemical abnormalities have been found to be implicated in the nigral degeneration observed in PD. However, limitations of long-term levodopa therapy for PD represent a major problem in the management of many of these patients; thus, new treatment strategies aim at slowing the progression of the disease. Tremors may cause significant disability; epidemiologic studies of essential tremor indicate 0.5–1.0% in the general population. Despite the recent discovery of the gene defect and its product, no curative therapy is available to date for Huntington's disease. Clinical trials on hypokinetic and hyperkinetic movement disorders are reviewed in Chapters 9 and 10 by Drs. Uc, DeLeo, Rodnitzky, Hristova, and Koller.

Multiple sclerosis (MS) is the most common central nervous system (CNS) demyelinating disease. The number of approved drugs available to treat MS exploded at the end of the twentieth century. These include three varieties of human interferon $\beta$ and glatiramer acetate. Drs. Schluep and Bogousslavsky review the revolutionary focus on major clinical trials of MS in Chapter 11.

Many human pathogens cause life-threatening CNS infections. Major advances in the treatment and chemoprophylaxis of a variety of CNS infections have occurred. Effective vaccination has significantly decreased the incidence of poliovirus infections of the CNS and postinfectious encephalitides. Advances in the treatment and prevention of bacterial meningitides, including potent bactericidal antibacterials and initial adjunctive therapy with dexamethasone, have

*Preface* xix

reduced the morbidity and mortality associated with these infections. In Chapter 12, Drs. Hingtgen and Roos address clinical trials in CNS infections.

Neuromuscular diseases comprise a varied and challenging collection of disorders that affect the final common pathways of the nervous system potentially leading to respiratory failure or inability to swallow or maintain adequate nutritional status. Muscle disorders, diseases of the peripheral nerves, and neuromuscular junction disorders are addressed in Chapters 13, 14, and 15 by Drs. Klein, Polydefkis, Chaudhry, Pascuzzi, Mantegazza, Antozzi, Cornelio, and Di Donato.

This monograph is obviously not an encyclopedic volume on clinical trials in the clinical neurosciences. A vast array of effective treatment options is currently available for the health care professional on the front line of care of the neurologically compromised patient. We hope this contribution will enhance evidence-based medicine decision algorithms, thereby protecting patients from ineffective or potentially harmful treatment.

We thank the authors for their authoritative contributions. We thank the publishers, particularly Susan Pioli, Jennifer Rhuda, and Sophia Battaglia, for their part in seeing this project through to fruition. We thank Phyllis Cowherd for her excellent administrative and clerical assistance. As always, the support and encouragement of family and friends have been appreciated.

José Biller, M.D.
Julien Bogousslavsky, M.D.

## REFERENCES

1. Sandercock PAG, Celani MG, Ricci S. The likely public health impact in Europe of simple treatments for acute ischaemic stroke (abstract). Cerebrovasc Dis 1992;2:236.

2. Field JH. Epidemiology of Head Injuries in England and Wales. London: Department of Health and Social Security, HM Stationery Office, 1976.

3. Annegers JF, Hauser WA, Elveback LR. Remission of seizures and relapses in patients with epilepsy. Epilepsia 1979;20:729–737.

**Clinical Trials in Neurologic Practice**

# 1
# Randomized Controlled Trials: Methodology, Outcomes, and Interpretation
Linda S. Williams

Neurology is a field that has always emphasized detailed observation and examination of patients, with the classic characterization of the neurologist's practice of "diagnose, then adiós." As advances in diagnostic techniques, molecular biology, and the genetic basis of disease have been realized, however, there has been a corresponding proliferation of clinical trials leading to new treatments for what were purely phenomenologic neurologic diseases.

The notion of experimenting on humans has its roots in the eighteenth century, with Lind's classic study of the treatment of scurvy, in which British sailors received various treatments, and only those who were given oranges and lemons experienced dramatic improvement of symptoms.[1] However, widespread use of systematic experimentation on humans for the purpose of testing therapies did not begin until the mid-1900s. The development of clinical trial techniques shares much ancestry with agronomy research, which began using scientific methods for comparing plant varieties well before this type of study was extrapolated to humans. What we now regard as a well-conducted clinical trial is a relatively recent occurrence, with most of the advances in clinical trial methodology occurring since the 1950s.

Before reviewing the methodology of clinical trials, it is critical to define what is meant by this sometimes misused term. A reasonable general definition of *clinical trial* for our purposes is that proposed by Friedman[2]: "... a *prospective* study comparing the effect and value of *intervention(s)* against a *control* in human beings [italics added]."

This definition introduces three critical components of a clinical trial: (1) the prospective nature of data collection, (2) the introduction of an intervention, and (3) the comparison of patients receiving the intervention to prospectively followed patients who do not receive the intervention (control subjects). The prospective nature of data collection separates a clinical trial from a case-control or retrospective cohort study. The presence of an intervention distinguishes a clinical trial from a

2   *Clinical Trials in Neurologic Practice*

prospective cohort study. The presence of a control group delineates a clinical trial from a case series. Although all of these other types of studies are aptly termed clinical *research*, they are not clinical *trials*.

Because of their ability to demonstrate clinically meaningful differences between interventions despite the biologic noise inevitable in human experimentation, randomized clinical trials (RCTs) have become the gold standard against which other clinical research is compared. Although the RCT is the clinical research design most closely resembling the tightly controlled experiment in the basic science laboratory, the complexity of experimenting on genetically and environmentally unique humans creates special challenges and necessitates extra care in research design and execution to avoid common and potentially disastrous pitfalls. The aim of this chapter is to provide an overview of the major issues in RCT design, implementation and interpretation, using examples from clinical trials in neurologic diseases when possible. Special emphasis on the emerging issue of patient-centered outcomes is included. The chapter concludes with a brief practical guide to reading and applying RCT data in daily practice.

## HYPOTHESIS

Like any experiment, an RCT should have a single, well-defined hypothesis around which the trial is designed. This question should be identified in advance and is the foundation of such critical issues as study population, sample size calculations, and design selection. Many RCTs hypothesize that a specific treatment is better than placebo; this type of study is the simplest RCT to design, conduct, and interpret. Other trials, often called *equivalency studies*, hypothesize that there is no difference between two treatments. It is important to recognize that demonstrating equivalency of two treatments is not the same as failing to demonstrate a difference between groups. Equivalency studies require different methods of sample size calculation; thus, they must be explicit about their prespecified hypotheses regarding the selection of the value below which any differences are considered not significant. Equivalency studies should also be preceded by a recent, well-designed RCT in a similar population that clearly demonstrates the efficacy of the standard treatment over placebo.

## CLINICAL TRIAL PHASES

The concept of different phases of clinical trials with different general objectives was first introduced by researchers at the National Cancer Institute in Bethesda, Maryland.[3] This classification has been widely accepted and now applies to RCTs in other disease conditions. Preclinical studies are typically in vitro or animal studies, the purpose of which is to demonstrate the mechanism of action of the compound and establish animal pharmacology and toxicology data. *Phase I* trials are typically tolerability studies in humans and serve to establish the maximum tolerated dose and side-effect profile of a compound by dose-escalation strategies. A typical strategy is to give a prespecified dose to a small number of subjects, often three to five, and then escalate to the next dose level until a prespecified proportion of patients experience toxicity. Some phase I trials use healthy volunteers, and some enroll patients with the disease for which the treatment purportedly may be effective. The subjects with disease are often the most severely affected, for whom no other effective treatment is known. As such, generalizing response to the compound from data at this stage of development is usually impossible. *Phase II* trials are meant to evaluate the biologic activity of the compound (early efficacy data) and may also be used to better estimate the rate and type of adverse effects. Phase II trials also serve to refine the choice of primary end point for the phase III trial. Most clinicians are familiar with *phase III* trials, because these are usually the types in which clinicians participate and the types most widely reported in the scientific literature. Phase III trials are designed to evaluate the efficacy of an intervention in a specific disease and population. Although phase III trials are the gold standard for demonstrating treatment efficacy in humans, pitfalls can include the selected nature of the subjects and the usually brief follow-up period. These deficiencies are addressed by a *phase IV* trial, which is an evaluation of outcomes in a wider range of subjects without a control group. This type of trial is sometimes called a *postmarketing study* and is valuable for its ability to help bridge the gap between efficacy (the benefit and risk of the intervention in an ideal setting) and effectiveness (the benefit and risk of the intervention in an unselected population receiving standard care).

## STUDY POPULATION

The population in which an RCT is conducted has a pervasive impact on the ability of the study to adequately test the stated hypothesis and on the interpretation of trial results. Figure 1.1 illustrates the select nature of participants in an RCT and is a reminder of the potential pitfalls when applying new interventions in individual patients.

Precisely because of this select nature of study participants, researchers designing an RCT must take special care to clearly define their study population. This allows the reader of the RCT to most accurately evaluate the intervention in light of his or her own patient(s). For the clinical trialist, there is a continual struggle to balance the internal and external validity of a study—that is, how valid the design of the particular study in that specific population is versus how valid the study is when applied to the more general population for whom the intervention is intended. It may be easier to show an effect of an intervention— for example, if the study population is homogeneous with respect to disease stage or severity. This homogeneity, however, may severely limit the generalizability of results. Despite this struggle, the principle that a study first must be internally valid is paramount; if it is not, the results cannot be reliably generalized to any population, regardless of how similar it is to the study population.

Even when carefully planned and described, participants in clinical trials have inherent differences compared to the experimental population. Geographic (either local, national, or international) and site (hospital-based, clinic-based, community sample) variables are usually unique to a particular study population and may introduce a variety of biases. One study of the potential magnitude of site-related

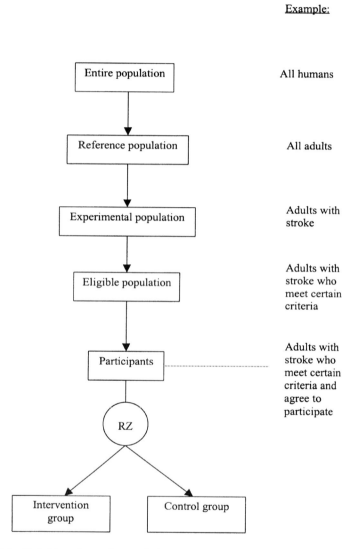

*Figure 1.1* Definition of a study population. (RZ = randomization.)

selection bias found that subjects from tertiary-care academic medical centers were different than the population-based subjects in a variety of ways.[4] Subjects from the academic centers were older and had different diseases than the population-based sample, and they also were more likely to desire aggressive care. The direction and magnitude of this potential bias can be difficult to estimate.

In addition to differences dependent on the site of recruitment, there are also systematic differences in study volunteers themselves: They are generally healthier, have less mortality, and are more likely to adhere to treatments than those who decline to participate.[5,6] These and other factors can make it difficult to generalize results from an RCT to clinical practice. Trialists should record, at a minimum, demographic information and reasons for exclusion on all potential subjects, and these differences should be reported. Comparing the study participants to nonparticipants can help to resolve the question of external validity of the RCT.

## TRIAL DESIGN

There are several general types of RCTs (Figure 1.2). All of them have unique statistical as well as practical considerations in design and interpretation. The most common type of RCT, which is exclusively described in subsequent sections on the considerations of sample size issues, is the *parallel* design. In this type of trial, two (or more) groups are enrolled and followed simultaneously, and subjects remain in the group into which they were initially randomized.

A variation of this type of trial is the *factorial* design, in which two or more interventions are compared with a control in a single experiment. When two interventions are tested, this is often referred to as a "2 × 2" design. One neurologic example of the factorial design is the Canadian Aspirin Sulfinpyrazone Transient Ischemic Attack (TIA) trial.[7] This trial enrolled patients with TIA and randomized them to receive either aspirin or placebo, then randomized subjects within these two groups to sulfinpyrazone or placebo. Thus, four treatments were tested for the prevention of subsequent stroke or TIA: aspirin only, aspirin plus sulfinpyrazone, sulfinpyrazone only, and no treatment. The advantage of this design is that two separate experiments can be conducted for only a small increase in sample size and, thus, cost. The difficulty of such a trial, however, is the possibility of an interaction between the two interventions—that is, the possibility that the effect of one intervention differs based on the presence or absence of the other intervention. This possibility is especially real if the two interventions act through similar pathways (e.g., platelet function, as in our example) or on the same response variable (e.g., bleeding time).

A third type of RCT design is the *crossover* design. This design allows each person to serve as his or her own control, which has the advantage of decreasing variability and thus requiring fewer subjects to demonstrate a given difference in treatments.[8,9] The simplest crossover study (see Figure 1.2) is the two-period crossover. In this design, randomization is not to treatment group but to order of treatment; thus, half of the subjects receive Treatment 1 first and half receive Treatment 2 (or placebo) first. After a prespecified time, the treatments are stopped and a washout period ensues. Then the treatments are reversed: Subjects who received Treatment 1 now receive Treatment 2 and vice versa. A run-in period may also be used before randomization to establish baseline disease characteristics, evaluate compliance, or allow washout of other medications. This type of study design is often used in headache research, in which a new antimigraine medication, for example, may be compared to placebo or to an established treatment. Crossover design is particularly well-suited to headache research, because the wide variability in individual headache patterns would require larger sample sizes for a parallel-design RCT to

### 2a. Parallel group design

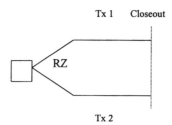

### 2b. Factorial design

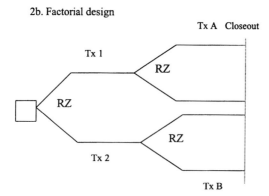

### 2c. Cross-over design

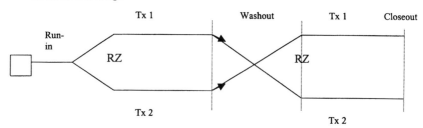

*Figure 1.2* Randomized controlled trial designs. (RZ = randomization; Tx = treatment.)

demonstrate a similar magnitude of difference between two treatments. Some of the disadvantages of crossover RCTs relate to the concept of the washout period and include (1) determining an appropriate washout period, (2) the assumption that washout does occur, and (3) the need to assess potential period-treatment interactions—that is, whether the treatment effect differs when given as the first treatment or as the second. Crossover trials also are more severely impacted by dropouts than are parallel trials. Further discussion of the advantages and disadvantages of crossover trials, especially as they apply to headache research, can be found in several references.[10–12]

*Randomized Controlled Trials: Methodology, Outcomes, and Interpretation* 7

*Table 1.1* Variables in the sample size calculation

| Parameter | Definition |
|-----------|-----------|
| α | Probability of a false-positive result (type I error), also called the *significance level* |
| β | Probability of a false-negative result (type II error) |
| δ | Difference between groups that is desired to be detected |

## Sample Size Calculation and Trial Power

Fundamental to the planning and the interpretation of RCTs is the issue of sample size calculation. Trialists must have a clear idea of the number of subjects needed to demonstrate a clinically meaningful difference in the intervention group. The reader of an RCT must have a clear idea of whether the trial was large enough to detect differences in outcomes that are reasonably expected to result from the intervention. Three main variables enter the sample size calculations (Table 1.1): (1) alpha (α), referred to as the *significance level*; (2) beta (β), the probability of a false-negative result, and (3) delta (δ), the expected difference in outcome between the two treatment groups. Three frequently used terms based on these variables also must be defined. *Type I error* is the false-positive occurrence of an observed difference in outcome between the intervention and control group. In other words, type I error refers to finding a difference when none really exists. The probability of this error is α. *Type II error* is the false-negative rejection of the null hypothesis. In other words, type II error refers to not finding a difference (a negative study) when a significant difference truly exists between the intervention and control groups. The probability of a type II error is β. The *power* of a study is defined as 1-β and is the probability of correctly rejecting the null hypothesis (the probability of finding a difference when one truly exists).

Before illustrating these parameters with an example from an RCT, it is important to realize that these three parameters are chosen by the investigators and should be clearly spelled out in any publication of trial results. Both α and β are typically based on convention: Investigators are usually more willing to fail to find a difference that truly exists than to find a difference that is false. Thus, β is typically larger than α. Most RCTs set β at 0.1–0.2 and set α at 0.05; therefore, the power of most trials (i.e., the probability of finding a difference that truly exists) is usually 0.8–0.9. The most malleable parameter specified by the investigators when planning an RCT is δ (the difference between the two groups that is desired to be detected). This parameter is critical to trialists, because it influences the overall number of subjects needed, and to clinicians, because it allows them to judge whether the difference the trial was powered to detect was reasonable and truly clinically meaningful. Investigators also must prespecify whether to look for differences in both directions (two-tailed, e.g., improvement or worsening) or in one direction only (one-tailed). Two-tailed tests are typically chosen, because it is difficult to justify not testing whether an intervention may be better or worse than the control.

These issues are illustrated by examining the Swedish Aspirin Low-Dose Trial.[13] This RCT was designed to assess the efficacy of low-dose aspirin (75 mg) as a secondary prevention of stroke and death after TIA or minor stroke. The pri-

8    *Clinical Trials in Neurologic Practice*

mary publication from this study defines the parameters entering into the sample size calculation as follows:

A preliminary conservative estimate of the necessary sample size was based on the expected incidence of stroke. With an incidence of 4% per year, *a 30% risk reduction*, 3-year inclusion in the study, and at least 2 years of follow up, a *type I error cut-off level of 0.05 (two-tailed)*, and a *type II error cut-off level of 0.20*, the required total number of patients was calculated to be 1,280 [italics added].

In this example, the authors have not only informed the reader what difference the trial was powered to detect (30% difference between treatment and control groups), they have also reported other pertinent estimates that influenced the trial planning. Many reports of RCTs do not clearly state these critical parameters.

The formulas for calculating sample sizes can be found in many statistical references.[2,14–16] Different sample size calculations are used for continuous variables (e.g., blood pressure) and proportions (e.g., the proportion of subjects who experience a recurrent stroke). Other equations are used for paired data, repeated measures, equivalency, and other types of outcomes. The equation given below, for sample size determination when the primary response variable is a proportion, is an example of one of the many sample size calculations. In any sample size calculation, $Z_\alpha$ and $Z_\beta$ are constants relating to the chosen $\alpha$ and $\beta$ levels and can be found in standard tables. The expected proportions of subjects are $-_I$ and $-_C$, with the outcome of interest in the intervention group $I$ and the control group $C$, given by $(-_I + -_C)/2$, while 2N is the total sample size required, and N is the sample size per group:

$$2N = 4(Z_\alpha + Z_\beta)^2 P(1 - P)/(P - C - P - I)^2$$

To illustrate, consider a trial with $\alpha = 0.05$ and $\beta = 0.2$, two-sided test, with the estimated proportion achieving the outcome of interest at 30% in the control group and 20% in the intervention group. The calculation would be the following:

$$2N = 4(1.96 + 0.84)^2((0.25(0.75))/(0.3 - 0.2)^2)$$

$$2N = 588(\text{round up to } 590)$$

$$N = 295 \text{ subjects per group}$$

The principles given below and in Table 1.2 illustrate the effects of varying any one of these components on the sample size requirements.

1.    *The smaller the difference the investigators want to detect, the more subjects are required.* The corollary is that the fewer the subjects, the larger the difference must be between groups for this difference to be detected. This principle has important implications. First, many trials are underpowered to detect differences that reasonably could be expected to be seen with the intervention (type II error). RCTs with too few subjects may, for example, only be able to detect a difference of greater than 50% between two groups, and few treatments are likely to produce

*Randomized Controlled Trials: Methodology, Outcomes, and Interpretation* 9

*Table 1.2*  Effects of varying parameters on sample size estimates

| Parameter change | Effect on sample size |
| --- | --- |
| Detect a smaller difference between groups | ↑ |
| Decrease the probability of a type I error (decrease α) | ↑ |
| Increase the power (decrease the probability of a type II error) | ↑ |
| Observe a higher event rate (more subjects with the outcome of interest) | ↓ |

↑ = increase; ↓ = decrease.

such dramatically different outcomes. One review of negative RCTs found that 94% had a greater than 10% probability of failing to detect a 25% difference between groups, and 70% had the same chance of missing a 50% difference in treatment effect.[17] Bigger is not always better, however, as trials that are very large may be able to detect statistical differences between groups that are of questionable clinical significance. For the clinician to balance these two aspects of an RCT, the difference the trial was powered to detect must be clearly stated.

2.  *The more certain the investigators want to be to only identify treatment that is truly beneficial (decrease the false-positive rate), the larger the sample size required.* Practically, this means that the investigators specify a smaller α (e.g., 0.01 instead of 0.05). This means that a difference is only considered significant if there is equal to or less than a 1% probability that the difference would be observed by chance. Trials with an extremely toxic investigational agent are examples of RCTs in which choosing a smaller α might be desired.

3.  *The more certain the investigators want to be about not missing a potentially beneficial treatment (decrease the false-negative rate, increase the study power), the larger the sample size required.* For example, β may be set at 0.1 instead of 0.2, giving the trial a power of 0.9 (1 – 0.1). This means that there is only a 10% probability that the trial will fail to identify a significant difference that truly exists between intervention and control groups. Investigators may choose lower levels of β (higher power) when conducting a trial in a disease with no other proven treatments. However, increases in power always come at the expense of more subjects required.

4.  *The more subjects that develop the outcome of interest, the fewer subjects needed overall.* This applies to secondary prevention trials such as the one in our example. If, using the Swedish Aspirin Low-Dose Trial example, the true incidence of secondary stroke or TIA was 8% instead of 4%, then fewer patients would be needed to achieve the number with the outcome of interest. It is easy to imagine how small variations in the estimated event rates can have serious implications for the length, and thus cost, of secondary prevention trials. Investigators must thoroughly search the available literature and their own proposed study populations for the best possible estimates to plan a study capable of providing efficacy data about two different treatments.

Other parameters that affect the sample size calculation often are not specified to the reader, including estimated dropout rates, losses to follow up, and noncompliance rates. Investigators must build in these estimates to ensure that an adequate number of subjects is enrolled.

10    *Clinical Trials in Neurologic Practice*

## RANDOMIZATION

Randomization was first reported in 1931, in a clinical trial of pulmonary tuberculosis treatment,[18] and was used at the National Institutes of Health beginning in the early 1950s.[3] In the ensuing decades, researchers have increasingly capitalized on the power of this technique in producing comparable groups.[19,20]

Randomization is a part of virtually all clinical trials, because it is powerful. This power is directly related to the tendency of randomization to produce groups that are alike in both measured and unmeasured characteristics. Thus, if the sample size is large enough, groups will have similar proportions with various risks for, or modifiers of, the disease in question, and they also will tend to have similar proportions of unmeasured (e.g., genetic, psychological, environmental) factors that may also modify treatment response. Another critical benefit of randomization is that it ensures that common statistical techniques can be used, because a probability distribution can be reliably assigned to each randomly allocated group, and associated significance levels can be constructed around the observed differences. The final benefit of randomization is that it removes the potential for bias in group allocation. This bias, usually termed *selection bias*, can be for or against the intervention and can occur consciously or subconsciously. Accordingly, proper methods of randomization must be used to ensure that group allocation is truly random—that is, that all subjects are equally likely to be assigned to either group. Proper randomization techniques also eliminate the potential for *accidental bias*, in which randomization fails to produce groups balanced for potential risk factors and covariates. Despite the critical influence of the randomization process, less than one-third of all trials adequately report their randomization procedures,[21] and some may actually use nonrandom allocation in a purportedly randomized design.[22] A critical search for mention of randomization methods should be part of every neurologist's checklist when evaluating an article about treatment.

Several randomization procedures have become widely used, and special computer software has been developed to aid in the randomization process. *Simple randomization* can be done in simple or more complex ways. One illustration of simple randomization is tossing an unbiased coin each time a person is eligible for randomization. It has been said that C. Miller Fisher kept one red marble and one blue marble in the pocket of his laboratory coat for the purposes of randomly assigning his patients to a variety of treatments. Assuming that the marbles were exactly the same size and weight, this is one illustration of a simple randomization technique. It is important to note that simply alternating treatment assignment is *not* a random method of group allocation. In an unblinded or single-blind study, alternating enrollment often leads to selection bias (e.g., delaying randomization so the preferred treatment will be assigned), and in a double-blind trial, unblinding results if the treatment allocation becomes known for any reason.

More commonly, a random table of numbers is used to allocate treatment groups. A typical strategy might include a random digit table, in which rows and columns contain the equally likely digits from 0 to 9. A row or column can then be randomly selected, and the sequence of digits in that row can be used to allocate treatment. Treatment A, for example, would be the assignment for those patients for whom the next digit was even, and Treatment B would be the assignment to those for whom the next digit was odd. For large RCTs, a computer-generated random number–producing algorithm is often used. The interval in which random numbers are to be produced is set (e.g., integers from 0–999). In this example, if the probability of treatment assignment is 0.5, then all subjects whose randomly generated number is between 0 and 499 would get Treatment A, and those with numbers from 500 to 999 would receive Treatment B.

Although this method of randomization is effective for large groups, at any one point during the trial there may be an imbalance of certain variables. This is especially problematic for smaller trials, as it can lead to a failure of randomization to produce balanced groups. To eliminate this potential pitfall, small trials often use *blocked randomization*. In this strategy, first described by Hill in 1951,[23] randomization occurs within even-numbered blocks (commonly 4 or 6) of subjects. This ensures that after every fourth randomized subject, for example, the number of participants in each group is equal. Another advantage of blocked randomization is that intervention groups are comparable even if the trial is terminated prematurely (e.g., for safety concerns). Multicenter RCTs also use blocked randomization because of the need to randomize within each site. This is done to eliminate the effects of site-specific patient mix and investigator practices. If one site has subjects with more severe disease, for example, and by chance has more patients randomized to the intervention group, the two groups may be unbalanced on critical variables affecting treatment response, thereby jeopardizing the ability of the RCT to demonstrate treatment efficacy.

Despite investigators' best efforts at successful randomization, subjects and investigators not infrequently find ways of subverting this process. Schulz et al.[24] analyzed the quality of randomization reporting and the estimated treatment effect in 250 controlled trials. Trials in which inadequate methods were used to ensure concealment of allocation consistently yielded larger estimates of treatment effects, with odds ratios exaggerated an average of 30–40%.[24] Because published accounts of actual instances of subverting randomization are understandably rare, Schulz related some anonymous examples of the lengths to which investigators and subjects may go to decipher randomization sequence or treatment assignment.[25] These accounts serve to remind us that, as Schulz says, "RCTs are an anathema to the human spirit," thus we should acknowledge the human elements of conducting RCTs and be vigilant in insisting on proper methods of randomization in controlled trials in neurology.


## BLINDING

*Blinding* refers not to the masking of randomization sequence, but to the masking of treatment group assignment. An *unblinded* study refers to one in which both patients and investigators are aware of group assignment. The major drawback to an unblinded study is the introduction of bias. This may result either from conscious or subconscious motivations of the subject (e.g., symptom reporting) or the investigator (e.g., outcome assessment). An elegant example of this subconscious bias is provided by Noseworthy and colleagues, in their report on the effects of blinding in an RCT in multiple sclerosis.[26] In the context of a randomized, placebo-controlled trial, patients were examined by both a blinded and an unblinded investigator. When the responses were compared, the unblinded neurologists' scores showed an erroneous treatment benefit at 6, 12, and 24 months,

12    *Clinical Trials in Neurologic Practice*

compared to the scores from the blinded neurologists. When the neurologist knew the patient was on active treatment, patients were scored higher than when known to be on placebo. This paper, as well as other examples,[27] reminds us of why unblinded treatment studies should be viewed with extreme caution. In situations in which it is not possible to blind patients or investigators, or both (e.g., a trial of surgery versus medical therapy), every attempt should be made to blind the investigators completing the outcome assessments for primary treatment efficacy. In a *single-blind* study, the investigators, but not the patients, are aware of treatment assignment. This type of design might be used when the intervention could have severe side effects necessitating physician knowledge of group assignment for participant safety. Although the problem of patient-introduced bias is obviated, the previous example illustrates why this is a suboptimal design. As described, this limitation can be partially overcome by having the outcome assessments completed by blinded investigators, although it does add to the complexity, and thus the cost, of the trial.

The preferred study design is a *double-blind* trial, meaning that both the investigators and the subjects are unaware of treatment assignment. This design has become the gold standard for questions of treatment efficacy, because it minimizes the introduction of bias more than other trial designs. It is important to note that, although double-blind trials minimize bias, they do not eliminate it. Bias in offering trial participation, concurrent treatment(s), and outcome adjudication may still occur, but these and other potential biases are less likely and have potentially less effect when randomization and blinding are well-executed.

Double-blind RCTs are most commonly used to test the efficacy of medical treatments. The new treatment is often compared to a placebo, or sham treatment. The decision to use a placebo instead of another treatment is supported when (1) no standard treatment is available for the condition, or (2) the condition in which the new treatment is being tested is self-limited (e.g., migraine headaches). In either case, subjects must be clearly informed that they may receive a placebo. Ethical arguments about the use of placebo in RCTs are not uncommon. These arguments often center on what constitutes "standard of care" and the informed consent process. An example of the debate over standard of care issues is the European Stroke Prevention Study 2, a randomized, double-blind $2 \times 2$ factorial design study, in which subjects with recent TIA or stroke were randomized to receive (1) aspirin alone, (2) dipyridamole alone, (3) aspirin plus dipyridamole, or (4) placebo for secondary stroke prevention.[28] This study was conducted from 1989 to 1995. Before this time, the efficacy of aspirin for the secondary prevention of stroke was clearly demonstrated in many studies and summarized in the Antiplatelet Trialists' Collaboration publication on antiplatelet therapy as secondary prevention.[29] The European Stroke Prevention Study 2 investigators wrote that, "In view of the conflicting data from the individual stroke prevention trials and the more recent debate with respect to the best dosing of aspirin, it was felt by the study group that a placebo control arm could not be avoided for assessing this low dose (25 mg twice daily) of aspirin."[28] This argument has been criticized by several authors, however, and remains difficult to defend in light of previous evidence.[30,31]

Another reason that it is critical to clearly define treatment and placebo groups is that placebo treatments may produce improvements that are at least measurable, if not equal, to the intervention. An informative example of the power of the placebo effect is Giang and colleagues' study of intravenous cyclophosphamide

*Randomized Controlled Trials: Methodology, Outcomes, and Interpretation*  13

for patients with progressive multiple sclerosis.[32] In this study, 10 patients received four treatments (intravenous cyclophosphamide) paired with a conditioned stimulus (an unusual taste). Patients received the treatment plus the stimulus or the stimulus alone in randomized, double-blind fashion in the next two treatment sessions. Eight of the 10 subjects had a decreased peripheral leukocyte count after the stimulus alone ($p = .04$), thus demonstrating the potential physiologic influences of a conditioned response.

Although double-blind trials increase the accuracy of treatment evaluations, there is a corresponding increase in trial complexity and expense. External committees must be formed for safety, data monitoring, and outcome adjudication. Emergency unblinding mechanisms must be established for patient safety. Extra personnel are sometimes needed for outcome assessment, especially if the treatment has unique physiologic effects that may unblind local investigators. Active drug and placebo must be formulated to look, taste, and smell as identical as possible; this is especially important for crossover studies, in which each subject takes both the active and control treatment. Adequate blinding may be impossible when two active treatments are being compared; in this instance, a "double-dummy" approach may be used, in which each treatment has an identical-appearing placebo. A subject would take Treatment A/placebo and Treatment B/placebo, with study medication bottles precoded so that no patient receives both treatments and no patient receives only placebo. A classic example of a failure to adequately blind two treatments is the trial involving vitamin C for the common cold; subjects found they could easily distinguish the ascorbic acid tablet from the sucrose-containing placebo by taste.[33] Some trials survey subjects or investigators, or both, about subject treatment assignment to determine the adequacy of blinding efforts.[34,35] If successful, demonstrating that no systematic unblinding occurred can strengthen readers' confidence in the trial results.

## OUTCOME ASSESSMENTS

Baseline data are usually collected at trial entry or during a prespecified interval before study entry. When prerandomization screenings are done, it is desirable to have the randomization take place as close to the screening period as is reasonably possible. Doing so ensures that no ensuing events make the patient ineligible or in other ways influence the likelihood of eventual outcomes. Once collected, these data have several important uses. First, the data are the source for determining whether study groups have equal distributions of variables (e.g., demographic and socioeconomic factors, disease risk factors, and severity indices). This comparison is critical because randomization *tends to produce* (not guarantees) balanced groups. Second, baseline data may identify variables on which randomization is to be stratified (e.g., a certain stage or severity of the disease under study). Even when not prespecified, baseline variables may identify important subgroups in which to perform secondary analyses. Third, baseline data may serve as the basis on which to gauge intersubject change (e.g., assess changes in health-related quality of life from study entry to exit).

Data may be collected from patient interviews, examinations, medical records, or laboratories. Although an often-unglamorous part of a trial, ensuring that data

## 14    Clinical Trials in Neurologic Practice

collection is of high quality is an essential component of high-quality output. This is especially critical for key types of data, such as baseline characteristics and primary outcomes.

The two main problems in data collection are incorrect data and missing data. Incorrect data may be randomly incorrect, or they may be systematically incorrect. Random data errors can be reduced by programming data entry systems to reject an entry outside a given range. Data forms should be designed for ease of data entry and accuracy. Computer entry of data from paper forms should use screens programmed to resemble the paper forms to reduce entry errors. Systematic errors can be assessed during the study—for example, to identify tendencies for the subjects of one interviewer to have higher scores on a depression scale than those of other interviewers. Variability of data is another component that may represent error in measurement or may be intrinsic to the variable being measured. Because increased variability results in a decreased ability to detect differences between groups, efforts to reduce measurement errors (e.g., using repeated measurements) and use measures that minimize intrinsic variability (e.g., well-validated questionnaires) are well spent. Missing data may be patient-related, as in loss to follow-up, or study-related (e.g., error in completing forms). Missing data create unique problems in data analysis, and strategies for dealing with missing data should be pre-specified. The percentage of missing data should be kept as low as possible and should be compared between groups. If significantly different, bias may be introduced, as the opportunity to observe outcome events is less in the group with more missing data. One common method of dealing with missing data is the "last observation carried forward" strategy.[36] In this case, sensitivity analyses can also be done in which analyses are completed as if all patients with missing data had the worst possible outcome and then as if all had the best possible outcome. This informs the reader about the effect of missing data on the trial results. Other methods of imputing missing data are more complicated.[37–40] Additional data may be found in a text by Little and Rubin.[41] It is important to note that many of these techniques assume that the data are randomly missing, meaning that the probability of missing data does not depend on the preceding measurement or on group assignment. Additional methods, all of which are less than ideal, must be used when data are missing nonrandomly.

Types of outcomes monitored include adverse events, compliance, and primary and secondary outcomes. Adverse events must be clearly defined before study initiation and should be systematically sought and recorded. The frequency of adverse event reporting is influenced by the ascertainment method. Open-ended questions tend to produce only the most recent or most severe symptoms. A checklist approach may identify many symptoms that are coincidental to treatment. These two methods have been compared in several trials, but no consistent relationship has been reported between method of ascertainment and frequency and severity of adverse events.[42–45] For ethical reasons, response variables indicating both benefit and harm must be measured throughout the trial, and stopping rules must be prespecified so that very efficacious or very harmful interventions can be identified and the risk to subsequent trial participants eliminated. Independent data and safety monitoring boards are usually constructed for this purpose. Rather than rely on a single test, several statistical methods are usually used

*Randomized Controlled Trials: Methodology, Outcomes, and Interpretation*    15

when monitoring data[46–49]; description of these diverse methodologies is beyond the scope of this chapter.

The degree to which participants complied with the study protocol informs the RCT reader about the validity of the results and the practicality of the intervention. Noncompliance tends to underestimate both benefit and risk associated with an intervention and thus increases the number of subjects needed to demonstrate a given difference in treatment effect. Methods of increasing compliance should be considered both before and during the study. Simplicity in study design, outcome assessment, and follow-up are key to maximizing compliance. During the trial, frequent contact with study personnel (nurses, research assistants), continuity of contact, telephone or mail reminders, family support, and keeping the subject well-informed enhance compliance. Compliance can be assessed in various ways, depending on the variable for which compliance is sought. Pill counts, patient diaries, laboratory assessments, and interviews are some of the common monitoring techniques. As described in the RCT Analysis section, noncompliers are often systematically different than compliers; this impacts the decision about which subjects to analyze.

Primary and secondary outcomes are critical to the validity of an RCT and must be chosen carefully. Both types of outcomes should be prespecified, and analysis strategies for these variables should be similarly preplanned. Special attention should be given before the trial starts to ensure the completeness and accuracy of data collection for these variables, as losses here can quickly doom a study.

Outcome variables may be continuous, categorical, or ordinal, and the sample size calculation and analyses vary for each type. Continuous variables are most often encountered as physiologic measurements (e.g., blood pressure). Continuous variables are simpler to analyze and usually (because of decreased variability) require fewer patients to document a given treatment effect; however, the clinical meaning of a change in the variable may be difficult to interpret. For example, a nerve conduction velocity of 43 meters per second may be statistically significantly different than 37 meters per second, but the clinical meaning of this difference may not be apparent to the patient. Categorical variables are those that fall into specific categories rather than numbers (e.g., gender or ethnicity). Global measures of outcome are often categorical (e.g., normal, mild disability, moderate disability, severe disability, or dead). Sometimes a multilevel categorical variable is collapsed into a dichotomous variable; this should be prespecified and based on pre-existing evidence so that it makes clinical or scale-related sense, or both. Ordinal variables are categorical variables that have a specific order; theoretically, this implies that the distance between each level is identical.

Sometimes the real variable of interest is difficult to measure or takes so long to develop that an RCT would take many years to observe the necessary number of outcome events. In this instance, surrogate outcome variables are sometimes used. Examples of surrogate outcome measures that are increasingly used in neurologic research are magnetic resonance image–based exacerbations in multiple sclerosis trials (which occur more frequently than clinical relapses) and infarct volume in acute stroke trials (which can be measured soon after the stroke rather than the typical 3- or 6-month follow-up). As demonstrated by the only modest correlation between stroke infarct volume and clinical outcome in one large RCT,[50] however, caution is warranted in extrapolating efficacy for a surrogate outcome measure to

16    *Clinical Trials in Neurologic Practice*

efficacy for the desired outcome. Ideally, the response of the surrogate to the intervention should be documented to be similar in magnitude and relation to other key outcome predictors as the primary outcome of interest. Practically, this validation is rarely performed. If a drug reduces the number of exacerbations on magnetic resonance image, is it valid to assume that it also reduces the number of clinical exacerbations and the long-term disability in patients with multiple sclerosis?[51] Questions like this will likely continue to confront both trialists and clinicians. Surrogate outcomes can be useful in identifying compounds with potential disease activity and thus are increasingly used in the drug discovery process.

The potential pitfalls of surrogate end points are illustrated by a study of cardiac arrhythmias. Before this study, the suppression of ventricular arrhythmias had been used as a surrogate for reducing the occurrence of sudden cardiac death, because it had been demonstrated that the presence of these arrhythmias correlated with an increased likelihood of sudden death.[52] The Cardiac Arrhythmia Suppression Trial showed, however, that the effective suppression of cardiac arrhythmias was not associated with decreased risk for sudden cardiac death but instead increased patient mortality.[53,54] Similar problems have been encountered in using CD-4 lymphocyte count as a surrogate outcome variable in Acquired Immune Deficiency Syndrome clinical trials,[55–57] and in tumor response as a surrogate outcome for survival in cancer trials.[57] Surrogate end points may be more appropriate in trials in which no other good therapy exists, because the need to rapidly identify potentially efficacious treatments may more easily outweigh the imprecision in knowing how the intervention directly relates to the primary outcome. Two helpful reviews of the uses of surrogate outcome measures are those by Prentice[58] and Gotzsche.[59]


## PATIENT-CENTERED OUTCOMES

Assessing the impact of health care interventions is increasingly shifting from biologic and physician-determined parameters (e.g., mortality, physiologic tests, physicians' global ratings) to patient-focused parameters. Although they can be more difficult to quantify, patient-centered outcomes such as functional status, life satisfaction, and health-related quality of life (HRQOL) are often more clinically relevant and, if adequately developed, as reliable as biologic or physiologic measures.

Because the most frequently measured patient-centered outcome is HRQOL, this discussion focuses on HRQOL assessment in RCTs. Although there may be semantic disagreements about what constructs underlie HRQOL, this concept broadly refers to the combination of physical, emotional, and social aspects of life that are or can be impacted by changes in health states.[60] Fundamental dimensions essential to HRQOL have been proposed and include the following: physical functioning, psychological functioning, social functioning and role activities, overall life satisfaction, and perceptions of health status.[61] Although each of these dimensions may not be an appropriate outcome to measure in every RCT, careful justification should be required before one of these elements is discarded from a standard instrument used in a particular study.

Once the decision to assess patients' HRQOL has been made, an investigator must choose which type of HRQOL assessment is most likely to help answer the research question. Guyatt and colleagues put forth a useful taxonomy for concep-

*Randomized Controlled Trials: Methodology, Outcomes, and Interpretation* 17

tualizing the different ways in which HRQOL outcomes may be measured.[62] In this classification, approaches to measuring HRQOL are divided into generic and disease-specific. Generic HRQOL can be assessed using a generic health profile instrument (e.g., the Medical Outcome Study Short Form-36) or with a utility measure (e.g., the Health Utilities Index). Disease-specific HRQOL is usually assessed with a measure designed to capture specific aspects of the disease in question and their impact on patients' HRQOLs.

Several key questions should be considered before deciding which HRQOL measure to use for a given RCT. First, the investigator must plan how the HRQOL results will be used. If the plan is to compare HRQOL in study patients to that of patients with another condition, then a generic HRQOL measure is appropriate. If the primary reason for collecting HRQOL data is so that a cost-effectiveness analysis can be performed, then a utility measure, which produces a single score from 0 to 1 representing the net impact of the condition on HRQOL, is needed. If within-patient change is the focus of the planned analyses, then a disease-specific instrument is advantageous, as responsiveness is usually greater in disease-specific than generic instruments.

After thinking about the use of HRQOL data, individual instruments must be inspected for their relevance for patients with the disease being studied. Disease-specific HRQOL measures are, by definition, more relevant in a given disease than generic measures; this translates into three key benefits of using disease-specific measures: (1) increased content validity of domains (e.g., inclusion of all relevant effects of the disease on HRQOL), (2) increased content validity of individual questionnaire items (e.g., asking questions in such a way as to capture disease impact and monitor disease activity), and (3) increased sensitivity to change.[63]

Once an idea about the content validity of individual instruments for the study population is formed, the reliability, validity, and responsiveness of the candidate instruments must be assessed. Reliability assessments usually are determined by internal consistency estimates, often Cronbach's alpha.[64] High internal consistency demonstrates that the instrument is relatively free of random error. Standards for what constitutes an acceptable reliability coefficient are arbitrary, but in general, an instrument used to measure within-patient change should have a higher coefficient than one used to measure between-group differences, and larger studies can tolerate less reliable measures than small studies.[65] These generalities are based on the fact that when scores are averaged across subjects, and when there are many subjects, the error of measurement is reduced in comparing group differences. Nunnally[66] advocated a reliability level of 0.9 for instruments measuring within-patient change, but practically this would require using longer instruments, as the reliability of a scale increases as the number of items increases. Other types of reliability that are commonly assessed but may be less applicable in a clinical trials setting are test-retest and inter-rater reliability.

Unlike reliability, scale validity is typically evaluated in a variety of ways, and, as Aaronson says, "involves perhaps as much art as it does science."[67] Different types of validity have confusing and somewhat overlapping names. Some common types of scale validity include the following: (1) *face validity* (do the items appear well-constructed and understandable?); (2) *content validity* (do the items cover the range of effects of the disease?); (3) *criterion-related validity* (does the instrument have the expected relationship to a gold standard measure of the construct [in this case, HRQOL]?); and (4) *construct validity* (does the instrument [or an individual

18    *Clinical Trials in Neurologic Practice*

*Table 1.3*    Responsiveness statistics

| Statistic | Calculation* |
|---|---|
| Standardized effect size | $\dfrac{\text{(mean score 2} - \text{mean score 1)}}{\text{sd (score 1)}}$ |
| Standardized response mean | $\dfrac{\text{(mean score 2} - \text{mean score 1)}}{\text{sd (mean score 2} - \text{mean score 1)}}$ |
| Minimally important difference | $\dfrac{\text{"minimal clinically important difference"}}{\text{sd (mean score 2} - \text{mean score 1)}}$ |

sd = standard deviation.

*Score 1 refers to score at time 1, *score 2* refers to score at time 2.

domain within the instrument] have the expected relationship to other outcome measures in the disease or to other measures of similar theoretical constructs?)

Scale responsiveness refers to the ability of the instrument to assess an individual's change over time. An instrument may be reliable and valid, but for clinical trial purposes may not be useful if it is not capable of detecting small but meaningful changes over time.[68] Obtaining useful information about an individual scale's responsiveness is complicated for two reasons: (1) Responsiveness is frequently not assessed as part of the development process, and (2) no standard method of measuring responsiveness or of comparing the responsiveness of different scales is agreed upon.

Because no standard measure exists, responsiveness is often measured in several ways; most of these statistics involve dividing change scores by some indicator of the precision of measurement (Table 1.3). One approach is to calculate the effect size, which can be done in one of two ways: (1) the mean change score divided by the standard deviation of the variable at baseline (referred to as *standardized effect size*)[69,70] or (2) the mean change score divided by the standard deviation of the change scores (referred to as the *standardized response mean*).[71] Guyatt and colleagues have suggested measuring change using the *minimal important difference* divided by the standard deviation of the change scores,[72–74] but the minimal important difference is not universally defined and probably varies between scales, populations, and diseases. Methods for determining the statistical significance of the difference in responsiveness of two instruments[75] and the clinical significance of differences in responsiveness[76] have also been proposed, but these methods are not yet widely used in RCT analysis.

Regardless of the statistic, change scores can be used for several different purposes, including the following: (1) measuring differences between individuals in the amount of change experienced, (2) identifying correlates of change, and (3) inferring treatment effects from group differences. A review of responsiveness statistics and an example of their use are provided in an analysis of the responsiveness of the Sickness Impact Profile (SIP) and the SIP68.[77] An overview of the psychometric aspects of HRQOL measures is Hays and colleagues' paper,[78] and other discussions of scale development and the uses of HRQOL measures in RCTs can be found in several manuscripts[60,62,66,79] and books.[80–83]

# RANDOMIZED CONTROLLED TRIAL ANALYSIS

Data analysis of RCTs is dependent on thorough planning before study initiation and on the quality of data collected during the trial. No analysis can satisfactorily correct for poor planning or sloppy data collection, and inappropriate analyses can mislead clinicians about the true benefit and risk of the intervention. Specific strategies for data analysis of RCTs, including multicenter RCTs, are beyond the scope of this chapter; references include a variety of texts and manuscripts.[84–88] Although there are many important topics in RCT data analysis, this section focuses on three of the most common issues: (1) intention to treat (ITT) versus efficacy analysis, (2) the problem of multiple comparisons, and (3) the proper use and interpretation of subgroup analyses.

Although seemingly straightforward, the question of which subjects to analyze is often raised.[89,90] Some authors advocate only analyzing patients who actually received the intervention, whereas many investigators believe that all subjects assigned to an intervention group should be analyzed as part of that group, regardless of the degree to which they received the intervention (ITT). Although at first glance it seems logical to only analyze those subjects who actually received the treatment, it is critical to understand that removing randomized subjects from the analysis can easily introduce bias, and this bias is often of unknown magnitude and direction. The reason that bias is often introduced when subjects are removed from their assigned group is that their reason for not receiving the intervention is not random. In other words, there is an association between the factors leading to their failure to receive the intervention and the outcome of interest. Common reasons for excluding patients from analysis are that they are noncompliant (i.e., they did not fully adhere to the study protocol), have critical missing data, or did not actually meet study entrance criteria. It is not difficult to see, however, how these factors may be systematically related to different outcomes: Sicker patients may have more difficulty adhering to treatment protocols, be more likely to be lost to follow-up, and be more likely to experience the outcome of interest. Retrospective identification of patients who did not actually meet study criteria can also introduce bias, especially if the methods for identifying these subjects are not systematic and are not done by someone blinded to primary and secondary end points. Even if the absolute number of subjects removed from analysis is the same in the intervention and the control groups, the reasons for removal may not be the same in each group and may not apply to the same type of subject in each group.

Several RCTs illustrate some of these potential biases. An example of the pitfalls of failing to account for patients lost to follow-up is the Joint Study of Extracranial Arterial Occlusion.[91] The study reported that the risk reduction for TIA, stroke, or death was significantly greater for patients receiving surgery. However, when all patients were accounted for (including those who were not available for follow-up because of stroke or death) the benefit of surgery was not significantly greater than medical therapy. Classic examples of potential biases resulting from removing subjects from analysis are illustrated with two cardiac trials.[92,93] Both of these trials demonstrate that noncompliance is associated with worse outcomes in both the intervention and the placebo group. The Coronary Drug Project[92] tested the effect of lipid-lowering drugs on mortality after myocardial infarction. There was an apparent benefit from taking clofibrate, as those

## 20    Clinical Trials in Neurologic Practice

with at least 80% compliance had a mortality of 15%, versus 24.6% for noncompliers. However, a similar relationship was seen in the placebo patients, in whom compliers had a mortality of 15%, versus 28% for noncompliers. The Aspirin Myocardial Infarction Study also showed that compliant subjects in both treatment and control groups had significantly lower mortality than noncompliers.[93] These studies serve as reminders that significant bias may be introduced when subjects are post hoc excluded from trial analyses and that noncompliers in RCTs often have worse outcomes than compliers, regardless of their treatment group. Including noncompliant subjects in the analysis thus tends to decrease the ability of the RCT to demonstrate a difference between groups; if nonadherence is expected to be substantial because of treatment- or subject-specific characteristics, the sample size should be increased accordingly to compensate for the dilution of treatment effect.

The problem of multiple comparisons is frequently encountered in RCTs. Most trials compare subjects on many variables, including baseline variables, primary and secondary outcome variables, and repeated comparisons over time on the same variable(s). An investigator's choosing a significance level of 0.05 translates to an average of 5 of every 100 statistical tests (1 of 20) being positive by chance. Investigators can best combat this problem by carefully preplanning the analyses and limiting the number of tests done on baseline and primary outcome variables. Alternatively, a more stringent significance level may be chosen (e.g., 0.01), but this often results in a prohibitively large sample size requirement. A number of strategies for adjusting the significance level when performing multiple tests have been suggested; the most conservative of these is to divide the significance level ($\alpha$) by the number of tests done.[94] In general, primary analyses should be specified *a priori* and limited in number to avoid this problem, and secondary analyses should be viewed primarily as hypothesis-generating, because RCTs are typically not powered to demonstrate meaningful differences in these variables.

This problem with secondary analyses is related to the third common analysis problem in RCTs—that is, the conduct and interpretation of subgroup analyses. It is important to identify, for both positive and negative RCTs, subgroups who are more likely to experience benefit or harm from the intervention. Although this is often a clinically relevant question, it is critical to remember that in most RCTs, randomization does not occur within these subgroups (this would imply a factorial design); thus the groups tend to be unbalanced on both measured and unmeasured variables. This imbalance can introduce bias, and because many potentially important variables are unmeasured or unmeasurable, the magnitude and direction of the bias may be difficult to ascertain. Even when subgroups are identified *a priori*, the RCT is not usually powered to detect differences in these smaller groups; thus the likelihood of type II error is great. If many subgroups are analyzed, the risk of finding a significant association by chance (type I error) also is increased. An example of this problem is illustrated by the Second International Study of Infarct Survival trial, in which a relationship between astrologic sign and treatment benefit was discovered.[95] The benefit of carotid endarterectomy for the secondary prevention of cerebrovascular events in women has also been questioned because of subgroup analysis in the Asymptomatic Carotid Atherosclerosis Study.[96] In general, subgroup analyses should be viewed as hypothesis-generating and should not by themselves influence therapy. Factors that may suggest increased validity of subgroup analyses are similarity to other well-conducted trials in that subgroup, similar subgroup findings at multiple sites within a multicenter trial, and biologic evidence of different treatment responses in the subgroups.

## Reporting Randomized Controlled Trial Results

Despite the proliferation of RCTs and their acceptance as the gold standard for evaluating interventions in humans, many studies are still inadequately designed and reported. Recognizing the persistent problem of type II error (RCTs too small to observe even moderate to large differences in treatments) and the lack of useful information about trial design, methods, and analysis in most published RCTs, the Standards of Reporting Trials group and the Asilomar Working Group on Recommendations for Reporting of Clinical Trials in the Biomedical Literature met to synthesize guidelines for the uniform reporting of RCTs.[97] This work, referred to as the *CONSORT statement* (Consolidated Standards of Reporting Trials), has become the standard by which many journals evaluate submitted RCT manuscripts. The CONSORT statement suggested six headings (title, abstract, introduction, methods, results, and comment) and five subheadings for greater manuscript clarity and completeness of reporting. The additional subheadings are: (1) protocol, (2) assignment, and (3) masking (blinding) subheadings in the methods section; and (4) participant flow and follow-up and (5) analysis subheadings in the results section. In addition, the groups suggested a flow diagram detailing the number of subjects eligible for, randomized to, and completing the study, as well as the reasons for nonrandomization and noncompletion. Many major journals have adopted these guidelines for all manuscripts describing an RCT. Although there is some evidence that the quality of RCTs is improving over time, as exemplified by a review of acute stroke trials,[98] there are not yet specific data regarding the impact of the CONSORT statement. Nonetheless, clinical trialists in neurology and readers of these trials would be well-served by paying close attention to these suggested reporting criteria.

## Interpreting Randomized Controlled Trial Results

In addition to the suggested criteria in the CONSORT statement, readers of clinical trials require some additional information from RCTs. This information, useful for assessing how trial results may impact individual patients, has been summarized as a series of six questions in the book *Clinical Epidemiology. A Basic Science for Clinical Medicine*[99]:

1. Was the assignment of patients to treatments really randomized?
2. Were all clinically relevant outcomes reported?
3. Were the study patients recognizably similar to your own?
4. Were both clinical and statistical significance considered?
5. Is the therapeutic maneuver feasible in your practice?
6. Were all the patients who entered the study accounted for at its conclusion?

The systematic use of such questions can aid in the difficult problem of translating RCT results into daily practice. In addition to these questions, clinicians may

## 22   Clinical Trials in Neurologic Practice

find it useful to calculate the number of patients needed to treat (NNT) to prevent one undesirable outcome.[99] This is a useful statistic for comparing two different treatments for the same disease and can be easily calculated from any RCT report. The NNT is the reciprocal of the *absolute* risk reduction, and it helps to put the magnitude of the *relative* risk reduction (often emphasized) into clinical perspective. An instructive example is the CAPRIE trial, in which 19,185 subjects with recent stroke, myocardial infarction, or symptomatic peripheral vascular disease were randomized to receive aspirin or clopidogrel for the prevention of secondary stroke, myocardial infarction, or vascular death.[100] One or more of these adverse outcomes was experienced by 5.83% of those receiving aspirin and 5.32% of those receiving clopidogrel. Although significant ($p = .043$), this translates to a relative risk reduction of 8.7% and an absolute risk reduction of 0.05%; thus, 200 patients (1/0.005) would have to be treated with clopidogrel rather than aspirin to prevent one more stroke, myocardial infarction or vascular death. A large NNT may not indicate less clinical relevance if the treatment is inexpensive or is significantly safer, but, if these conditions are not met, the NNT helps to put the real benefit from the treatment into sharper clinical perspective.

The interpretation of HRQOL outcomes is less standardized. The crucial question that remains unanswered is "What level of difference in scores is clinically meaningful?" One approach to answering this question has been suggested by Guyatt and colleagues in their concept of the "minimally important difference."[72–74] Their research suggests that for HRQOL measures with 7-point response scales (e.g., 7 levels ranging from "a lot worse" to "a lot better"), a difference in scale score of 0.5 points tends to correlate with patient reports of meaningful improvement. Although this is a useful theoretical concept, the technique needs to be tested using other instruments (including those with different response scales) and in other diseases. General guidelines for interpreting HRQOL data in RCTs have been suggested.[101] Important issues addressed are (1) how to assess the validity of the HRQOL measures used, (2) whether the HRQOL measures performed as expected, (3) how to evaluate the magnitude of effect on HRQOL outcomes, and (4) how to translate HRQOL data from an RCT to daily clinical practice.

## CONCLUSIONS

The efforts invested by both physicians and patients to plan, conduct or participate in, analyze, and report results from an RCT are enormous. Despite these difficulties, RCTs have proliferated because there is no better way to answer the question of whether an intervention truly benefits the people for whom it is intended. Although the fundamental design of RCTs has remained constant, the methods for assessing outcomes, analyzing results, and interpreting clinical meaningfulness continue to evolve. Whether involved in RCTs as a trialist, a co-investigator in a multicenter trial, or as a front-line implementer of trial results, an understanding of the basic issues in the design, conduct, analysis, and interpretation of RCTs is fundamental to success in our ultimate goal: improving the lives of our patients.

## Acknowledgments

Dr. Williams is supported by a Research Career Development Award from the Office of Research and Development, Health Services Research and Development, Department of Veterans Affairs.

## REFERENCES

1. Bull JP. The historical development of clinical therapeutic trials. J Chronic Dis 1959;10:218–248.
2. Friedman LM, Furberg CD, DeMets DL (eds). Fundamentals of Clinical Trials (3rd ed). St. Louis: Mosby-Year Book, Inc., 1996.
3. Byar DP. Discussion of papers on "historical and methodological developments in clinical trials at the National Institutes of Health." Stat Med 1990;9:903–906.
4. Layde PM, Broste SK, Desbiens N, et al. Generalizability of clinical studies conducted at tertiary care medical centers: a population-based analysis. J Clin Epidemiol 1996;49:835–841.
5. Smith P, Anesen H. Mortality in non-consenters in a post-myocardial infarction trial. J Intern Med 1990;228:253–256.
6. Wilhelmsen L, Ljungberg S, Wedel H, Werko L. A comparison between participants and non-participants in a primary preventive trial. J Chron Dis 1976;29:331–339.
7. The Canadian Cooperative Study Group. A randomized trial of aspirin and sulfinpyrazone in threatened stroke. N Engl J Med 1978;299:53–59.
8. Louis TA, Lavori PW, Bailar JC III, Polansky M. Crossover and self-controlled designs in clinical research. N Engl J Med 1984;310:24–31.
9. Woods JR, Williams JG, Tavel M. The two-period crossover design in medical research. Ann Intern Med 1989;110:560–566.
10. Jones B, Kenward MG. Design and Analysis of Cross-Over Trials. London: Dhapman and Hall, 1989.
11. Jones B, Lewis JA. The case for crossover trials in phase III trials. Stat Med 1995;14:1025–1038.
12. Olesen J, Tfelt-Hansen P. Headache. In RJ Porter, BS Schoenberg (eds), Control Clin Trials In Neurological Disease. Boston: Kluwer Academic Publishers, 1990;185–201.
13. The SALT Collaborative Group. Swedish aspirin low-dose trial (SALT) of 75 mg aspirin as secondary prophylaxis after cerebrovascular ischemic events. Lancet 1991;338:1345–1349.
14. Donner A. Approaches to sample size estimation in the design of clinical trials—a review. Stat Med 1984;3:199–214.
15. Lachin JM. Introduction to sample size determination and power analysis for clinical trials. Control Clin Trials 1981;2:93–113.
16. Phillips AN, Pocock SJ. Sample size requirements for prospective studies, with examples for coronary heart disease. J Clin Epidemiol 1989;42:639–648.
17. Frieman JA, Chalmers TC, Smith H Jr, et al. The importance of beta, the type II error and sample size in the design and interpretation of the randomized controlled trial: survey of 71 "negative" trials. N Engl J Med 1978;299:690–694.
18. Amberson JB Jr, McMahon BT, Pinner M. A clinical trial of sancroysin in pulmonary tuberculosis. Am Rev Tuberc 1931;24:401–435.
19. Kalish LA, Begg CB. Treatment allocation methods in clinical trials: a review. Stat Med 1985; 4:129–144.
20. Pocock SJ. Allocation of patients to treatment in clinical trials. Biometrics 1979;35:183–197.
21. Williams DS, Davis CE. Reporting of assignment methods in clinical trials. Control Clin Trials 1994;15:294–298.
22. Altman D, Doré CJ. Randomization and baseline comparisons in clinical trials. Lancet 1985; 335:149–155.
23. Hill AB. The clinical trial. Br Med Bull 1951;7:278–282.
24. Schulz KF, Chalmers I, Hayes RJ, Altman DG. Empirical evidence of bias: dimensions of methodological quality associated with estimates of treatment effects in controlled trials. JAMA 1995;273:408–412.
25. Schulz KF. Subverting randomization in controlled trials. JAMA 1995;274:1456–1458.

## 24   Clinical Trials in Neurologic Practice

26. Noseworthy JH, Ebers GC, Vandervoort MK, et al. The impact of blinding on the results of a randomized, placebo-controlled multiple sclerosis clinical trial. Neurology 1994;44:16–20.
27. Pascuzzi RM. Blinded and seeing the light (John Noseworthy, Lou Gehrig and other tales of enlightenment). Semin Neurol 1998;18:415–418.
28. Diener HC, Cunha L, Forbes C, et al. European Stroke Prevention Study 2. Dipyridamole and acetylsalicylic acid in the secondary prevention of stroke. J Neurol Sci 1996;143:1–13.
29. Antiplatelet Trialists' Collaboration. Secondary prevention of vascular disease by prolonged antiplatelet treatment. BMJ 1988;296:320–331.
30. Enserink M. Fraud and ethics charges hit stroke drug trial. Science 1996;274:2004–2005.
31. Barner A. Aspirin and stroke. Science 1997;275(5304):1246–1247.
32. Giang DW, Goodman AD, Schiffer RB, et al. Conditioning of cyclophosphamide-induced leukopenia in humans. J Neuropsychiatry Clin Neurosci 1996;8:194–201.
33. Karlowski TR, Chalmers TC, Grenkel LD, et al. Ascorbic acid for the common cold: a prophylactic and therapeutic trial. JAMA 1975;231:1038–1042.
34. Howard J, Whittemore AS, Hoover JJ, et al. How blind was the patient blind in AMIS? Clin Pharmacol Ther 1982;13:543–553.
35. Mosucci M, Byrne L, Weintraub M, Cox C. Blinding, unblinding, and the placebo effect: an analysis of patients' guesses of treatment assignment in a double-blind clinical trial. Clin Pharmacol Ther 1987;41:256–265.
36. Greenless JS, Reece WS, Zieschang KD. Imputation of missing values when the probability of response depends on the variable being imputed. J Am Stat Assoc 1982;77:251–261.
37. Espeland MA, Byington RP, Hire D, Davis VG, et al. Analysis strategies for serial multivariate ultrasonographic data that are incomplete. Stat Med 1992;11:1041–1056.
38. Efron B. Missing data and the bootstrap. J Am Stat Assoc 1994;89:463–474.
39. Downey RG, King, C. Missing data in Likert ratings: a comparison of replacement methods. J Gen Psychol 1998;125:175–191.
40. Fayers PM, Curran D, Machin D. Incomplete quality of life data in randomized trials: missing items. Stat Med 1998;15:679–696.
41. Little RJA, Rubin DB. Statistical Analysis with Missing Data. New York: John Wiley & Sons, 1987.
42. Avery CW, Ibelle BP, Allison B, Mandell N. Systematic errors in the evaluation of side effects. Am J Psychiatry 1967;123:875–878.
43. Downing RW, Rickels K, Meyers F. Side reactions in neurotics: 1. A comparison of two methods of assessment. J Clin Pharmacol 1970;10:289–297.
44. Simpson RJ, Tiplady B, Skegg DCG. Event recording in a clinical trial of a new medicine. BMJ 1980;280:1133–1134.
45. Canner PL. Monitoring of the data for evidence of adverse or beneficial treatment effects. Control Clin Trials 1983;4:467–483.
46. Fleming T. DeMets DL. Monitoring of clinical trials: issues and recommendations. Control Clin Trials 1993;14:183–197.
47. Pocock SJ. Statistical and ethical issues in monitoring clinical trials. Stat Med 1993;12:1459–1469.
48. Baum M, Houghton J, Abrams K. Early stopping rules—clinical perspectives and ethical considerations. Stats Med 1994;13:1459–1470.
49. Green SB, Freedman LS. Early stopping of prevention trials when multiple outcomes are of interest: a discussion. Stats Med 1994;13:1479–1484.
50. Saver JL, Johnston KC, Homer D, et al. Infarct volume as a surrogate or auxiliary outcome measure in ischemic stroke clinical trials. Stroke 1999;30:293–298.
51. Rudick RR, Antel J, Confavreux C, et al. Clinical outcomes assessment in multiple sclerosis. Ann Neurol 1996;40:469–479.
52. Bigger JT Jr, Fleiss JL, Kleiger R, et al. The relationships among ventricular arrhythmias, left ventricular dysfunction, and mortality in the 2 years after myocardial infarction. Circulation 1984; 69:250–258.
53. The Cardiac Arrhythmia Suppression Trial (CAST) Investigators. Preliminary report: effect of encainide and flecainide on mortality in a randomized trial of arrhythmia suppression after myocardial infarction. N Engl J Med 1989;321:406–412.
54. The Cardiac Arrhythmia Suppression Trial II Investigators. Effect of the antiarrhythmic agent moricizine on survival after myocardial infarction. N Engl J Med 1992;327:227–233.
55. Aboulker J-P, Swart AM. Preliminary analysis of the Concorde trial. Lancet 1993;341:889–890.
56. Fischl MA, Olson RM, Follansbee SE, et al. Zalcitabine compared with zidovudine in patients with advanced HIV-1 infection who received previous zidovudine therapy. Ann Intern Med 1993; 118:762–769.

## Randomized Controlled Trials: Methodology, Outcomes, and Interpretation 25

57. Fleming TR. Surrogate markers in AIDS and cancer trials. Stat Med 1995;13:1423–1435.
58. Prentice RL. Surrogate end points in clinical trials: definition and operational criteria. Stat Med 1989;8:431–440.
59. Gotzsche PC, Liberati A, Torri V, Rossetti L. Beware of surrogate outcome measures. Int J Technology Assess Health Care. 1996;12:238–246.
60. Guyatt G, Feeny D, Patrick D. Issues in quality-of-life measurement in clinical trials. Control Clin Trials 1991;12:81S–90S.
61. Berzon R, Hays RD, Shumaker SA. International use, application and performance of health-related quality of life instruments. Qual Life Res 1993;2:367–368.
62. Guyatt GH, Veldhuyzen Van Zanten SJO, Feeny DH, Patrick DL. Measuring quality of life in clinical trials: a taxonomy and review. Can Med Ass J 1989;140:1441–1448.
63. Williams LS. Health-related quality of life outcomes in stroke. Neuroepidemiology 1998;17:116–120.
64. Cronbach LJ. Coefficient alpha and the internal structure of tests. Psychometrika 1951;16:297–334.
65. Streiner DL, Norman GR. Health Measurement Scales. A Practical Guide to Their Development and Use (2nd ed). Oxford, UK: Oxford University Press, 1995.
66. Nunnaly J. Psychometric Theory (2nd ed). New York: McGraw-Hill, 1978.
67. Aaronson NK. Quality of life assessment in clinical trials: methodologic issues. Control Clin Trials 1989;10:195S–208S.
68. Guyatt G, Walter S, Norman G. Measuring change over time: assessing the usefulness of evaluative instruments. J Chron Dis 1987;40:171–178.
69. Cohen J. Statistical Power Analysis for the Behavioral Sciences. New York: Academic Press; 1977.
70. Kazis LE, Anerson JJ, Meenan RF. Effect sizes for interpreting changes in health status. Med Care 1989;27(Suppl):S178–S189.
71. Liang MH, Larson MG, Cullen KE, et al. Comparative measurement of efficiency and sensitivity of five health status instruments for arthritis research. Arthritis Rheum 1985;28:545–547.
72. Jaeschke R, Guyatt G, Keller J, Singer J. Measurement of health status: ascertaining the meaning of a change in quality-of-life questionnaire score. Control Clin Trials 1989;10:407–415.
73. Juniper EF, Guyatt GH, Willan A, Griffith LE. Determining a minimal important change in a disease-specific quality of life questionnaire. J Clin Epidemiol 1994;47:81–87.
74. Redelmeier DA, Goldstein RS, Guyatt GH. Assessing the minimal important difference in symptoms: a comparison of two techniques. J Clin Epidemiol 1996;49:1215–1219.
75. Tuley MR, Mulrow CD, McMahan CA. Estimating and testing an index of responsiveness and the relationship to power. J Clin Epidemiol 1991;44:417–421.
76. Jacobson NS, Truax P. Clinical Significance: A Statistical Approach to Defining Meaningful Change in Psychotherapy Research. In AE Kazdin (ed), Methodological Issues and Strategies in Clinical Research. Washington: American Psychological Association, 1992.
77. deBruin AF, Diederiks JPM, de Witte AP, et al. Assessing the responsiveness of a functional status measure: the Sickness Impact Profile versus the SIP68. J Clin Epidemiol 1997;50:529–540.
78. Hays RD, Anderson R, Revicki D. Psychometric considerations in evaluating health-related quality of life measures. Quality of Life Research 1993;2:441–449.
79. Pocock SJ. A perspective on the role of quality of life assessment in clincal trials. Control Clin Trials 1991;12:257S–265S.
80. Gelber RD, Gelber S. Quality-Of-Life Assessment in Clinical Trials. In PF Thall (ed), Recent Advances in Clinical Trial Design and Analysis. Boston: Kluwer Academic Publishers, 1995.
81. DeVellis RF. Scale Development: Theory and Applications. In L Bickman, DJ Rob (eds), Applied Social Research Methods Series, vol. 26. Newbury Park, CA: Sage Publications Inc., 1991.
82. Spilker B (ed). Quality of Life Assessment in Clinical Trials. New York: Raven Press, 1990.
83. Stewart AL, Ware JE (eds). Measuring Functioning and Well-Being. Durham, NC: Duke University Press, 1992.
84. Armitage P. Statistical Methods in Medical Research. New York: John Wiley & Sons, 1977.
85. Colton T. Statistics in Medicine. Boston: Little, Brown, 1974.
86. Fisher L, Van Belle G. Biostatistics—A Methodology for the Health Sciences. New York: John Wiley & Sons, 1993.
87. Fleiss JL. Analysis of data from multiclinic trials. Control Clin Trials 1986;7:267–275.
88. Woolson R. Statistical Methods for the Analysis of Biomedical Data. New York: John Wiley & Sons, 1987.
89. Peto R, Pike MC, Armitage P, et al. Design and analysis of randomized clinical trials requiring prolonged observation of each patient. 1. Introduction and design. Br J Cancer 1976;34:585–612.
90. May GS, DeMets DL, Friedman LM, et al. The randomized clinical trial: bias in analysis. Circulation 1981;64:669–673.

## 26　Clinical Trials in Neurologic Practice

91. Fields WS, Maslenikov V, Meyer JS, et al. Joint study of extracranial arterial occlusion: V. Progress report of prognosis following surgical or nonsurgical tests for transient ischemic attacks and cervical carotid artery lesions. JAMA 1970;211:1993–2003.
92. Coronary Drug Project Research Group. Influence of adherence to treatment and response of cholesterol on mortality in the Coronary Drug Project. N Engl J Med 1980;303:1038–1041.
93. Mattson ME, Friedman LM. Issues in medication adherence assessment in clinical trials of the National Heart, Lung, and Blood Institute. Control Clin Trials 1984;5(4Suppl):488–496.
94. Tukey JW. Some thoughts on clinical trials, especially problems of multiplicity. Science 1977;198:679–684.
95. ISIS-2 (Second International Study of Infarct Survival) Collaborative Group. Randomized trial of intravenous streptokinase, oral aspirin, both or neither, among 17187 cases of suspected acute myocardial infarction: ISIS-2. Lancet 1988;ii:349–360.
96. Executive Committee for the Asymptomatic Carotid Atherosclerosis (ACAS) Study. Endarterectomy for asymptomatic carotid artery stenosis. JAMA 1995;273:1421–1428.
97. Begg C, Cho M, Eastwood S, et al. Improving the quality of reporting of randomized controlled trials. The CONSORT Statement. JAMA 1996;276:637–639.
98. Bath FJ, Owen VE, Bath PMW. Quality of full and final publications reporting acute stroke trials: a systematic review. Stroke 1998;29:2203–2210.
99. Sackett DL, Haynes RB, Guyatt GH, Tugwell P (eds). Clinical Epidemiology: A Basic Science for Clinical Medicine (2nd ed). Boston: Little, Brown, 1991.
100. CAPRIE Steering Committee. A randomised, blinded, trial of clopidogrel versus aspirin in patients at risk of ischaemic events (CAPRIE). Lancet 1996;348:1329–1339.
101. Guyatt GH, Naylor D, Juniper E, et al. Users' guides to the medical literature. XII. How to use articles about health-related quality of life. JAMA 1997;277:1232–1237.

# 2
# Clinical Trials in Stroke

John R. Marler

In 1980, few of the treatments used to prevent or treat stroke had been proven beneficial in clinical trials. Since then, several large, major multicenter trials have been completed, and most of the common stroke therapies have been evaluated in one or more clinical trials. Progress has been made in stroke prevention with the repeated demonstration for patients in several risk categories of the value of carotid endarterectomy, platelet antiaggregants, and warfarin. New prevention strategies under evaluation in clinical trials include folate, estrogen, and carotid angioplasty with stenting. For the treatment of acute stroke, trials have demonstrated the benefit of tissue plasminogen activator given within three hours of stroke onset and the value of nimodipine for the prevention of vasospasm after aneurysmal subarachnoid hemorrhage.[1] There are reports suggesting potential benefit for ancrod within four hours of,[2] and intra-arterial pro-urokinase as late as 6 hours after, stroke onset in a few carefully selected patients.[3] Numerous trials have been done in an attempt to demonstrate the value of cytoprotective agents.[4] Most of the cytoprotective trials failed to demonstrate any benefit. The failure of these trials is explained by a lack of adequate dose finding and safety studies. It is also explained by the use of a time window for neuronal recovery from reversible ischemia in humans that is five to six times longer than that used in laboratory models of stroke.

Most stroke prevention trials are designed to measure benefit by reducing the number of strokes, transient ischemic attacks (TIAs), or deaths. Kaplan-Meier graphs compare the percentage of patients surviving at different times from randomization without the occurrence of a prespecified end point event. The results are easy to understand and have obvious relevance to the patient. Counting strokes, however, does not measure many of the neuropsychological difficulties that follow a stroke. Carotid endarterectomy and platelet antiaggregants may have benefits or adverse effects not accounted for in trials that focus on counting strokes and deaths. Although these neuropsychological outcomes may show more effects from the drugs used, they have not yet been tested sufficiently to be the primary outcomes for stroke prevention trials. They could

28   *Clinical Trials in Neurologic Practice*

*Table 2.1*   Different types of control groups used in clinical trials

| Types of controls for clinical trials |
| --- |
| Placebo concurrent control |
| No-treatment concurrent control |
| Dose-response concurrent control |
| Active (positive) concurrent control |
| External control (including historical control) |
| Multiple control groups |

Source: U.S. Food and Drug Administration. International Conference on Harmonisation: choice of control group in clinical trials. Federal Register 1999;64(185):51767–51780.

begin to be used as secondary outcomes so that more insight into the effects of different treatment strategies on a broader range of neurologic function can be acquired.

Developing treatments to prevent stroke is an incremental process. Clearly, treating hypertension and cessation of smoking are the most significant steps an individual can take to prevent stroke. After these steps are taken, the gains for further intervention are smaller. To detect a small difference between two treatment groups in a clinical trial, a much larger sample size is needed. The smaller the effect that is to be detected, the larger, and hence more expensive, the clinical trial to detect the effect. Several methods of reducing the expense of clinical trials are discussed in this chapter. Nevertheless, to add more treatments to the standard regimen being developed, larger and more complex trials will need to be performed. This requires the involvement of all who provide care for patients at risk for stroke, not just neurologists at academic medical centers.

Reading a report of a clinical trial in a medical journal is like reading a 10-page summary of a novel by Charles Dickens. The process of carrying out a large, multicenter clinical trial involves hundreds, if not thousands, of different people besides the patients themselves. The organizational structure is particularly complex. The protocol for a clinical trial is usually 10–20 pages long. The manual of operations can fill one or more thick notebooks. There may be 20 or more different data collection forms for each patient. It is impossible to fully describe a clinical trial in the limited space provided by major journals (Table 2.1).

Each of the inclusion and exclusion criteria must be considered for its relevance to clinical practice. For example, patients in several of the trials of carotid endarterectomy were excluded if they had evidence of atrial fibrillation.[5,6] Does this mean that a patient with atrial fibrillation and recent TIAs found to have greater than 90% stenosis of the symptomatic carotid artery would or would not benefit from carotid endarterectomy? By excluding atrial fibrillation patients, the trial left this question unanswered. The reason for the exclusion was to ensure that the surgery was only performed on patients who had symptoms caused by the carotid lesion. If atrial fibrillation was present and there had been an ischemic episode, it could have been caused by a blood clot formed in the fibrillating heart and not by an event related to the more distal carotid stenosis. Because the patients with atrial fibrillation are probably at even higher risk of stroke when they have carotid stenosis, the reader may conclude that there is likely some benefit to carotid endarterectomy. However, because of the design of the trials, there is some question.

When a clinical trial is being planned, the inclusion and exclusion criteria should be kept to a minimum. If a clinical investigator suspects that a particular patient characteristic will affect the patient's response to a treatment, then that characteristic could be made the basis of a secondary analysis to be performed after the trial is completed. Then there will be data to determine whether the patient characteristic actually does predict the response to the treatment being tested. The reader of a clinical trial report must decide whether the selection of patients is practical. If there are extensive tests to be done and many criteria to be followed before a treatment can be used, then the results of the trial are applicable to only a few patients. To increase their applicability, clinical trials are designed to include a broad range of patients. To some, broad inclusion criteria may seem to lack precision or engender a lack of concern for the individual patient. Actually, the reverse is true. To treat every patient as well as possible, it would be helpful to have a large number of different treatments, each with a known benefit in relation to the particular characteristics of the one patient being treated at a given time. For example, to know whether a particular subtype of stroke responds better to one treatment than another, information is needed from clinical trials that include patients with all stroke types. If patients are excluded from the trials, then the information needed to make important decisions for a particular patient may not be available. Individual patients benefit from clinical trials that include as many different patients as possible.

Readers also need to know exactly what the reported benefits and risks mean when translated to practice. More important, physicians need to know the meaning of trial results from the point of view of the patient. This is more difficult when the treatment has known risks. For example, carotid endarterectomy has a well-known 2% or greater incidence of major stroke or death during the procedure or within 30 days. The incidence of any stroke or death may be as high as 6%. The initial risk of the surgery is eventually offset by the reduced incidence of subsequent strokes. In the use of thrombolytic therapy for acute stroke, many physicians focus on the 6% serious complication rate due to intracranial bleeding. However, there is at least a 12% absolute difference after accounting for any adverse effect of the thrombolytic therapy. The thought of causing an intracranial hemorrhage with a treatment is difficult for the treating physician to accept, just as surgical complications are unwanted but unavoidable consequences that must be accepted by the surgeon. However, the clinical trials that have been done make it clear to the patient in which treatment group he or she would rather be. The physician's role then becomes participation in further research efforts to reduce the adverse and increase the beneficial effects of the treatment.

Intuition is a poor guide when deciding what outcome in a stroke clinical trial is acceptable for a particular therapeutic agent. Although the desire of the physician is that there be a dramatic benefit for every patient who receives a particular drug, the reality is that only a subset of patients will experience this anticipated benefit. The result of expecting too much from a treatment is that

30   *Clinical Trials in Neurologic Practice*

many stroke trials are designed to detect a major change in outcomes, such as 30% or 50%. In reality, few drugs for stroke prevention or treatment can have this large an effect in every patient treated. The fact is that even changes of a few percentage points for the large group in a clinical trial can mean a large benefit for some of the patients treated. One of the major flaws in stroke trials has been the design to look for a "penicillin" effect, when actually a much smaller effect would be accepted as significant. The result has been that many trials have been designed that could not detect smaller and clinically meaningful benefits from a particular treatment. Because few trials can be repeated, effective treatments are not being developed because there is not sufficient power in the trial to detect smaller and more realistic effects. Several examples are discussed below, in the sections on acute stroke treatment.

Several stroke trials are discussed in detail. They were chosen for discussion because they had a major impact on medical practice and demonstrate a particularly interesting finding or example of problems encountered in clinical trial methodology. For each trial, the advances in treatment and clinical trial methodology are discussed. The trials are classified as prevention or acute treatment, and within those groups by the specific intervention.

## STROKE PREVENTION

Epidemiologic studies define factors that independently predict an increased risk of stroke. Often, there are treatments that alter risk factors. A clinical trial is needed to determine whether the alteration in risk factors has a beneficial result on the health of the individual taking the treatment. Because very few individuals with a given risk factor will actually have a stroke, trials with a large number of patients are needed to detect a small change in the absolute rate of stroke. An extensive series of trials has been performed to evaluate platelet antiaggregants, warfarin, and surgery to prevent stroke. Most of the trials have been secondary prevention treatments started after a patient has already demonstrated symptoms of cerebrovascular disease.

### Platelet Antiaggregants

Aspirin

The prevention of ischemic stroke begins with the use of aspirin. Aspirin has been demonstrated to be effective for the prevention of ischemic stroke in several secondary prevention studies. A primary prevention study has not yet demonstrated its effectiveness for stroke prevention, although it has been shown effective in the primary prevention of heart attack.[7]

The results of the Canadian Cooperative Study Group's Randomized Trial of Aspirin and Sulfinpyrazone in Threatened Stroke was published in 1978.[8] The study was a multicenter, double-blind, factorial, randomized clinical trial. In total, 585 patients with one or more episodes of cerebral ischemic attack within the previous 3 months were randomized. Patients received 325 mg of aspirin or identical placebo and 200 mg of sulfinpyrazone or identical placebo four times per day. Patients were evaluated at one month and every three months after randomization. The outcomes of the trial were TIA, stroke, and death. Events were reported between the seventh day and the end of the trial, or 6 months after a patient withdrew from the study because of stopping the study medication, starting contaminating medications, moving away from a center, or submitting to operation (carotid endarterectomy). Among patients who withdrew due to drug side effects, 72% were taking aspirin. The results of the trial for aspirin were that 15.9% of patients who received aspirin either had a stroke or died from 7 days until the end of the trial or 6 months after being withdrawn from the study. This compares to 23.1% in the group that did not receive aspirin. This was a 7.2% absolute, and 31% relative, reduction in the stroke and death rate. This difference is statistically significant. Another result is that the 30% of the female patients did not appear to benefit from the aspirin; in fact, there was a 5% absolute increase in the number of strokes and deaths in the female aspirin group. However, this difference was not statistically significant. The effect of aspirin was not as great when patients who received neither aspirin nor sulfinpyrazone were compared to patients who received aspirin alone (Table 2.2).

The most perplexing issue about aspirin is the dose. Doses ranging from 81 to 1,300 mg, a 16-fold difference, have been used and compared in different trials. All doses seem to provide some benefit, so no dosage is clearly better than any other. The complications tend to increase, and the compliance tends to decrease, as the dose becomes larger. Whether there is increased benefit if the patient can tolerate a higher dose has not been established. It is also not clear whether aspirin is equally effective in the prevention of all the different manifestations of atherosclerosis. The effect in myocardial infarction may have a different mechanism of action than for stroke. All trials agree that aspirin is better than placebo for the secondary prevention of stroke in patients with a much higher risk of stroke than the rest of the population. Starting with a higher dose has advantages, as was done in the Canadian trial, it is disappointing to complete a clinical trial and, if it was negative, suspect that there was no effect seen because the dosage was too low.

Careful reading of this trial report points out many interesting features. After the first year of the trial, the entry criteria were changed to include patients with single as well as multiple cerebral ischemic episodes. The study randomized patients in different strata according to the presumed site of ischemia and by the presence or

*Table 2.2*  The Canadian Cooperative Study Group Randomized Trial of Aspirin and Sulfinpyrazone in Threatened Stroke*

|        | Aspirin (%) | No aspirin (%) | Difference (%) |
|--------|-------------|----------------|----------------|
| Stroke | 3.4         | 6.4            | 3              |
| Death  | 12.4        | 16.6           | 4.2            |
| All    | 15.9        | 23.1           | 7.2            |

*Percentage of patients with stroke or death between 7 days and end of trial or 6 months after withdrawal from trial

Source: This table is derived from data presented in Table 5 of the primary report of the trial results (The Canadian Cooperative Study Group. A randomized trial of aspirin and sulfinpyrazone in threatened stroke. N Engl J Med 1978;299:53–59).

32   *Clinical Trials in Neurologic Practice*

absence of a residual deficit at the time of randomization. Six hundred and forty-nine patients were entered. Sixty-four were later found to be ineligible, resulting in a study population of 585. There was some imbalance in the treatment assignment of the 64 ineligible patients. Eligibility was determined before the results of the trial were analyzed, but excluding patients after randomization is controversial. The investigators in this trial were apparently more focused on determining whether the drug worked if it was taken by a patient than on determining how different therapeutic strategies compared with each other. The comparison of therapeutic strategies must take into account those patients who cannot tolerate the drug and stop taking it. This type of comparison reflects actual practice, because it accepts the variation that is inevitable in the interpretation of the inclusion and exclusion criteria. The focus on drug activity by the investigators in this trial was further demonstrated when they did not count all events occurring in the first week after randomization in all four study groups. Sulfinpyrazone was thought to have little or no effect during the first week after treatment started. The focus on the drug, rather than the entire treatment strategy, probably had minimal effect on the overall outcome of the trial. The compliance rate was 92%. Another fact for consideration is that 74% of the patients had cerebral angiography before randomization, which prevented the risks of angiography affecting the results of the trial. This is appropriate because angiography was not required to determine eligibility for the trial.

There are often surprising findings in the subgroup analyses of trials. It is difficult to determine their significance, because the number of patients may be too small to perform an appropriate statistical test. In addition, unless a hypothesis is stated prospectively, it is not known whether the finding is not just due to chance after many different subgroup comparisons are made. In the Canadian Cooperative Study, there was a statistically significant difference in the response to aspirin by men and women. The actual meaning of this is still not entirely clear, nor is its clinical implication.

## Ticlopidine

Aspirin has many side effects, including gastric irritation and ulceration. In addition, aspirin may have less benefit in females than in males. Alternative platelet antiaggregants currently approved for use to prevent stroke include ticlopidine and clopidogrel. In August 1989, the Ticlopidine Aspirin Stroke Study Group reported the results of a major randomized, controlled double-blind clinical trial.[9] The trial compared ticlopidine to aspirin for its ability to reduce the incidence of stroke and death in 3,069 patients who had a recent TIA (transient stroke) or minor stroke. Because aspirin was considered standard care for the patients selected for the trial, an active control design was chosen to compare two active agents.[10] The designers of the trial had to make a decision: Would they attempt to demonstrate equivalence of the two active agents, aspirin and ticlopidine, or would they seek to demonstrate the superiority of one of the active agents? The ticlopidine trial was designed to test for the superiority of ticlopidine as compared to aspirin. The dose of aspirin used was 1,300 mg per day, given as two tablets twice daily. This is the same dose of aspirin used in the study done by the Canadian Cooperative Study Group discussed above, and later used in the North American Symptomatic Carotid Endarterectomy Trial (NASCET) of carotid endarterectomy in symptomatic patients.[5] Ticlopidine was administered twice daily as one 250-mg tablet. The results of the trial were published in August 1989. The follow-up of all patients was completed December 31, 1987. The trial showed a lower incidence of stroke and death in the group of patients treated with ticlopidine. The methodology is notable for the careful medical monitoring and the efforts to reduce bias in the trial by carefully masking knowledge of the treatment assignment from the patient, treating physician, and clinical investigators.

The credibility of a clinical trial determines the ability of its results to have an effect on medical practice. By using randomization and blinding, the effect of patient and investigator expectation can be minimized, because patients and investigators know that some subjects will not receive the agent being tested in the trial. By equalizing the expectation by the patient and the treating physician for each treatment, blinding and randomization increase the ability of a clinical trial to detect true drug effects.[10] In the ticlopidine aspirin trial being discussed here, the only groups who knew the treatment received by a patient were the independent external safety monitoring committee and the staff at the data management center for the study. Outcomes for each patient were monitored by blinded adjudicators, expert in their fields, to assure patient safety and to ensure diagnostic accuracy and consistency across all the clinical centers for the trial.

The term *intention to treat* has several different meanings. One level of meaning is that in a clinical trial, once a patient is randomized to a particular treatment group, then all adverse events and outcome measures for that patient are attributed to the assigned treatment, regardless of whether the patient actually receives the treatment. This was true for the ticlopidine trial. However, although a trial may analyze patients in their assigned group, regardless of the actual treatment received, all randomized patients may not be in the final analysis regardless of the original "intent" to treat the patients. This adds a second level of meaning to the term *intention to treat*. In the Extracranial/Intracranial Bypass Trial,[11] and the Canadian Aspirin-Sulfinpyrazone Trial,[8] the primary analysis excluded patients who were found ineligible after being randomized by a blinded panel of adjudicators who did not know the treatment assignment for the patients. In the Ticlopidine-Aspirin Stroke Trial,[9] eligibility for all patients randomized was reviewed centrally, but all randomized patients were included in the final analysis. The adjudicators concluded that 12 patients included in the final analysis were ineligible because they did not meet the inclusion and exclusion criteria of the trial. This small number indicates that the selection criteria are robust in a variety of clinical sites. This additional level of intention to treat adds to the credibility of the trial, because the results more accurately reflect how the treatment will be used in actual clinical practice.

Safety monitoring is important to protect patients in a randomized clinical trial, especially when there is blinding of investigators and patients to the treatment assignment. To reduce bias and increase scientific credibility, a safety monitoring committee should be independent of the clinical investigators and the trial sponsors. The safety monitoring committee in the ticlopidine-aspirin trial received summary reports of adverse events prepared by the statistical center for the trial.[9] The investigators were not aware of treatment assignment and did not participate in the decision to continue or stop the trial.

The primary analysis of the ticlopidine aspirin trial showed a statistically significant difference for the primary end point of death from any cause or nonfatal

34  *Clinical Trials in Neurologic Practice*

stroke.[9] The event rate in the ticlopidine-treated group was 17%, for the aspirin-treated group, it was 19%. Although ticlopidine had a lower event rate, 62.3% of treated patients experienced adverse events of any type, compared to 53.2% of patients treated with aspirin. Diarrhea was reported by 20% of patients receiving ticlopidine, compared to 10% of patients receiving aspirin. Reports of gastrointestinal hemorrhage, gastritis, and peptic ulcer were significantly higher among patients receiving aspirin. However, ticlopidine had significantly higher incidences of urticaria, rash, and severe neutropenia. Neutropenia occurred in fewer than 1% of patients, 13 cases, but all cases occurred in the group treated with ticlopidine. All cases of neutropenia were reversed when the drug was stopped, but one of the 13 patients died. Nevertheless, the small risk of neutropenia and the resulting requirement for monitoring has limited use of the drug.

## Clopidogrel

Clopidogrel is another platelet antiaggregant. It is similar to ticlopidine but has a broader antiplatelet effect. Clopidogrel reduces venous as well as arterial thrombosis and reduces atherogenesis in some laboratory models. A large multicenter trial comparing aspirin to clopidogrel in patients who had recent stroke, intermittent claudication, or myocardial infarction was performed. The results of the Clopidogrel versus Aspirin in Patients at Risk of Ischemic Events (CAPRIE) trial were reported in 1996.[12] The trial design called for 15,000 patients to be recruited, with 5,000 in each of the three risk groups. The recruitment was planned to last for three years. Follow-up was to continue for one year after the last patient was recruited, to achieve a total of 35,000 years of patient follow-up. To estimate the required years of follow-up, it was assumed that the three-year incidence of primary end points would be 25% for patients with myocardial infarction or stroke and 14% for patients with intermittent claudication. A two-sided statistical test was chosen, as either aspirin or clopidogrel could be superior. With a two-sided alpha value of 0.05, it was expected that the study would have 90% power to detect a relative risk reduction of 11.6%. When patients were recruited more quickly than anticipated, the power of the study was threatened because the number of patient-years of follow-up was reduced. Therefore, the steering committee of the study, blind to any results, decided to increase the number of patients recruited so that the desired power of the study could be achieved. Although the focus of a clinical trial is often the number of patients and the number of events, the real objective is to reduce the rate of events. Therefore, the total number of events per year of a patient's life is the most important outcome. In recognition of this important principle of stroke prevention, most trials are designed to have a minimum number of years of observation for each patient.

Understanding the results of the CAPRIE trial was complicated by the fact that there were three groups of patients and three outcome events: myocardial infarction, stroke, or vascular death. There were 2,800 different validated outcome events: 1,353 in the clopidogrel study and 1,447 in the aspirin group. These were not all end point events, because any one patient could have many outcome events but only one end point event, which would be the first outcome event to occur. The most common end point event was stroke, which occurred in

38% of all events. As a first event, stroke was also the most common event. There were 1,960 first events. Of these, stroke was the first event in 46%, myocardial infarction in 31%, and vascular death in 23%. In the patients who were enrolled in the trial because of stroke, 5.43% had a stroke at some time during the study. The yearly primary event rate was approximately 7% per year for stroke, myocardial infarction, or vascular death. There were 976 nonfatal and 79 fatal stroke events. Although death is a very specific end point, vascular death is more difficult to ascertain. In the CAPRIE trial, a central validation committee reviewed all deaths to ascertain the cause. Only deaths caused by vascular disease were counted as outcome events.

Statistical analysis showed an overall difference between clopidogrel and aspirin when all patients were considered. In those patients enrolled because they had a stroke, the yearly event rate (stroke, myocardial infarction, or vascular death) was 7.15% per year in the clopidogrel group and 7.71% in the aspirin group. This difference was not statistically significant ($p = .26$). There was a very significant difference between clopidogrel and aspirin in the patients with peripheral vascular disease. This difference in the peripheral vascular disease group carried the entire intent to treat group. Does this mean that clopidogrel gives no benefit for prevention of myocardial infarction, second stroke, or vascular death in stroke patients? The answer requires some discipline on the part of the reader, because common sense is not always the best guide. Although there is no statistical significance to the difference between aspirin and clopidogrel in the stroke subgroup, this subgroup analysis does not have the power necessary to rule out any benefit of clopidogrel. It is not a valid conclusion that there is no benefit of clopidogrel for patients with stroke. The valid conclusion is that there is not enough data to determine whether clopidogrel has more or less benefit than aspirin for patients with stroke. Overall, however, the therapeutic strategy of using clopidogrel instead of aspirin for patients with stroke, myocardial infarction, or peripheral vascular disease does have an increased benefit when compared to aspirin (Table 2.3).

The choice of a two-sided test of the primary outcome could have had significant implications if aspirin and clopidogrel were equivalent, or if clopidogrel had been less effective than aspirin. When beginning a trial, investigators need to know that if they use a two-sided test, they express a desire to show that either of the two treatments might be superior to the other.


Dipyridamole Combined with Aspirin

Aspirin has been demonstrated to reduce the stroke rate in several secondary prevention trials. Better stroke prevention requires either a more effective agent, such as clopidogrel, or the addition of a second agent, preferably one with a completely different mechanism of action. The European Stroke Prevention Study (ESPS) Group has reported two trials, ESPS1[13] and ESPS2,[14] which evaluated the combination of dipyridamole and aspirin for stroke prevention. In ESPS1, dipyridamole, 75 mg three times per day, was given with aspirin, 330 mg three times per day. There was a 38% reduction in secondary stroke compared to the group treated with placebo. This risk reduction was substantially higher than when aspirin was used alone.

36    *Clinical Trials in Neurologic Practice*

*Table 2.3*    Outcome events in Clopidogrel Aspirin Trial (CAPRIE)

| | Clopidogrel | | Aspirin | | Total | |
|---|---|---|---|---|---|---|
| *Validated outcome events* | *No.* | *%* | *No.* | *%* | *No.* | *%* |
| **Nonfatal events** | 793 | 28.32 | 876 | 31.29 | 1,669 | 59.61 |
| Ischemic stroke | 472 | 16.86 | 504 | 18 | 976 | 34.86 |
| Myocardial infarction (MI) | 255 | 9.11 | 301 | 10.75 | 556 | 19.86 |
| Intracerebral hemorrhage | 14 | 0.5 | 24 | 0.86 | 38 | 1.36 |
| Amputation | 52 | 1.86 | 47 | 1.68 | 99 | 3.54 |
| **Fatal events** | 560 | 20 | 571 | 20.39 | 1,131 | 40.39 |
| Ischemic stroke | 37 | 1.32 | 42 | 1.5 | 79 | 2.82 |
| MI | 53 | 1.89 | 75 | 2.68 | 128 | 4.57 |
| Hemorrhagic death | 23 | 0.82 | 27 | 0.96 | 50 | 1.79 |
| Other vascular death | 260 | 9.29 | 261 | 9.32 | 521 | 18.61 |
| Nonvascular death | 187 | 6.68 | 166 | 5.93 | 353 | 12.61 |
| **Total events** | 1,353 | 48.32 | 1,447 | 51.68 | 2,800 | 100 |
| **Fatal and nonfatal ischemic stroke** | 509 | 18.18 | 546 | 19.50 | 1,055 | 37.68 |
| **Fatal and nonfatal ischemic MI** | 308 | 11 | 376 | 13.43 | 684 | 24.43 |
| **Other nonfatal events** | 66 | 2.36 | 71 | 2.54 | 137 | 4.89 |
| **Other deaths** | 470 | 16.79 | 454 | 16.21 | 924 | 33 |

Source: Adapted from CAPRIE Steering Committee. A randomised, blinded, trial of clopidogrel versus aspirin in patients at risk of ischaemic events (CAPRIE). Lancet 1996;348:1329–1339.

In ESPS2, patients were eligible if they were 18 years or older and had had a transient or permanent stroke within the preceding 3 months. Patients with a recent history of gastrointestinal bleeding or peptic ulcer were excluded. Eligible patients were randomized to one of four groups: (1) aspirin alone, (2) matched placebo, (3) aspirin plus modified release dipyridamole, and (4) modified-release dipyridamole alone. There were three specified primary outcomes: stroke, death, and stroke or death, whichever came first. The statistical design was a $2 \times 2$ factorial design that would detect the contribution of each single agent to any observed difference for the combination. The study was designed to have 80% power to detect a 25% relative risk reduction based on the observed rates in the preceding ESPS1 trial. Intention-to-treat analysis was based on all patients randomized, regardless of whether they were found eligible when the central Morbidity and Mortality Assessment Group reviewed eligibility. Despite the intention to perform an intent-to-treat analysis, it was discovered that randomization assignments were issued for 14 patients who did not exist. For this reason, the 438 patients from one center were not included in the final analysis. The absence of these patients did not change the results of the trial. Thus, the results are based on 6,602 patients rather than the 7,054 patients randomized.

During ESPS2, results from other trials provided evidence about the treatment of certain subgroups of patients. In particular, the benefit of warfarin compared to aspirin for patients with atrial fibrillation became known during the course of ESPS2.[15] The investigators in ESPS2 were told that, if they believed it was indicated, they could switch ESPS2 patients with atrial fibrillation from the study treatment to warfarin. When randomization was complete, there was no difference in the proportion of patients who had atrial fibrillation in each of the four treatment groups.

The results of the ESPS2 trial demonstrated that all three treatments—aspirin, dipyridamole, and aspirin combined with dipyridamole—had a beneficial effect and reduced the two-year rate of stroke. The absolute reduction over two years was 5.9% for the combination of aspirin and dipyridamole compared to placebo. This 5.9% compares to 2.9% for aspirin alone and 2.6% for dipyridamole alone in the ESPS2 trial. Recall that there was a 7.1% absolute reduction in stroke rate for aspirin compared to placebo in the Canadian Cooperative Study Group,[8] in a similar group of patients. In ESPS2, bleeding from any site was increased in both treatment groups that received any aspirin (4.5% [placebo] and 4.7% [DYP] compared to 8.2% [ASA] and 8.7% [ASA and DYP]). The benefit of the drug was measured by the prevention of stroke. The risks were not all apparent in the primary outcomes of stroke and death, except for the few fatal intracerebral hemorrhages. Because the increased risk of bleeding from aspirin is not accounted for, the absolute difference in stroke rate does not accurately reflect the use of the treatment; however, increase in the rate of severe hemorrhage is very small.

Comparing the results of two clinical trials is difficult, even if the selection criteria and primary outcomes are similar. The major reason is that there is usually a difference in the baseline characteristics of the patients who are randomized in the trial that appears to be a difference in the overall rate of stroke. When comparing trials that observe patients over a long period of time, the observation periods may be different; thus, absolute differences in the observed rate are not as relevant as absolute differences in the yearly incidence of stroke or differences in the overall relative risk reduction.

## Anticoagulants

### Warfarin

Warfarin is an oral anticoagulant that was first investigated for stroke prevention by Siekert et al.,[16] who defined the concept of TIA and demonstrated that it was a significant risk factor for "permanent," nontransient stroke. Warfarin's use for prevention of stroke for patients who have had a TIA remains unproven, but it has been shown to be effective in the prevention of stroke for patients with nonvalvular atrial fibrillation. When compared to placebo, there is little doubt that warfarin prevents stroke. However, as is discussed in the following paragraph, when compared to aspirin, use of warfarin raises a number of issues.

The evaluation of warfarin as a stroke prevention treatment is an example of changing medical practice during the course of a clinical trial or a series of clinical trials. Warfarin treatment must be highly individualized. Frequent blood tests, especially at the time treatment is started, are required to adjust dosage to an effective, but safe, dose. In earlier studies, such as SPAF I (discussed below), the prothrombin time was compared to a laboratory standard time, and the prothrombin time ratio was used. This test varied from laboratory to laboratory. To provide better standardization, the international normalized ratio (INR) was developed. The INR is an important value in stroke prevention studies and an essential feature of any trial's protocol. If the INR is too low, the risk exists that warfarin may have limited effectiveness. If the INR is too high, then there is the risk of serious hemorrhage, including intracranial hemorrhage. In addition, treat-

## 38    Clinical Trials in Neurologic Practice

ment with warfarin has to be discontinued at times when hemostasis must be maintained, such as during dental procedures or surgery.

Because of the frequent blood tests, most trials of anticoagulants, including warfarin, have been unblinded trials in which the treating physician and patient knew what drug the patient was receiving. Methodology has recently been developed for blinding long-term treatment with anticoagulants. Most trials have blinded observers when outcome determinations are made. Blinding the outcome determination reduces bias, but it does not account for the bias introduced into the study by having the treatment administered by an unblinded physician. There is no way to account for this bias when reading the results of the trial. Perhaps the reader will choose to demand a higher standard of statistical significance than the usual $p$ value of .05 when the trial is not completely blinded.

The value of warfarin in stroke prevention depends not only on the intensity of treatment, but also on the mechanism of stroke. Warfarin is used for stroke prevention after a first stroke, after a TIA, and in patients with nonvalvular atrial fibrillation. The use for patients with nonvalvular atrial fibrillation has been the use best evaluated in clinical trials.

The Stroke Prevention in Atrial Fibrillation (SPAF) investigators reported the first of a series of three clinical trials in 1991.[15] The first SPAF trial had three treatment groups: aspirin, warfarin, and placebo. Not all patients were eligible for warfarin; those who were not were randomized separately to placebo or aspirin treatment.

Therefore, there were two groups of patients treated with aspirin and two placebo groups. The dose of aspirin used was 325 mg given once per day. The warfarin dose was adjusted to maintain a prothrombin time ratio between 1.3 and 1.8. It is estimated that this corresponded to an INR between 2.0 and 4.5. Patients in the SPAF Trial were randomized to one of five treatment arms (Figure 2.1). Patients who were anticoagulation candidates received warfarin, aspirin, or placebo. Patients who were not anticoagulation candidates received either aspirin or placebo. Randomization to the placebo treatment was stopped early by the independent monitoring committee for the trial. Both warfarin and aspirin were found highly beneficial in stroke prevention compared to placebo. The yearly rate of stroke or systemic embolism was 2.3% in the warfarin-treated group and 7.4% in the comparable placebo group ($p = .01$). There was one intracerebral hemorrhage among the warfarin-treated patients. The yearly rate of stroke or systemic embolism was 3.6% in the aspirin group and 6.3% in the comparable placebo group ($p = .02$).

## Surgery to Prevent Stroke

### Extracranial/Intracranial Arterial Bypass

Several nonmedical interventions have been proposed for the prevention of ischemic stroke. These include extracranial-intracranial (EC/IC) arterial bypass, carotid endarterectomy, and carotid angioplasty with stenting.

The EC/IC Bypass Study Group published the primary results of their trial in 1985.[11] This trial evaluated a new procedure for stroke prevention: extracranial-intracranial bypass. In this procedure, an anastomosis through the skull of a superficial temporal artery to the distal ipsilateral middle cerebral artery is created to

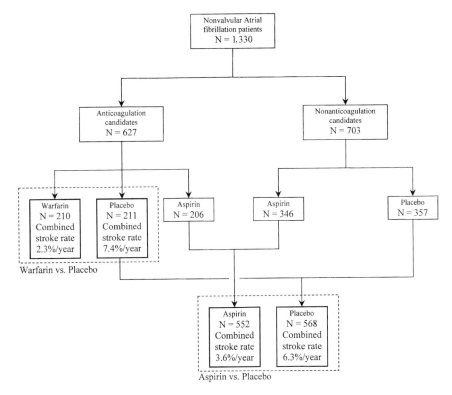

*Figure 2.1* Randomization in the Stroke Prevention in Atrial Fibrillation Trial.[15] Eligible patients were first classified as warfarin candidates or as not, according to standard criteria. The patients then were randomized to aspirin or placebo if they were not anticoagulation candidates. Candidates for warfarin were randomized to warfarin, aspirin, or placebo. The two main results compared warfarin to placebo and aspirin to placebo. There was not sufficient statistical power to compare aspirin to warfarin in the warfarin candidates.

provide a blood flow bypass around stenotic or occlusive lesions in brain arteries. The lesions treated in the trial were (1) occlusion or stenosis of the trunk or major branches before the bifurcation or trifurcation of the middle cerebral artery, (2) stenosis or occlusion of the carotid artery above the C2 vertebral body (a lesion that is not approachable through carotid endarterectomy), or (3) occlusion of the internal carotid artery. After randomization, each patient's baseline data were reviewed by a group of investigators at the coordinating center who were blinded to the treatment group assignment of the patient. In the trial, 1,485 patients were randomized. Subsequent review made 118 (7.9%) of these patients ineligible. The primary analysis of the study was performed on the remaining 1,377 patients. Of these, 714 were assigned to receive no surgical treatment; 663 were assigned to surgical therapy. All patients received the best possible medical treatment to reduce stroke, including aspirin and management of hypertension. No patients were lost to follow-up. Fifteen patients randomized to the nonsurgical group crossed over from one treatment arm to the other when they had EC/IC bypass done. Nine had

40    *Clinical Trials in Neurologic Practice*

*Table 2.4*    Outcome events in the EC/IC Bypass Trial[a]

| | Percent of patients | |
|---|---|---|
| *Type of event*[b] | *Extracranial/intracranial bypass (EC/IC)* | *No bypass* |
| No event | 57 | 56 |
| Nonfatal stroke | 26 | 24 |
| Minor | 19 | 19 |
| Major | 7 | 5 |
| Death | 17 | 20 |

[a]The EC/IC Bypass Study Group. Failure of extracranial-intracranial arterial bypass to reduce the risk of ischemic stroke. N Engl J Med 1985;313:1191–1200.

[b]There was no statistically significant difference between any of the outcomes. Subgroup analysis did not reveal any convincing data to suggest that surgery might be beneficial for any subgroup of patients.

the procedure on the same side as the lesion; six had the procedure on the contralateral side. Of the 663 surgical patients, 652 received the surgery. For the primary analysis, after exclusion of ineligible patients, the intent-to-treat principle was followed. Regardless of actual treatment received, the outcome for each patient was counted for the initial treatment group assigned.

The risk of EC/IC bypass occurs early. Any benefit comes later. Hence, the trial is designed to see if the initial risk of serious complication, such as stroke or death, is balanced by a decreased rate of stroke and death in the future. The success of a surgical procedure depends on a low complication rate. In the EC/IC bypass trial, the *perioperative period* was defined as the time from randomization until 30 days after the bypass procedure. In total, 12.2% of the 663 surgical patients had some type of cerebral ischemic event. Most of these were minor. Major stroke occurred in 30, or 4.5% of the surgical patients in the perioperative period. Of these 30 major strokes, seven (1.1%) were fatal. Ten of these 30 perioperative strokes occurred before the surgery could be performed, and three were fatal. In patients who received surgery, the perioperative morbidity for major stroke and death was 2.5% and 0.6%, respectively. In the nonsurgical group, during a comparable perioperative period, major stroke occurred in 1.3%, and death in 0.1%, of the patients. Subtracting these rates, the burden of EC/IC bypass was 3.2% for major stroke or death and 1% for death alone.

The primary analysis showed no benefit for EC/IC bypass. Fatal and nonfatal stroke occurred earlier in the patients who had bypass surgery. Table 2.4 shows that, over the length of the trial, there was a similar number of events in the two treatment groups. There was convincing evidence of a lack of benefit. Subgroup analysis did not suggest benefit of the procedure in any subgroup of the surgical patients when compared to a comparable subgroup of the nonsurgical patients.

## Carotid Endarterectomy

The purpose of carotid endarterectomy is to prevent stroke by removing atherosclerotic plaques in the internal carotid artery. The risk of stroke for patients with atherosclerotic plaques is much greater for those who have recently had such symptoms as a TIA or minor stroke. The NASCET[5] evaluated carotid endarterectomy for patients who had prior symptoms of stroke or transient stroke. The Asymptomatic Carotid Atherosclerosis Study (ACAS)[6] evaluated carotid endarterectomy for patients who had no prior symptoms attributed to the affected artery.

NASCET was stratified by degree of stenosis of the carotid artery. Severe stenosis was stenosis from 70% to 99%, and moderate stenosis was stenosis from 30% to 69%. This stratification created two parallel trials: one for severe stenosis, another for moderate stenosis. Both trials required angiographic measurement of the degree of stenosis. Patients were initially randomized according to the reading of the angiogram done at the clinical site. Later, the angiograms were read and measured a second time at the central coordinating center for the trial. Patients found to be ineligible because they did not have an appropriate carotid lesion or appropriate symptoms were excluded from the primary analysis. For the severe stenosis strata, 662 patients were randomized. Three patients were later excluded from the primary analysis after central review determined that they were ineligible. No patient was lost to follow-up, and none withdrew. Three hundred twenty-eight patients with severe stenosis were assigned to receive surgery in addition to the best-known medical treatment to prevent stroke. Three hundred thirty-one patients received the best-known medical treatment but no surgery.

Of 328 patients with severe stenosis, one did not receive carotid endarterectomy. In the 30-day perioperative period, 5.8% of the patients had a stroke or died. Major stroke and death occurred in 2.1% of patients. Perioperative death occurred in 0.6% of patients. During a comparable 32-day period from randomization, 3.3% of patients in the nonsurgical group had stroke or death, 0.9% had major stroke or death, and 0.3% died.

The severe stenosis component of NASCET was stopped before the planned completion. Before NASCET investigators began to randomize patients, a plan for interim analysis had been established. Two years after the randomization of the first patient, monthly interim analyses were performed. The protocol specified that if any of the monthly interim analyses showed a significant difference between treatment groups at the 0.001 level of significance, then the chairperson of the performance and safety monitoring board was to be notified. If the difference persisted for 6 months, then the entire monitoring committee was convened. Three years after the start of the NASCET trial, the monitoring committee recommended to the National Institute of Neurological Disorders and Stroke (NINDS) that the trial should stop randomization of patients with severe stenosis. The estimate of the risk of ipsilateral fatal and nonfatal stroke two years after randomization was 26% for patients who did not receive surgical treatment and 9% for those who did. The $p$ value for this difference was less than .001. Patients with severe stenosis in the nonsurgical group who were still eligible for carotid endarterectomy were informed of the trial outcome.

Randomization in NASCET continued for patients with moderate stenosis (less than 70%). This component of the trial continued until the planned end of follow-up. Eventually, 2,267 patients with moderate carotid stenosis were randomized to receive surgery or not to receive surgery. All patients received the best-known medical care to prevent subsequent stroke. A blinded review panel excluded 41 patients from the final analysis due to moderate ineligibility for not

42    *Clinical Trials in Neurologic Practice*

meeting the trial entry criteria. Within this group, 858 patients had stenosis between 50% and 70%, and 1,368 patients had stenosis less than 50%. The average length of follow-up for all patients was 5 years.

The Asymptomatic Carotid Atherosclerosis Study (ACAS) was a clinical trial that evaluated the efficacy of endarterectomy in patients with at least 60% stenosis of a carotid artery and no history of ischemic symptoms (TIA or minor stroke) in the territory of the stenotic artery.[6] Patients who had a previous TIA or minor stroke could be randomized in the ACAS trial if the symptoms were not attributable to the stenotic artery. A total of 1,662 patients were randomized, 825 to surgery as well as medical treatment and 834 to medical treatment alone. Of the 825 patients randomized to surgery, 101 did not have ipsilateral arteriography or carotid endarterectomy; 45 patients refused surgery after randomization, 12 patients were rejected because of severe cardiac disease, 3 had a stroke or died before surgery was performed, 8 were rejected for miscellaneous reasons, and 33 patients were rejected because they were not eligible due to arteriographic findings. In ACAS, a patient could be randomized when a carotid ultrasound result made it likely that the patient would have more than 60% stenosis. The ultrasound finding was checked with an arteriogram after randomization, and surgery was not performed if the degree of stenosis was less than 60% or if there was severe intracranial stenosis. In the group of ACAS patients randomized to receive no surgery, 45 patients received carotid endarterectomy. Nine patients in the surgery group and eleven in the nonsurgical group dropped out from follow-up. The overall trial result for ACAS was that after a median follow-up of 2.7 years, the estimate of the aggregate risk over 5 years for ipsilateral stroke and any perioperative stroke or death was estimated to be 5.1% for patients who received surgery and 11% for patients who did not. The aggregate risk reduction was 53% (95% confidence interval, 22–72%).

The ACAS trial evaluated two treatment strategies. One strategy was to provide optimum medical care until a TIA, if any, occurred. Because the results of NASCET for severe stenosis became known early in the ACAS trial, any patient who had a TIA and still had severe stenosis became a candidate for carotid endarterectomy. The other strategy was to perform an arteriogram and, if the degree of stenosis was 60% or greater, perform carotid endarterectomy. In the group randomized to surgery, the patients received surgery immediately. The advantage of early surgery in preventing stroke in asymptomatic patients was for patients who would have had a stroke before they would have had a warning TIA. Having surgery early, rather than delaying treatment until after a TIA, results in a lower overall stroke rate, because many patients present with a stroke before any warning TIA. One interesting finding in the ACAS was that women had a higher rate of perioperative stroke and death (3.6%) than men (1.7%). The overall risk reduction for men was estimated to be 66%, whereas that for women was only 17%. There was no statistical significance to the difference between men and women ($p = .1$).

ACAS was one of few trials to include the risk of angiography in the evaluation of carotid endarterectomy. In NASCET, all patients had angiography, but because the angiography was required before randomization, any complications were not included in the result of the NASCET trial. Neither ACAS nor NASCET accounted for the risk of angiography performed on patients who were found to be ineligible for surgery.

## TREATMENT OF ACUTE STROKE

### Anticoagulants

Heparin anticoagulation has been widely used for decades during hospitalization after acute stroke. Although heparin had not been demonstrated to be effective in clinical trials, the intention was to prevent stroke progression and recurrence by preventing the formation of blood clots and, perhaps, by promoting endogenous mechanisms of clot lysis. In 1997, the results of a large international randomized multicenter trial comparing subcutaneous heparin to aspirin were published.[17] This trial showed some benefit for prevention of recurrent stroke but no long-term benefit for subcutaneous heparin. The Trial of Organon 10172 in Acute Stroke Treatment (TOAST), published in 1998, compared an intravenous low-molecular-weight heparinoid, ORG10172 (also known as *danaparoid*), to placebo.[18] Patients were included who had symptoms of acute or progressing ischemic stroke of all types and could start treatment within 1 to 24 hours of stroke onset. Patients were excluded if they had evidence on computed tomography scan of midline shift or any intracranial hemorrhage. The primary outcome was defined as a Glasgow Outcome score of I or II and a Barthel Index score between 12 and 20. The intention-to-treat analysis required that patients have at least one clinical evaluation after the baseline examination. One thousand two hundred eighty-one patients were enrolled in the trial. Six of these patients were not included in the intent-to-treat analysis because no Glasgow or Barthel evaluation was done after baseline examination. The primary analysis showed no statistically significant benefit. Of the patients treated with ORG10172, 75.2% had a favorable outcome, compared to 73.7% of the patients treated with placebo ($p = .49$). The estimated odds ratio for favorable outcome was 1.09, with a confidence interval of 0.85–1.41.

Numerous secondary analyses were done with different outcomes. Only the secondary analysis comparing very favorable outcomes at seven days showed a statistically significant increase in favorable outcomes in the group treated with ORG10172. At seven days, 33.9% of patients treated with danaparoid had a very favorable outcome, compared to 27.8% of patients treated with placebo. This benefit was not apparent at three months.

Danaparoid did have the expected adverse effects on some patients. Serious bleeding occurred in 34 patients (5.3%) who received danaparoid and in 17 patients (2.6%) who received placebo. Serious intracranial bleeding occurred at a higher rate in patients with more severe strokes. Eleven patients had a NINDS Stroke Scale score greater than 15 and also had serious bleeding within 10 days of starting treatment. Ten of the 11 patients had received danaparoid. Partway through the trial, the safety monitoring committee recommended that those patients with a stroke scale greater than 15 not be enrolled in the trial for safety reasons.

Recurrent ischemic events during the treatment period occurred in 1.2% of patients, a much smaller proportion of patients than had been expected. Consistent with the expected benefits of danaparoid, recurrent ischemic events occurred less frequently in the group that received danaparoid, but the difference was not statistically significant, primarily because of the small number of events.

The TOAST trial had been preceded by a small clinical study[19] to determine the maximal safe and potentially effective dose for danaparoid. Although the

44    *Clinical Trials in Neurologic Practice*

negative results of the trial are disappointing, there is little doubt that the drug was given at a sufficient dose.

## Tissue Plasminogen Activator

From 1986 to 1995, the National Institute of Neurological Disorders and Stroke sponsored a series of clinical research studies that led to the approval of tissue plasminogen activator as a treatment for acute ischemic stroke by the U.S. Food and Drug Administration. The report of the phase three clinical trial was published in 1995.[20] One very important aspect of this trial is that it was the culmination of a series of carefully planned studies done in a sequence, each building on the previous study's experience. In this way, a drug with a very low therapeutic index was made available to treat stroke. The overarching theme of the trial was rapid treatment with minimal delay to perform diagnostic tests and clinical evaluations. Acute stroke was treated as a rapidly evolving process that required immediate intervention before additional brain tissue became irreversibly injured. In the first of the five studies, a phase II dose escalation and safety study without placebo controls, patients were treated within 90 minutes of the onset of symptoms at seven different intravenous doses of the drug, ranging from 20 to 90 mg/kg of body weight.[21] The early treatment time was chosen because it would be the time when the drug could have the most effect—that is, the time before most brain cells were irreversibly injured by ischemia. The next study was a similar dose escalation and safety study that included patients who could be treated between 90 and 180 minutes from symptom onset.[22] The third study was a very small study, with only 20 patients, that tested methods for randomization in the acute care setting.[23] The fourth study (Part I) was a 291-patient phase IIB study designed to detect drug activity at 24 hours after treatment.[20] The primary outcome was a 4-point or greater improvement from baseline in the National Institutes of Health (NIH) Stroke Scale. Secondary outcome measures included the NIH Stroke Scale, the Modified Rankin Scale, the Barthel Index, and the Glasgow Outcome Scale at 3 months after treatment with tissue plasminogen activator (tPA). The treatment effect as measured by the primary outcome was not statistically significant. However, other outcomes at 24 hours were significant, as were each of the four major clinical outcomes at 3 months. The Performance and Safety Monitoring Board recommended that a phase three trial begin as soon as possible.

The fifth and final study (reported as Part 2) was a 333-patient phase III randomized controlled clinical trial.[20] The primary outcome measure was a consistent and persuasive difference between the tPA and placebo group for each of the three-month outcome variables: NIH Stroke Scale, Barthel, Rankin, and Glasgow Outcome Scale. Patients were stratified by the time from stroke treatment to start of drug infusion. One-half of the patients were treated at 90 or fewer minutes from stroke onset. The other half was treated between 90 and 180 minutes after stroke onset. Special statistical methodology was used to test for a consistent and persuasive difference between four different outcome measurements. A global analysis of the four outcomes was developed to analyze the primary outcome. The trial showed a statistically significant increase in the number of patients with minimal or no disability. The odds ratio for this good outcome was 1.7, equivalent to a relative risk in this trial of 1.3 in favor of tPA. There was also a statistically significant increase in good outcome (minimal or no disability) on each of the four outcome measures used in the trial. This benefit was evident beyond any bad effects from symptomatic intracerebral hemorrhage, which occurred in 6% of the tPA-treated patients compared to 1% of the placebo-treated patients. The analysis of the primary outcome for this phase III trial showed almost exactly the same drug effect for tPA as had been shown in the fourth study which had been only a phase IIB trial of drug activity. Together, these two trials comprised the NINDS tPA Stroke Study, Parts 1 and 2.[20] Six hundred twenty-four patients were treated in these two trials. On first examination, there were no differences between the treatment effects for those patients treated early and those treated later. Further analysis demonstrated that there was a decrease in the benefit of the drug in patients treated later in the three-hour time interval compared to those treated earlier. Extensive statistical modeling was done to determine whether there were potential patient selection criteria that would make it possible to reduce the rate of symptomatic intracerebral hemorrhage and to exclude patients who would not benefit from treatment. No group of patients could be identified who could not potentially benefit from treatment with tPA.[24,25]

The NINDS tPA trials demonstrate the importance of including as many patients as possible in clinical trials. Before reviewing the results of the trial, many stroke experts had predicted that patients with stroke caused by small vessel disease would not benefit from thrombolysis with tPA. The results demonstrate that the patients with strokes attributed at the baseline examination to small vessel disease actually had a higher rate of positive response to the treatment than patients with baseline stroke type of any other category. Before a trial, clinicians are often capable of predicting the baseline characteristics of patients who will have a poor outcome. These characteristics include age, heart disease, and diabetes. Rather than exclude these patients, they should be included and a secondary analysis performed after the trial to determine whether this subgroup may have benefited from the treatment.

Since 1980, more complete data have been obtained on effectiveness of most treatments used for the treatment or prevention of ischemic stroke. Only a few of a multitude of trials that were performed have been selected for discussion in this chapter; they are summarized in Table 2.5. The trials discussed here have been strengthened by other trials testing the same, or similar, treatments. Several trials have been conducted to evaluate aspirin, warfarin, carotid endarterectomy, dipyridamole, and tPA. Each trial has added more information and included a different subset of stroke patients, adding to the completeness of knowledge about treating and preventing stroke. Trials in the future will increasingly evaluate new treatments. Clinical researchers will take on the more daunting task of evaluating strategies for the primary prevention of stroke. So far, cytoprotective drugs have failed to reduce brain injury when given six hours after stroke.[26] More aggressive approaches to stroke treatment will evaluate the same and new drugs even earlier and in combination with thrombolytic therapy. Presentations of cerebrovascular disease other than stroke, such as cerebrovascular dementia, will become the subject of intervention trials. New treatments for intracerebral hemorrhage will be found and tested. Trials will evolve from counting events, such as stroke and death in a few patients, to measuring the functional outcomes of all patients in a trial.

## 46  Clinical Trials in Neurologic Practice

*Table 2.5*   Selected Trials for the Treatment or Prevention of Ischemic Stroke

| Trial name | Active agents | Primary outcome |
|---|---|---|
| Canadian Aspirin-Sulfinpyrazone Trial[8] | Aspirin and sulfinpyrazone | Continuing transient ischemic attack, stroke, or death[a] |
| Ticlopidine Aspirin Trial[9] | Ticlopidine, 500 mg qd | Stroke and all deaths[a] |
| CAPRIE[12] | Clopidogrel, 75 mg qd vs. aspirin, 325 mg qd | Ischemic stroke, myocardial infarction, or vascular death |
| TOAST[18] | ORG10172-danaparoid | Favorable outcome at 3 months (GOS I or II and Barthel 12–20) |
| NINDS (phase IIB)[20] | Recombinant tissue plasminogen activator (rt-PA) | Percentage with improvement of ≥4 points on the 24-hour NIH Stroke Scale. |
| NINDS tPA Stroke Trial (phase III)[20] | Recombinant tissue plasminogen activator (rt-PA) | Global outcome (NIHSS, Rankin, Barthel, and Glasgow) |
| ESPS2 [14] | Aspirin, 25 mg twice daily | Stroke or death, whichever occurred first, during 2 years of observation |
|  | Dipyridamole, 200 mg twice daily |  |
|  | Aspirin plus dipyridamole |  |
| SPAF [15] | Aspirin, 325 mg daily | Stroke or systemic embolism |
|  | Warfarin, PT 1.3–1.8 |  |
| EC/IC Bypass Trial[11] | EC/IC temporal-middle cerebral artery anastomosis | Perioperative stroke and death and subsequent stroke and stroke death |
| ACAS[6] | Carotid endarterectomy in arteries with no symptoms | Ipsilateral stroke or any perioperative stroke or death |
| NASCET severe stenosis (≥70%)[5] | Carotid endarterectomy in patients with symptoms | Any fatal or nonfatal ipsilateral stroke |
| NASCET moderate stenosis (<70%) | Carotid endarterectomy | Any fatal or nonfatal ipsilateral stroke |

ACAS, Asymptomatic Carotid Atherosclerosis Study; CAPRIE, Clopidogrel versus Aspirin in Patients at Risk of Ischemic Events; EC/IC, Extracranial-Intracranial; ESPS2, European Stroke Prevention Study Group 2; GOS, Glasgow outcome score; NASCET, North American Symptomatic Carotid Endarterectomy Trial; NIH, National Institutes of Health; NINDS, National Institute of Neurological Disorders and Stroke; SPAF, Stroke Prevention in Atrial Fibrillation; TOAST, Trial of ORG10172 in Acute Stroke Treatment.

[a]Good outcome is the absence of the primary outcome.

[b]Percentage of all patients receiving aspirin alone or both aspirin and sulfinpyrazone.

[c]Percentage of all patients receiving sulfinpyrazone alone or both aspirin and sulfinpyrazone.

[d]Sufficient gastrointestinal bleeding to produce hematemesis or melena during the trial.

| n | Control[8] | Good outcome (%) | | Adverse events (%) | | Number to treat | Absolute difference (%) |
|---|---|---|---|---|---|---|---|
| | | Active | Control | Active | Control | | |
| 585 | Placebo | 41[b] | 34[c] | 2[d] | 3 | 14.1 | 7.1 |
| | | 38 | 38 | 3 | 1 | n/a | 0.1 |
| 3,069 | Active | 83 | 81 | 2.4 | 3.1 | 50 | 2 |
| 19,185 | Active | 94.68 | 94.17 | 3.75 | 4.22 | 196[e] | 0.51 |
| 1,281 | Placebo | 75.2 | 73.7 | 8.5 | 5.4 | — | 1.5 |
| 291 | Placebo | 47[f] | 27[f] | 6 | 0 | 5 | 20 |
| | | 47[g] | 39[g] | — | — | 12.5 | 8 |
| 333 | Placebo | 39[f] | 26[f] | 7 | 1 | 7 | 13 |
| 6,602 | Placebo | 80.07[h] | 77.03 | 8.2 | 4.5 | 32.8 | 3.04 |
| | | 80.56 | | 4.7 | 4.5 | 28.32 | 3.53 |
| | | 82.63 | | 8.7 | 4.5 | 18.76 | 5.33 |
| 1,330 | Placebo | 96.4/yr | 93.7/yr | — | — | 37 | 2.7/yr |
| | | 97.7/yr | 92.6/yr | — | — | 19.6 | 5.1/yr |
| 1,377 | No treatment | 57 | 56 | — | — | — | — |
| 1,662 | No treatment | 89 | 95 | 2.3[i] | 0.4 | 19 | 6 |
| 659 | No treatment | 91 | 74 | 5.8 | 3.3 | 6 | 17 |
| 858[j] | No treatment | 78[j] | 84[j] | 6.7[k] | 2.4[k] | 15[j] | 6[j] |
| 1,368[l] | | 85[l] | 81[l] | — | — | 26[l] | 4[l] |

[e]Number of patients to treat to prevent one additional event that would not be prevented by aspirin.

[f]Good Outcome is modified Rankin scale 0 or 1 (minimal or no disability) at 3 months.

[g]Percentage with NIHSS improvement by 4 or more points at 24 hours.

[h]Percentage of patients surviving 2 years without stroke or death.

[i]Includes any stroke or perioperative death, including those due to angiography (1.2%).

[j]Patients with 50–69% carotid stenosis.

[k]Patients with less than 70% carotid stenosis.

[l]Patients with less than 50% carotid stenosis.

# 48 *Clinical Trials in Neurologic Practice*

## REFERENCES

1. Pickard JD, Murray GD, Illingworth R, et al. Effect of oral nimodipine on cerebral infarction and outcome after subarachnoid haemorrhage: British aneurysm nimodipine trial. BMJ 1989;298:636–642.
2. Sherman DG for the STAT Writers Group. Defibrinogenation with viprinex (ancrod) for the treatment of acute ischemic stroke. Stroke 1999;30(1):234.
3. Furlan A, Higashida R, Wechsler L, et al. for the PROACT Investigators. Intra-arterial prourokinase for acute ischemic stroke. JAMA 1999;282:2003–2011.
4. DeKeyser J, Sulter G, Luiten PG. Clinical trials with neuroprotective drugs in acute ischaemic stroke: are we doing the right thing? Trends Neurosci 1999;22:535–540.
5. North American Symptomatic Carotid Endarterectomy Trial Collaborators. Beneficial effect of carotid endarterectomy in symptomatic patients with high-grade carotid stenosis. N Engl J Med 1991;325:445–453.
6. Executive Committee for the Asymptomatic Carotid Atherosclerosis Study. Endarterectomy for asymptomatic carotid artery stenosis. JAMA 1995;273:1421–1428.
7. Findings from the aspirin component of the ongoing Physician's Health Study. N Engl J Med 1988;318:262–264.
8. The Canadian Cooperative Study Group. A randomized trial of aspirin and sulfinpyrazone in threatened stroke. N Engl J Med 1978;299:53–59.
9. Hass WK, Easton JD, Adams HP Jr, et al. for the Ticlipidine Aspirin Study Group. A randomized trial comparing ticolopidine hydrochloride with aspirin for the prevention of stroke in high risk patients. N Engl J Med 1989;321:501–507.
10. Food and Drug Administration. International Conference on Harmonisation: choice of control group in clinical trials. Federal Register 1999;64(185):51767–51780.
11. The EC/IC Bypass Study Group. Failure of extracranial-intracranial arterial bypass to reduce the risk of ischemic stroke. N Engl J Med 1985;313:1191–1200.
12. CAPRIE Steering Committee. A randomised, blinded, trial of clopidogrel versus aspirin in patients at risk of ischaemic events (CAPRIE). Lancet 1996;348:1329–1339.
13. ESPS Group. The European Stroke Prevention Study (ESPS): principal endpoints. Lancet 1987;ii:1351–1354.
14. Diener HC, Cunha L, Forbes C, et al. European Stroke Prevention Study 2. Dipyridamole and acetylsalicylic acid in the secondary prevention of stroke. J Neuro Sci 1996;143:1–13.
15. Stroke Prevention in Atrial Fibrillation Investigators. Stroke prevention in atrial fibrillation study final results. Circulation 1991;84:527–539.
16. Siekert, RG. Anticoagulant therapy in cerebrovascular disease. Clin Neurosurg 1963;9:131–141.
17. International Stroke Trial Collaborative Group. The International Stroke Trial (IST): A randomised trial of aspirin, subcutaneous heparin, both, or neither among 19435 patients with acute ischemic stroke. Lancet 1997;349:1569–1581.
18. The Publications Committee for the Trial of ORG10172 in Acute Stroke Treatment (TOAST) Investigators. Low molecular weight heparinoid, ORG 10172 (danaparoid), and outcome after acute ischemic stroke. JAMA 1998;279:1265–1272.
19. Biller J, Massey EW, Marler JR, et al. A dose escalation study of ORG10172 (low molecular weight heparinoid) in stroke. Neurology 1989;39:262–265.
20. The National Institute of Neurological Disorders and Stroke rt-PA Stroke Study Group. Tissue plasminogen activator for acute ischemic stroke. N Engl J Med 1995;333(14):1581–1587.
21. Brott TG, Haley EC, Levy DE. Urgent therapy for stroke. Part I. Pilot study of tissue plasminogen activator administered within 90 minutes. Stroke 1992;23(5):632–640.
22. Haley EC, Levt DE, Brott TG, et al. Urgent therapy for stroke. Part II. Pilot study of tissue plasminogen activator administered 91–180 minutes from onset. Stroke 1992;23(5):641–645.
23. Haley EC, Brott TG, Sheppard GL, et al. Pilot randomized trial of tissue plasminogen activator in acute ischemic stroke. The TPA Bridging Group. Stroke 1993;24(7):1000–1004.
24. The National Institute of Neurological Disorders and Stroke rt-PA Stroke Study Group. Intracerebral hemorrhage after intravenous rt-PA therapy for ischemic stroke. Stroke 1997;28:2109–2118.
25. The National Institute of Neurological Disorders and Stroke rt-PA Stroke Study Group. Generalized efficacy of rt-PA for acute stroke: subgroup analysis of the NINDS rt-PA stroke trial. Stroke 1997;28:2119–2125.
26. De Keyser J, Sulter G, Luiten P. Clinical trials with neuroprotective drugs in acute ischemic stroke: are we doing the right thing? Trends Neurosci 1999;22:535–540.

# 3
# Intracerebral Hemorrhage

Carlos S. Kase

The management of patients with intracerebral hemorrhage (ICH) involves a number of complex issues, including the prevention and treatment of increased intracranial pressure (ICP), the choice between surgical and nonsurgical approaches, and the use of novel surgical techniques. The difficulties in selecting the proper approach to these are due mainly to a paucity of prospective controlled clinical trials for the assessment of various interventions, resulting in treatment decisions that are guided by personal opinion or preference, generally based on the results of small clinical series or nonrandomized prospective observations, with their inherent biases.[1] This is in stark contrast to the abundant data from randomized clinical trials (RCTs) that currently direct the management of acute ischemic stroke and subarachnoid hemorrhage.[2] The following sections review the studies that have attempted to address the various therapeutic issues in ICH, pointing to their strengths and weaknesses as well as to the clinical usefulness of the data they have generated.

## PREVENTION AND TREATMENT OF INCREASED INTRACRANIAL PRESSURE

Intracranial pressure is directly related to the volume of the intracranial contents that include brain volume, cerebrospinal fluid volume, and cerebral blood volume. In the presence of a cerebral mass lesion such as ICH, the increased brain volume may result in raised ICP, unless a concomitant reduction in the volume of the other compartments takes place, either physiologically or through therapeutic intervention. The management of increased ICP in patients with ICH has been approached in a number of ways, but the only measures that have been evaluated in controlled clinical trials have been the use of corticosteroids[3,4] and glycerol[5] for the reduction of brain edema, and hemodilution for improving microcirculatory function in areas surrounding the ICH[6] (Table 3.1).

49

50    *Clinical Trials in Neurologic Practice*

*Table 3.1*    Anti-edema agents tested in randomized, placebo-controlled clinical trials in intracerebral hemorrhage

| Agent | Dose | Mortality (%) |
|---|---|---|
| Dexamethasone[3] | 120 mg IV/IM over 10 days | 74[a] |
| Placebo | — | 71 |
| Dexamethasone[4] | 150 mg IV over 9 days | 48[b] |
| Placebo | — | 45 |
| Glycerol[5] | 500 cc 10% glycerol/day for 6 days | 34.5[c] |
| Placebo | — | 30.2 |

[a]At 14 days.
[b]At 21 days.
[c]At 6 months.

## Corticosteroids in the Management of Acute Intracerebral Hemorrhage

Corticosteroids are of proven value in reducing peritumoral edema in patients with metastatic or primary brain tumors,[7] but their role in the treatment of acute stroke patients is controversial.[8,9] In supratentorial ICH in particular, the evidence from two controlled clinical trials points to a lack of benefit,[3] or even harm,[4] from the use of this therapy.

Tellez and Bauer[3] compared the outcome of 40 ICH patients who received either 120 mg of dexamethasone over a 10-day period (initial dose, 12 mg intravenously [IV], then 4 mg IM intramuscularly every 6 hours for 3 days, 4 mg IM every 8 hours for 3 days, 4 mg IM every 12 hours for 2 days, and 4 mg IM per day for 2 days) with a group of 21 patients who received placebo. The treatment was started within 48 hours of stroke onset. The first 17 patients were openly assigned to treatment or control groups, whereas the remaining 23 patients entered a double-blind randomized assignment to dexamethasone or placebo. Figures of mortality at 14 days were similar for the two groups, with 74% for the dexamethasone-treated group (n = 19) and 71% for those who received placebo (n = 21). This study was conducted in the days preceding computed tomography (CT), thus not allowing for the evaluation of potentially important differences between the two groups, such as location and size of the hematoma—variables known to have a major impact in mortality.[1] In addition, the treatment group had more severe deficits at baseline, and patients with hemorrhagic infarction were also included, suggesting that the relatively small sample was a heterogeneous group of patients with an unknown distribution of diagnoses and stroke severity; this adds further doubt to the validity of the results obtained.

Similarly negative results were obtained by Poungvarin et al.,[4] who conducted a randomized, double-blind trial of the use of dexamethasone in 93 patients with CT-diagnosed ICH treated within 48 hours of stroke onset. The design included stratification of patients by admission level of consciousness (Glasgow coma score [GCS] 3–7, 8–11, and 12–14), and the use of IV dexamethasone for a period of 9 days at an initial dose of 10 mg, followed by 5 mg every 6 hours for 6 days, 5 mg every 12 hours for 2 days, and 5 mg for 1 day. The baseline variables were well balanced between the two groups; neither group was treated with mannitol or glycerol, and hyperventilation was attempted in all patients who developed signs of brain herniation. At the time of a third interim analysis with 93 subjects enrolled (dexamethasone, 46; placebo, 47), the mortality rate after 21 days from onset was 48% for the dexamethasone-treated group and 45% for the placebo ($p = .93$). Among patients with a GCS greater than or equal to 8, the 7-day mortality was significantly lower ($p = .01$) for the treatment group, but no differences in mortality were detected subsequently (at 21 days) in this subgroup. The rate of complications (infections, complications of diabetes) was significantly higher ($p < .001$) in the dexamethasone-treated patients (20 of 46, or 43%) than in the controls (6 of 47, or 13%). Although the number of diabetics was the same in the two groups, the blood glucose levels after 24 hours of treatment were $191.5 \pm 9.9$ mg/dl in the treatment group and $155.0 \pm 7.7$ mg/dl in the control group ($p = .04$). It is possible that hyperglycemia was an additional factor correlated with the poor outcome observed in the treated group, as the presence of hyperglycemia has been shown to correlate with worse outcome in patients with acute ischemic stroke than with those who are normoglycemic at presentation.[10,11] These interim analysis results of equal mortality and higher complication rates in the treated group led to early termination of the trial because of a significantly poorer outcome in the dexamethasone-treated patients. These data suggest that dexamethasone at the doses tested in this study is not to be recommended for the treatment of acute ICH.

## Intravenous Glycerol in the Management of Acute Intracerebral Hemorrhage

The apparent value of IV glycerol as an anti-edema agent in experimental animals prompted Yu et al.[5] to test this agent in patients with ICH. In a double-blind, randomized, placebo-controlled design, they enrolled 216 patients with CT-documented ICH who were treated within 24 hours from onset with IV glycerol (500 ml of 10% glycerol) or 500 ml of physiologic saline placebo given over 4 hours for 6 consecutive days. The baseline characteristics of the two groups (glycerol, 107; placebo, 109) were well balanced, including stratification of patients to GCS levels of 3–7, 8–11, and 12–15. The outcome data included mortality and functional outcome comparisons in the two groups at various intervals from treatment onset. At 6 months, there were no differences in mortality (glycerol, 34.5%; placebo, 30.2%), or increases in Barthel index score (glycerol, $21.18 \pm 21.2$; placebo, $23.81 \pm 20$) and reduction in GCS score (glycerol, $0.81 \pm 1.5$; placebo, $1.16 \pm 1.7$) in 6-month survivors. The main complication of therapy, hemolysis, was severe enough to warrant discontinuation of therapy in nine glycerol-treated patients. The results of this trial indicate no benefits of IV glycerol in patients with ICH in terms of either survival or improved functional outcome at 6 months, at the same time showing substantial treatment-related side effects.

## Hemodilution in the Management of Acute Intracerebral Hemorrhage

Hemodilution, by decreasing blood viscosity without reducing its oxygen-carrying capacity, leads to an improvement in cerebral blood flow in acute

52   *Clinical Trials in Neurologic Practice*

stroke. The Italian Haemodilution Trial[6] evaluated the effects of therapeutic hemodilution when administered within 12 hours of onset to patients with acute stroke in a randomized controlled design. A total of 633 patients were treated with hemodilution by the combination of venesection followed by volume replacement with Dextran-40 (i.e., isovolemic hemodilution), with the purpose of lowering the hematocrit to an intended 35%. This group was then compared with a control group (n = 634) managed with conventional measures for acute stroke. The entry criteria included patients with ischemic and hemorrhagic strokes, the latter including 83 patients in the treatment group and 81 controls. The overall results were negative, as mortality and disability at 6 months were equal in the two groups, the same as in the ischemic and hemorrhagic stroke subgroups. Outcome measures in the group with ICH were almost identical in the hemodilution and control groups, with 30% and 31% mortality, 39% and 33% severe disability, and 31% and 35% functional independence, respectively.

### Other Nonsurgical Interventions in the Management of Acute Intracerebral Hemorrhage

A number of measures are of importance in the management of patients with an acute ICH, but few have been evaluated in a controlled fashion. Most of these treatments are supported in their use by data from clinical series and generally reflect the experience in the management of ICH in the intensive care unit setting.[2] As a result of the lack of controlled data, these recommendations are reviewed only briefly.

*Head position* plays an important role in the management of increased ICP, as minor changes in head position can result in substantial variations of ICP, due to impairment in venous drainage from the cranial cavity. A head position to be avoided is horizontal with hyper-rotation, as it is associated with the most consistent elevations in ICP. The position that most effectively facilitates cranial venous drainage is head elevation to 20–30 degrees.[12] Because *hyperthermia* increases cerebral blood flow and ICP, the use of cooling blankets and antipyretics is essential in the management of patients with ICH. Although *hypothermia* is known to reduce the cerebral metabolic rate by as much as 50% at a body temperature of 30°C,[13] the therapeutic value of induced hypothermia in patients with intracranial masses and elevated ICP has not been demonstrated.[14] *Hypoxia* leads to raised ICP in patients with poor intracranial compliance. The maintenance of adequate oxygenation is thus essential in this setting, and it often requires the use of endotracheal intubation, which is recommended in patients with $PO_2$ below 60 mm Hg, or $PCO_2$ greater than 50 mm Hg, or who are at risk for aspiration.[2] *Hypertension* in patients with ICH contributes to increased ICP, promotes the formation of brain edema, and may be associated with continued growth of the hematoma.[2] However, precise guidelines for blood pressure control are not available, and the current recommendation, based on uncontrolled observations, is to maintain a mean arterial pressure below 130 mm Hg with the use of the alpha- and beta-blocker labetalol in combination with diuretics (furosemide), or nitroprusside in patients who fail to respond to the former agent.[15] *Seizures* in patients with ICH should be treated promptly, as they are associated with transient increase in ICP, even in paralyzed patients.[14]

The specific measures used to control elevated ICP in patients with ICH have not been tested in RCTs,[16] and their use is based on the observed improved outcome of patients treated aggressively in the intensive care unit setting. *Hyperventilation* to a $PCO_2$ of 30–35 mm Hg effectively reduces ICP by inducing cerebral vasoconstriction. Whether this effect is transient or sustained over several days is still a matter of controversy.[2] Because its effects are rapid and are maximal early after its institution, hyperventilation is particularly valuable in instances of acutely elevated ICP with impending cerebral herniation or midline displacement. *Osmotic diuretics*, such as mannitol, also rapidly and reliably lower ICP. Their effect is probably via a combination of a shifting of water from the brain substance into the intravascular space, a reduction in cerebrospinal fluid production and volume, and an improvement in cerebral microcirculation.[15] Their use in patients with ICH has been associated with improved outcomes in uncontrolled clinical series.[17] *High-dose intravenous barbiturates*, such as thiopental (1–5 mg/kg), lower ICP but have the disadvantage of promoting hypotension and infections, along with a resulting coma that renders the clinical neurologic examination impossible to follow.

## Continuous Intracranial Pressure Monitoring

The use of continuous monitoring of ICP in patients with ICH has improved our understanding of the course and consequences of elevated ICP in patients with ICH. The early observations of Janny et al.[18] on continuous ICP monitoring via a ventricular catheter indicated that the highest levels of increased ICP occur early in the course of patients with ICH, with subsequent gradual decline in ICP until normalization in 20–30 days. They suggested that continuous ICP monitoring is a valuable tool in the management of patients with ICH, serving as a guide to the need to subject to surgical therapy those patients in whom the initially raised ICP fails to decline with use of maximal medical therapy. Subsequently, Papo et al.[19] documented an inconsistent correlation between ICP and level of consciousness in relationship to outcome. Although a good correlation of level of consciousness and ICP was observed at the two extremes of ICP (alert patients had normal or slightly elevated ICP, whereas those in coma had markedly elevated ICP), in those with intermediate levels of ICP, the correlation was poor. In their series, the 22 patients who had surgical drainage of ICH on the basis of their clinical and ICP parameters had the same mortality (32%) as the 44 patients treated nonsurgically (29%). Ropper and King[20] reported their experience with the ICP monitoring of 10 consecutive comatose patients with supratentorial ICH. Using a subarachnoid screw device for ICP monitoring, they found that all four patients who remained with ICPs consistently above 20 mm Hg, and did not undergo surgical evacuation of the hematoma, died. The three patients with similar ICP-recording patterns who underwent surgery survived; one of these patients died 1 month later from causes unrelated to stroke. These results led the authors to suggest that continuous ICP measurement in comatose patients with supratentorial ICH is a potentially valuable tool to help make the decision of whether to subject these critically ill patients to surgical drainage of the hematoma.

## 54 *Clinical Trials in Neurologic Practice*

*Table 3.2*   Nonrandomized clinical series of surgical management of intracerebral hemorrhage: precomputed tomography scan series

| Author(s) | Year | No. of patients | | Mortality (%) | |
|---|---|---|---|---|---|
| | | Surgical group | Medical group | Surgical group | Medical group |
| Cuatico et al.[21] | 1965 | 102 | 0 | 8 | — |
| Cook et al.[22] | 1965 | 57 | 0 | 51 | — |
| Luessenhop et al.[23] | 1967 | 37 | 27 | 32 | 44 |
| Paillas and Alliez[24] | 1973 | 250 | 0 | 36 | — |
| Pásztor et al.[25] | 1980 | 156 | 0 | 17 | — |
| Kaneko et al.[26] | 1977 | 38 | 0 | 8 | — |

## CHOICE BETWEEN SURGICAL AND NONSURGICAL MANAGEMENT OF INTRACEREBRAL HEMORRHAGE

This continues to be a most difficult treatment decision in patients with ICH, as there are only scarce data available to help the clinician in the management of individual patients. This is largely the result of a remarkable paucity of prospective randomized treatment trials in ICH. In addition, the information gathered from nonrandomized clinical series has been predictably inconsistent among studies, and the amount of useful information derived from them has been meager. The following section contains a review of the results of nonrandomized clinical series and of RCTs in ICH.

### Nonrandomized Clinical Series

Before the introduction of CT scan, six uncontrolled studies[21–26] addressed the issue of surgical treatment of ICH (Table 3.2). Cuatico et al.[21] reported 102 patients treated surgically with a remarkably low mortality of 8%. However, the report did not state the distribution of patients by degree of preoperative clinical severity or the criteria for the selection of surgical therapy, suggesting that the low mortality figures may have simply reflected the selection of patients by their low surgical risk. These authors made the observation of a more favorable outcome in operated patients with lobar hematomas than in those with deep hemispheric hemorrhages. Cook et al.[22] reported their experience with 57 surgically treated patients with supratentorial ICH and documented the best results in those who had less severe clinical deficits at presentation and were clinically stable or improving. These authors pointed out the biases of selected surgical series, as only one-third of their patients were in a poor preoperative prognostic category, and wondered about a potentially equally favorable outcome for those in the better preoperative prognostic category, should they have been treated nonsurgically. Luessenhop et al.[23] reported 64 patients with supratentorial ICH, 37 treated with craniotomy, performed in the majority of them, within 24 hours from stroke onset, and 27 treated nonsurgically. The mortality for the surgical group was 32% (12 of 37), whereas that of the nonsurgical group was 44% (12 of 27). As in other nonrandomized studies, the decision regarding assignment to surgical or nonsurgical treatment was made by the surgeon, on the basis of the preoperative clinical condition. These authors also observed a much lower mortality rate in patients with lobar (11%) than with deep basal ganglionic (92%) hemorrhages, who had operative mortalities of 4% and 89%, respectively. Paillas and Alliez[24] reported a 30-day mortality of 36% in a group of 250 patients with ICH treated surgically. The selection biases in the series included the exclusion of elderly patients (only 18% were older than 60 years) and a tendency to delay surgery until the fifth to tenth day after onset, the latter strategy taking advantage of the exclusion of patients who present with severely compromised condition and have attendant early mortality.[27] Pásztor et al.[25] reported a 17% operative mortality in a group of 156 patients with supratentorial ICH, but most operations were delayed (56% after 2 weeks from onset). As expected, the number of comatose or stuporous patients at the time of operation declined from 65% to 11% for those operated within 3 days, and after 1 month, from onset, respectively. Kaneko et al.[26] reported their initial experience with 38 patients with putaminal hemorrhage who had early (within 7 hours from onset) evacuation of ICH. A low mortality of 8% was attributed to the ability to surgically obliterate the bleeding artery, thus preventing the reaccumulation of the hematoma. In addition, the authors stated that early surgery allows for the removal of the clot before the full development of cerebral edema, a feature that they related to the improved outcome in their series.

Since the introduction of CT, the understanding of prognostic variables related to the hematoma itself has stimulated an interest in defining subgroups of patients who may benefit from surgical drainage of the ICH and in evaluating the results of surgical and nonsurgical treatment of comparable groups of patients. The main nonrandomized studies of surgical and nonsurgical treatment of CT-defined ICH are listed in Table 3.3. Kanaya et al.[28] found no differences in outcome in patients who are alert or somnolent on one hand, or comatose on the other, suggesting that surgery offers no therapeutic benefit for patients with putaminal hemorrhage at either end of the spectrum of clinical severity. In the group of intermediate clinical severity, the surgical mortality was 18%, in comparison with 52% for patients treated nonsurgically. The authors concluded that patients with putaminal hemorrhage who were alert or somnolent should be treated nonsurgically, whereas surgery should be considered in those who have a more severely depressed level of consciousness. Similarly encouraging results were reported from the retrospective series of Kaneko et al.[29] These authors reported their experience with early (within 7 hours of onset) surgery in 100 patients who were either "stuporous" (GCS scores of 10–12) or "semicomatose" (GCS scores of 6–9), with hematomas of more than 20 to 30 $cm^3$ in volume, and with more than 5 mm of midline shift. Patients with "mild symptoms" and those in coma with GCS scores of 5 or lower were treated nonsurgically. The surgical mortality was remarkably low at 7%, and the long-term outcome was highly satisfactory, with 89% of the 93 survivors being ambulatory after 6 months from surgery. However, these results should be interpreted with caution, as there was no control group treated nonsurgically, and the preoperative level of consciousness was relatively good for the group overall, as 78% of the patients had GCS scores of 10–13, and only 22% had GCS scores in the 6–9 range. Other nonrandomized trials have generally shown lack of superiority of one form of therapy over the other. Waga and Yamamoto[30] compared 18 patients with putaminal hemorrhage treated surgically with 56 patients treated nonsurgically, and the 30-day

## 56  Clinical Trials in Neurologic Practice

*Table 3.3*  Nonrandomized clinical series of surgical management of intracerebral hemorrhage: computed tomography scan series

| Author(s) | Year | No. of patients | | Mortality (%) | |
|---|---|---|---|---|---|
| | | Surgical group | Medical group | Surgical group | Medical group |
| Kanaya et al.[28] | 1980 | 410 | 204 | 18[a] | 58[a] |
| Kaneko et al.[29] | 1983 | 100 | 0 | 7 | — |
| Waga and Yamamoto[30] | 1983 | 18 | 56 | 28 | 14 |
| Bolander et al.[31] | 1983 | 39 | 35 | 13 | 20 |
| Volpin et al.[32] | 1984 | 32[b] | 34[b] | 19 | 44 |
| Kanno et al.[33] | 1984 | Total of 265 patients with putaminal intracerebral hemorrhage | | 4[c,d] | 8 |
| | | | | 17[a,c] | 25[a,c] |
| | | | | 86[c,e] | 96[c,e] |
| Piotrowski and Rochowanski[35] | 1996 | 300 | 0 | 31 | — |
| Schwarz et al.[36,f] | 1997 | 24 | 24 | 42[c] | 54[c] |

[a]Patients with moderate putaminal hemorrhage.
[b]Patients with hematoma volumes of 26–85 cc.
[c]Dead or vegetative.
[d]Patients with mild putaminal hemorrhage.
[e]Patients with severe putaminal hemorrhage.
[f]Retrospective, case-control series.

mortality rate was 28% and 14%, respectively, a statistically significant difference in favor of nonsurgical treatment. However, these results are difficult to interpret because the two treatment groups were markedly different in size, noncontemporaneous, and with marked differences in the preoperative level of consciousness; 44% of the surgical patients were in poor clinical grades, whereas only 20% were in those categories in the nonsurgical group. Bolander et al.[31] found no differences in mortality at 3 months between their 39 surgical (13% mortality) and 35 nonsurgical (20% mortality) patients with supratentorial ICH. However, they found that patients with hematoma volumes of 40–80 cm$^3$ did better in the surgical group (6% mortality) than in the nonsurgical group (25% mortality). Similar conclusions were reached by Volpin et al.[32] after the analysis of 132 patients with basal ganglionic and lobar hemorrhages. These authors found no mortality among 39 patients with volumes below 26 cm$^3$, all treated nonsurgically, whereas 34 comatose patients with hematoma volumes of 85 cm$^3$ or more (23 treated surgically, 11 nonsurgically) had 100% mortality. In the intermediate group of 59 patients with hematoma volumes between 26 and 85 cm$^3$, the 32 who had surgery had significantly better survival rates than the 34 who did not. Kanno et al.[33] analyzed their results of treatment of 265 patients with putaminal hemorrhage and found differences in outcome between the surgical and nonsurgical group that depended on the severity of the initial clinical picture and the degree of extension and mass effect of the hematoma on CT: Patients with large hematomas that displaced the midline and extended into the

Intracerebral Hemorrhage    57

diencephalon and midbrain had poor outcomes regardless of the form of treatment used; those with small hematomas with minimal mass effect and no ventricular extension did well irrespective of the treatment modality used; and those in the intermediate category had slightly better outcomes after surgery, especially when performed within 6 hours of ICH onset. Similar conclusions were reached by Fujitsu et al.,[34] based on their analysis of 180 patients with putaminal hemorrhage: In patients with either nonprogressive or fulminant clinical course, surgery offered no advantage over nonsurgical treatment; in those with a rapidly progressive course, surgical treatment was superior to nonsurgical treatment. The retrospective study of Piotrowski and Rochowanski[35] documented an operative mortality of 31% in 300 patients older than 60 years of age who underwent surgical drainage of hematomas 3 cm in diameter or larger on CT scan. This study did not include a nonsurgically treated comparison group. Using a retrospective case-control design, Schwarz et al.[36] compared the outcome of 24 surgical patients with ICH of lobar or ganglionic location with 24 matched, unoperated patients. The outcome, labeled as *dead* or *vegetative*, was achieved by a similar proportion of surgically treated (42%) and nonsurgically treated (54%) patients at hospital discharge.

The biased, imprecise, and at times contradictory data generated by these non-randomized clinical series have failed to clarify the issue of whether surgical treatment is superior to nonsurgical management of ICH. Some of the observations, such as that of the possible benefit of surgery in intermediate-size hematomas and in those of lobar location, are useful as testable hypotheses that deserve analysis in properly designed and conducted prospective RCTs.

## Randomized Clinical Trials

A relatively small number of patients have been enrolled in RCTs for the assessment of the benefits of surgical or nonsurgical treatment of ICH (Table 3.4). The first trial was conducted by McKissock et al.[37] in 1961, before the introduction of CT scan. One hundred eighty patients, 91 treated nonsurgically and 89 treated by surgery, were comparable in regard to baseline characteristics, and the majority was treated within 48 hours of ICH onset. The mortality rates were similar in the two groups, 51% for the nonsurgical group and 65% for the surgical group, and the level of functional disability on follow-up was virtually the same. These authors reported that patients with lobar hematomas had a better outcome than those with basal ganglionic or thalamic hemorrhages, but in neither group was surgery superior to nonsurgical treatment. Juvela et al.[38] reported the results of randomization of 52 patients with supratentorial ICH to surgical (n = 26) or non-surgical (n = 26) treatment within 48 hours from onset. Patients were enrolled if they had a GCS score less than 9 and/or severe hemiparesis or aphasia, and were admitted to the hospital within 24 hours from ICH onset. The mortality rates were the same for the two groups, both acutely and after long-term follow-up. When patients were stratified according to their prerandomization clinical status, those who were "stuporous" or "semicomatose" with GCS scores of 7–10 did better when treated surgically, but the numbers of patients in the groups were small (four surgical, five nonsurgical), and the quality of life of the five survivors (four surgical, one nonsurgical) was poor; all being totally disabled at 1 year after ICH. These authors found no differences in outcome in the surgical group

## 58    Clinical Trials in Neurologic Practice

*Table 3.4*    Randomized clinical trials of surgical management of intracerebral hemorrhage

| Author(s) | Year | No. of patients | | Mortality (%) | |
|---|---|---|---|---|---|
| | | Surgical group | Medical group | Surgical group | Medical group |
| McKissock et al.[37] | 1961 | 89 | 91 | 65 | 51 |
| Juvela et al.[38] | 1989 | 26 | 26 | 46 | 38 |
| Batjer et al.[39] | 1990 | 8 | 13 | 50[a] | 85[a] |
| Morgenstern et al.[40] | 1998 | 17 | 17 | 19[b] | 24[b] |
| Zuccarello et al.[41] | 1999 | 9 | 11 | 22[c] | 27[c] |
| Auer et al.[45,d] | 1989 | 50 | 50 | 42[b] | 70[b] |

[a]Dead or vegetative.
[b]Mortality at 6 months.
[c]Mortality at 3 months.
[d]Surgical arm was endoscopic surgery.

based on early or late operations during the initial 24 hours. Their conclusion, based on an overall mortality of 42% at 6 months and the poor quality of life in the survivors (irrespective of the treatment modality used), was that supratentorial ICH should be treated conservatively. Batjer et al.[39] randomized patients with putaminal hemorrhage to three treatment groups: (1) "Best medical management," which included endotracheal intubation and hyperventilation, osmotic diuretics and furosemide, dexamethasone, and appropriate treatment of hypertension and other medical complications; (2) Best medical management plus ICP monitoring by frontal ventriculostomy, aimed at maintaining ICP below 20 mm Hg, with the use of medical therapy, at times with the addition of intermittent CSF drainage; and (3) Surgical evacuation of the hematoma using microsurgical technique. After randomizing only 21 patients over a period of 5.5 years, an interim analysis showed that patients fared very poorly, regardless of treatment group assignment: 15 patients (71%) had died or remained in a vegetative state at 6 months after treatment, and only four (19%) were at home and living independently. Due to these poor results, the trial was terminated. Although the GCS scores were not used to assess preoperative level of consciousness and hematoma volumes were not provided, it appears that the majority of the patients (14 of 21, or 67%) were in an intermediate level of neurologic involvement. Although this trial suffered from methodological flaws (incomplete characterization of the clinical and CT features of the treatment groups), its results failed to suggest that any one treatment modality is favorable in the management of patients with putaminal ICH. In a meta-analysis that included all patients enrolled in these three randomized trials of open craniotomy for ICH, Hankey and Hon[16] concluded that the odds of being "dead or dependent" at 6 months were 2.1 times greater among patients treated surgically than among those treated nonsurgically.

In a recent communication, Morgenstern et al.[40] demonstrated the feasibility of performing a randomized clinical trial of surgical versus nonsurgical treatment of ICH by randomizing 17 patients to each group over a 3-year period at a

*Intracerebral Hemorrhage* 59

single institution. Surgery (conventional open craniotomy with hematoma drainage by suction) was performed within 12 hours of ICH onset, and the series included patients with lobar and putaminal hemorrhage. The randomization process resulted in comparable data on ICH volume (surgical group, 49 cm$^3$; nonsurgical group, 44 cm$^3$) and GCS score (surgical group, 11; nonsurgical group, 10), but there was an imbalance with regard to hematoma location, as there was a higher proportion of putaminal than lobar hemorrhages in the surgical group. The results indicated a nonsignificant trend toward decreased mortality in the surgical group at 1 month (surgical group, 5.9%; nonsurgical group, 23.5%), but at 6 months the benefit of surgery essentially disappeared (mortality: surgical group, 18.9%; nonsurgical group, 23.5%) (see Table 3.4). It is possible that a true beneficial effect of surgery in this group of patients could not be demonstrated because of the small numbers of patients included.

In a similar single-institution feasibility study, Zuccarello et al.[41] randomized 20 patients with supratentorial (lobar, putaminal, thalamic) ICH to surgery within 8 hours of onset or nonsurgical treatment. The surgical group (n = 9) was comparable to the nonsurgical group (n = 11) in terms of baseline variables (age, National Institutes of Health Stroke Scale [NIHSS] and GCS score, ICH volume), but there was an imbalance with regard to intraventricular extension of the ICH, which was present in 73% of the nonsurgical group and 33% of the surgical group. Because intraventricular extension of ICH is a powerful predictor of poor outcome in ICH,[42] this imbalance may have played a role in biasing the results against the nonsurgical group. The surgical procedure was either conventional craniotomy (n = 7) or stereotactic drainage with local instillation of a thrombolytic agent (urokinase). The overall results showed a nonsignificant trend toward better outcome at 3 months in the surgical group, as measured by functional outcome scales (favorable Glasgow Outcome Scale in 56% of surgical and 36% of nonsurgical patients; Barthel Index greater than 75 in 44% and 27%, respectively; Rankin Scale score of 2 and 4, respectively), whereas mortality was not significantly different between the two groups (surgical group, 22%; nonsurgical group, 27%) (see Table 3.4).

These two studies have provided similar data that suggest the following: (1) A randomized trial of early (within 12 hours from onset) surgery is feasible in patients with supratentorial ICH; (2) a potential benefit of surgical treatment may have been missed on account of the small numbers of patients included; and (3) the various surgical options (open craniotomy, stereotactic hematoma removal) should be compared with nonsurgical treatment in a large-scale, multicenter randomized clinical trial. The calculations of sample size included in the study of Zuccarello et al.[41] suggest that slightly more than 100 patients per group would be needed to test whether a statistically significant difference exists between treatment groups.

## NOVEL SURGICAL TECHNIQUES FOR THE MANAGEMENT OF INTRACEREBRAL HEMORRHAGE

The surgical trauma associated with conventional hematoma evacuation by craniotomy has stimulated the interest to develop new, less traumatic options for hematoma drainage. The first such effort was the introduction of a new instrument

60    *Clinical Trials in Neurologic Practice*

for the stereotactic evacuation of intracerebral hematomas by Backlund and von Holst in 1978.[43] The technique involved the use of a rotating drill and an aspiration cannula that were introduced through a burr hole into the center of the hematoma, a procedure usually performed under local anesthesia and using CT guidance for the location of the aspiration cannula. This procedure has often been used along with local instillation of a fibrinolytic agent (urokinase or rt-PA) for the purpose of liquifying the clot before its removal by suction. This has allowed the gradual removal of the hematoma over periods of several days by repeating the procedure every 6–12 hours through a silicone tube that remains in place until the clot has been completely removed. The procedure has been applied to patients with putaminal, thalamic, and lobar hematomas, and the results have been reported as usually satisfactory, with a low rate of postoperative complications. Although comparisons of this technique with hematoma removal by conventional craniotomy have shown similar rates of postoperative mortality and better functional outcome in patients who had the stereotactic procedure,[44] a prospective randomized trial for testing of the two techniques has not been performed.

Another novel approach to hematoma drainage was reported by Auer et al.,[45] who used an endoscopic surgical technique. The procedure was performed with a "neuroendoscope" that was introduced into the hematoma by an ultrasound-assisted stereotactic technique, and the hematoma was evacuated under direct visual control via a miniature video camera attached to the endoscope. The authors conducted a randomized trial that evaluated this technique in 50 patients, compared with an equal number treated nonsurgically (see Table 3.4). Patients treated had putaminal, lobar, and thalamic hemorrhages. The reported mortality figures favored the surgically treated over the nonsurgically treated at 1 week (14% versus 28%; $p < .01$), 3 weeks (28% versus 45%), and 6 months (42% versus 70%; $p < .01$). The best results were obtained in patients younger than 60 years of age who were either alert or somnolent preoperatively. Hematoma size was another factor related to outcome: In patients with hemorrhages larger than 50 $cm^3$ in volume, mortality was significantly lower in the surgical group (45% versus 86%; $p < .01$), whereas those with hematomas smaller than 50 $cm^3$ had no differences in mortality; their functional outcome, however, was better, as 25% of operated patients were fully independent, a state not achieved by any patients in the nonsurgical group. In addition, hematoma location was of major importance in determining outcome, as the overall benefit of surgical treatment appeared to be restricted to those with lobar hematomas: This group had a mortality rate of approximately 33%, in comparison with 70% for the nonsurgical group ($p < .05$). Differences in mortality were nonsignificant for patients with putaminal and thalamic hemorrhages. On the basis of this preliminary experience, Auer et al.[45] concluded that the endoscopic technique of surgical evacuation of ICH offers an advantage over nonsurgical treatment in a subgroup of patients who are younger than 60 years of age, have a subcortical (lobar) hemorrhage, and have a preoperative state of consciousness in the alert or somnolent level. From these data, Hankey and Hon[16] calculated that the odds of being "dead or dependent" at 6 months were 0.45 times less among patients treated surgically than among those treated nonsurgically.

These promising surgical techniques should be tested in properly selected subgroups of patients in a prospective randomized trial, in comparison with conventional craniotomy and nonsurgical management of ICH. Until such trial is

*Intracerebral Hemorrhage*    61

performed, clinical decisions about the management of this condition with high mortality and morbidity will continue to be based on personal opinion, biased data, and faulty conclusions.

## REFERENCES

1. Kase CS, Crowell RM. Prognosis and treatment of patients with intracerebral hemorrhage. In CS Kase, LR Caplan (eds), Intracerebral Hemorrhage. Boston: Butterworth–Heinemann, 1994;467–489.
2. Broderick JP, Adams HP, Barsan W, et al. Guidelines for the management of spontaneous intracerebral hemorrhage: a statement for healthcare professionals from a special writing group of the Stroke Council, American Heart Association. Stroke 1999;30:905–915.
3. Tellez H, Bauer RB. Dexamethasone as treatment in cerebrovascular disease, 1: a controlled study in intracerebral hemorrhage. Stroke 1973;4:541–546.
4. Poungvarin N, Bhoopat W, Viriyavejakul A, et al. Effects of dexamethasone in primary supratentorial intracerebral hemorrhage. N Engl J Med 1987;316:1229–1233.
5. Yu YL, Kumana CR, Lauder IJ, et al. Treatment of acute cerebral hemorrhage with intravenous glycerol: a double-blind, placebo-controlled, randomized trial. Stroke 1992;23:967–971.
6. Italian Acute Stroke Study Group. Haemodilution in acute stroke: results of the Italian haemodilution trial. Lancet 1988;1:318–321.
7. Patchell RA, Posner JB. Neurologic complications of systemic cancer. Neurol Clin 1985;3:729–750.
8. Norris JW. Steroid therapy in acute cerebral infarction. Arch Neurol 1976;33:69–71.
9. Norris JW, Hachinski VC. High dose steroid treatment in cerebral infarction. Br Med J 1986;292:21–23.
10. Pulsinelli WA, Levy DE, Sigsbee B, et al. Increased damage after ischemic stroke in patients with hyperglycemia with or without established diabetes mellitus. Am J Med 1983;74:540–544.
11. Weir CJ, Murray GD, Dyker AG, Lees KR. Is hyperglycemia an independent predictor of poor outcome after acute stroke?: results of a long term follow up study. Br Med J 1997;314:1303–1306.
12. Feldman Z, Kanter MJ, Robertson CS, et al. Effect of head elevation on intracranial pressure, cerebral perfusion pressure, and cerebral blood flow in head injured patients. J Neurosurg 1992;76:207–211.
13. Vandam LD, Burnap TK. Hypothermia. N Engl J Med 1959;261:546–553,595-603.
14. Ropper AH. Treatment of intracranial hypertension. In AH Ropper (ed), Neurological and Neurosurgical Intensive Care (3rd ed). New York: Raven Press, 1993;29–52.
15. Diringer MN. Intracerebral hemorrhage: pathophysiology and management. Crit Care Med 1993;21:1591–1603.
16. Hankey GJ, Hon C. Surgery for primary intracerebral hemorrhage: is it safe and effective?: a systematic review of case series and randomized trials. Stroke 1997;28:2126–2132.
17. Duff TA, Ayeni S, Levin AB, Javid M. Nonsurgical management of spontaneous intracerebral hematoma. Neurosurgery 1981;9:387–393.
18. Janny P, Colnet G, Georget A-M, Chazal J. Intracranial pressure with intracerebral hemorrhages. Surg Neurol 1978;10:371–375.
19. Papo I, Janny P, Caruselli G, et al. Intracranial pressure time course in primary intracerebral hemorrhage. Neurosurgery 1979;4:504–511.
20. Ropper AH, King RB. Intracranial pressure monitoring in comatose patients with cerebral hemorrhage. Arch Neurol 1984;41:725–728.
21. Cuatico W, Adib S, Gaston P. Spontaneous intracerebral hematomas: a surgical appraisal. J Neurosurg 1965;22:569–575.
22. Cook AW, Plaut M, Browder J. Spontaneous intracerebral hemorrhage: factors related to surgical results. Arch Neurol 1965;13:25–29.
23. Luessenhop AJ, Shevlin WA, Ferrero AA, et al. Surgical management of primary intracerebral hemorrhage. J Neurosurg 1967;27:419–427.
24. Paillas JE, Alliez B. Surgical treatment of spontaneous intracerebral hemorrhage: immediate and long-term results in 250 cases. J Neurosurg 1973;39:145–151.
25. Pásztor E, Afra D, Orosz É. Experiences with the surgical treatment of 156 ICH (1955-1977). In HW Pia, C Langmaid, J Zierski (eds), Spontaneous Intracerebral Haematomas: Advances in Diagnosis and Therapy. Heidelberg, Germany: Springer-Verlag, 1980;251–257.

## 62   Clinical Trials in Neurologic Practice

26. Kaneko M, Koba T, Yokoyama T. Early surgical treatment for hypertensive intracerebral hemorrhage. J Neurosurg 1977;46:579–583.
27. Silver FL, Norris JW, Lewis AJ, Hachinski VC. Early mortality following stroke: a prospective review. Stroke 1984;15:492–496.
28. Kanaya H, Yukawa H, Itoh Z, et al. Grading and the Indications for Treatment in ICH of the Basal Ganglia (Cooperative Study in Japan). In HW Pia, C Langmaid, J Zierski (eds), Spontaneous Intracerebral Haematomas: Advances in Diagnosis and Therapy, Heidelberg, Germany: Springer-Verlag, 1980;268–274.
29. Kaneko M, Tanaka K, Shimada T, et al. Long-term evaluation of ultra-early operation for hypertensive intracerebral hemorrhage in 100 cases. J Neurosurg 1983;58:838–842.
30. Waga S, Yamamoto Y. Hypertensive putaminal hemorrhage: treatment and results: is surgical treatment superior to conservative one? Stroke 1983;14:480–485.
31. Bolander HG, Kourtopoulos H, Liliequist B, Wittboldt S. Treatment of spontaneous intracerebral haemorrhage: a retrospective analysis of 74 consecutive cases with special reference to computer tomographic data. Acta Neurochir 1983;67:19–28.
32. Volpin L, Cervellini P, Colombo F, et al. Spontaneous intracerebral hematomas: a new proposal about the usefulness and limits of surgical treatment. Neurosurgery 1984;15:663–666.
33. Kanno T, Sano H, Shinomiya Y, et al. Role of surgery in hypertensive intracerebral hematoma: a comparative study of 305 nonsurgical and 154 surgical cases. J Neurosurg 1984;61:1091–1099.
34. Fujitsu K, Muramoto M, Ikeda Y, et al. Indications for surgical treatment of putaminal hemorrhage: comparative study based on serial CT and time-course analysis. J Neurosurg 1990;73:518–525.
35. Piotrowski WP, Rochowanski E. Operative results in hypertensive intracerebral hematomas in patients over 60. Gerontology 1996;42:339–347.
36. Schwarz S, Jauss M, Krieger D, et al. Haematoma evacuation does not improve outcome in spontaneous supratentorial intracerebral haemorrhage: a case-control study. Acta Neurochir 1997;139:897–904.
37. McKissock W, Richardson A, Taylor J. Primary intracerebral haemorrhage: a controlled trial of surgical and conservative treatment in 180 unselected cases. Lancet 1961;2:221–226.
38. Juvela S, Heiskanen O, Poranen A, et al. The treatment of spontaneous intracerebral hemorrhage: a prospective randomized trial of surgical and conservative treatment. J Neurosurg 1989;70:755–758.
39. Batjer HH, Reisch JS, Allen BC, et al. Failure of surgery to improve outcome in hypertensive putaminal hemorrhage: a prospective randomized trial. Arch Neurol 1990;47:1103–1106.
40. Morgenstern LB, Frankowski RF, Shedden P, et al. Surgical treatment for intracerebral hemorrhage (STICH): a single-center, randomized clinical trial. Neurology 1998;51.1359–1363.
41. Zuccarello M, Brott T, Derex L, et al. Early surgical treatment for supratentorial intracerebral hemorrhage: a randomized feasibility study. Stroke 1999;30:1833–1839.
42. Broderick JP, Brott TG, Duldner JE, et al. Volume of intracerebral hemorrhage: a powerful and easy-to-use predictor of 30-day mortality. Stroke 1993;24:987–993.
43. Backlund E-O, von Holst H. Controlled subtotal evacuation of intracerebral haematomas by stereotactic technique. Surg Neurol 1978;9:99–101.
44. Matsumoto K, Hondo H. CT-guided stereotaxic evacuation of hypertensive intracerebral hematomas. J Neurosurg 1984;61:440–448.
45. Auer LM, Deinsberger W, Niederkorn K, et al. Endoscopic surgery versus medical treatment for spontaneous intracerebral hematoma: a randomized study. J Neurosurg 1989;70:530–535.

# 4
# Aneurysmal Subarachnoid Hemorrhage Trials

Luca Regli and Bernhard Walder

Subarachnoid hemorrhage (SAH) continues to be a common cause of worldwide morbidity and mortality among young adults of both genders. Intracranial aneurysm rupture is the most common identifiable cause of nontraumatic SAH. Although the case-fatality rates from SAH have progressively declined,[1] the incidence of SAH, unlike other types of stroke, has not declined over time.[2] The outcome of patients remains poor, despite rapidly evolving research regarding diagnosis, causes, and treatment of SAH. The overall mortality rate is estimated to be 25%. Approximately 50% of patients who survive the aneurysmal rupture will have significant morbidity,[3] for approximately 30% of which secondary ischemia is responsible.[4,5]

Cerebral vasospasm after aneurysmal SAH is a major cause of disability and death. Therefore, because little can be done to ameliorate the immediate deleterious effect of aneurysm rupture, rebleeding and vasospasm are the major problems for which clinical trials have been designed. Large, multicenter prospective cohort analyses and multicenter prospective randomized trials have influenced considerably the treatment protocols for SAH patients. Nevertheless, many currently accepted treatment options are not supported by rigorous clinical scientific evidence. Some specific treatments for SAH are not amenable to testing by randomized, prospective trials because of practical or ethical considerations.

In 1994, the Stroke Council of the American Heart Association published practice guidelines for the management of aneurysmal SAH to precisely address these issues.[6] The reading of these guidelines is strongly recommended, as it is not the purpose of this chapter to repeat them. They can also be found on the website of the American Heart Association (www.americanheart.org).

Despite these guidelines, controversies around treatment protocols for patients with SAH are ongoing. The beneficial role of calcium antagonists, the role of prophylactic treatment with hypervolemia, and the role of transluminal balloon angioplasty are just some of the controversial issues. Recent multicenter prospective randomized trials have addressed the efficacy of antioxidant and

63

64    *Clinical Trials in Neurologic Practice*

anti-inflammatory agents, mainly tirilazad mesylate. The technical development and advancement of interventional endovascular surgery has opened new avenues in aneurysm and cerebral vasospasm treatment. An international multicenter prospective randomized trial comparing treatment of ruptured aneurysm with surgical clipping versus endovascular coiling began in 1999 and is ongoing.

## PREVENTION OF REBLEEDING

### Treatment of Ruptured Aneurysms

The most extensive data on the results of modern management of ruptured aneurysms have been provided by the International Cooperative Study on Timing of Aneurysm Surgery, in which more than 3,000 patients were entered in a prospective observational study from 1980 to 1983.[4,7] Surgical repair is today the first-line treatment option for ruptured aneurysms. Endovascular techniques for the treatment of intracranial aneurysms have been evolving since 1973.[8] The Guglielmi detachable coil device has been in use in North America since 1991 and in Europe since 1992.[9] Significant improvement in coiling has an increased occlusion rate and a reduced complication rate. This has fueled the belief that aneurysm coiling could become the first-line treatment. The International Subarachnoid Aneurysm Trial (ISAT) compared surgery and endovascular coil treatment of ruptured aneurysms and is the largest ever randomized clinical trial in SAH management.[10] The study had randomized more than 1,300 patients by mid-2000 and has planned to recruit more than 2,500 patients. The results of the ISAT study will answer two main questions. First, is aneurysm coiling as effective as clipping to protect against rebleeding? Second, is patient outcome improved with endovascular treatment? The results of this large, multicenter prospective randomized trial will have an impact on the management strategies in patients with aneurysmal subarachnoid hemorrhage.

### Antifibrinolytics

Early clipping or coiling of the ruptured aneurysm is the most efficacious prevention of rebleeding and is becoming increasingly common in neurosurgical centers. In patients with delayed surgery the use of antifibrinolytic treatment has been recommended.[11] Systematic reviews have shown that antifibrinolytics reduce the rebleeding rate by approximately 45% but do not affect overall outcome because of an increase in the rate of delayed cerebral ischemia due to cerebral vasospasm.[6] The trials on antifibrinolytic therapy date from over 10 years, when triple-H therapy (hypervolemia, hypertension, hemodilution) and nimodipine were not used routinely to decrease the incidence of symptomatic vasospasm. Members of the STAR study group recently conducted a prospective double-blind, placebo-controlled multicenter clinical trial[12] to investigate whether antifibrinolytics, in combination with treatment to prevent cerebral ischemia, improve outcome in patients with subarachnoid hemorrhage and delayed (longer than 48 hours) occlusion of the aneurysm. The overall results of this study show no beneficial effect on outcome despite reduction in rebleeding rate. Actually, in patients with impaired level of consciousness on admission (World Federation of Neurological Surgeons [WFNS] grade IV or V), antifibrinolytics adversely affected outcome. In patients with normal level of consciousness (WFNS grade I–III) there was a clear trend toward beneficial effect of this treatment. However, patients with normal levels of consciousness are ideal candidates for early surgery or coiling to prevent rebleeding. Antifibrinolytic treatment needs no consideration for SAH patients, even if combined with treatment to prevent cerebral ischemia.

## PREVENTION AND TREATMENT OF SYMPTOMATIC VASOSPASM

### Calcium Antagonists in Aneurysmal Subarachnoid Hemorrhage

Several controlled randomized clinical trials have studied calcium antagonists, mainly nimodipine, in patients with aneurysmal SAH and were published between 1983 and 1993.[13–23] In two trials not using nimodipine, one used AT877,[23] and the other nicardipine.[19] According to the AHA guidelines, these trials can be summarized as follows: (1) Oral nimodipine consistently reduced poor outcome due to vasospasm in all grades of patients; (2) the incidence of symptomatic vasospasm was not affected by nimodipine; (3) angiographic vasospasm was not affected by nimodipine; and (4) complications and side effects of the drug were minimal. Despite these recommendations supported by level I and II evidence from the individual trials, some recent reports have called the use of calcium antagonists into question,[24] and controversy about their beneficial effect exists.

To determine whether calcium antagonists improve outcome in patients with aneurysmal SAH and whether these drugs reduce the frequency of secondary cerebral ischemia, structured reviews have been published in which the authors performed a meta-analysis of all the controlled clinical trials.[25–27]

In their meta-analysis including seven trials and 1,202 patients, Barker and Ogilvy[28] demonstrated that prophylactic nimodipine is *effective* in increasing the odds of good outcome after aneurysmal SAH. Efficacy was both statistically significant ($p = .004$) and clinically significant in magnitude, with one additional good outcome expected for every seventh patient treated. The meta-analysis also showed that nimodipine significantly increased the odds of good or fair outcome and reduced the odds of radiographically detectable infarction and permanent deficit and death from secondary ischemia. A slight decrease in overall mortality or rebleeding-related death or deficit with nimodipine was demonstrated but was not statistically significant. Due to limitation of the data in the original trials, they declined to perform a meta-analysis of the potential effect of nimodipine on arteriographic vasospasm. They failed to show significant differences in other subgroup analyses comparing oral versus intravenous administration, and low dose versus high dose. They also analyzed the potential sources of bias in such observational studies.[28] The meta-analysis was not weakened by publication bias or the undue influence of any single trial. As the trials included in the meta-analysis did not specify the use of prophylactic hypervolemic-hypertensive ther-

66    *Clinical Trials in Neurologic Practice*

apy, the efficacy of nimodipine in such a setting cannot be analyzed. Barker and Ogilvy[28] concluded that the efficacy of prophylactic nimodipine in improving outcome after SAH is demonstrated by meta-analysis and that isolated retrospective trials[24] that fail to show efficacy under specific conditions should not weigh heavily in decisions regarding its use.

Similarly, Feigin et al.[27] demonstrate in their meta-analysis, including 10 controlled trials with 2,756 patients, significant reduction of poor outcome after SAH with nimodipine treatment (27% relative risk reduction; 95% confidence interval, 13–39%), as well as secondary ischemia (33% relative risk reduction; 95% confidence interval, 25–41%). Again, there was no significant difference between route or dosage of nimodipine administration.

The clinical trials and their meta-analysis demonstrate that nimodipine improves overall outcome after aneurysmal SAH. Oral administration of nimodipine 60 mg every 4 hours can be advocated.

## Triple-H Therapy (Hypervolemia, Hypertension, Hemodilution)

A popular concept of cerebral vasospasm prevention, as well as of cerebral vasospasm treatment in patients experiencing SAH, is the induction of a hypervolemic, hemodiluted, and hypertensive/hyperdynamic state (triple-H therapy). Triple-H therapy can be used in prevention of cerebral vasospasm or as a treatment of symptomatic vasospasm and is based on the hypothesis that an increase in arterial pressure and cardiac output and a decrease of blood viscosity optimize cerebral blood flow, thereby decreasing the incidence of symptomatic vasospasm. However, it is not clear in the literature which component of triple-H therapy impacts prevention or treatment of cerebral vasospasm. Similarly, it is not well established how to define an induced hypertensive, hypervolemic, and hemodiluted state.

### Triple-H Therapy as Prevention

Clinically relevant reduction of cerebral vasospasm was reported in observational studies using preventive triple-H therapy compared with observational studies not using preventive therapy.[29] Only small randomized, controlled studies were conducted of triple-H therapy as a preventive treatment analyzing clinically relevant end points, such as symptomatic cerebral vasospasm, neurologic disability, and mortality.[30–32] Rosenwasser et al.[31] compared preoperative hypervolemia (n = 15) (administering blood [aim: hematocrit 45%], albumin, and crystalloid) with preoperative normovolemia (n = 15) in patients scheduled for late surgical aneurysm treatment. Their results showed that the incidence of symptomatic cerebral vasospasm was significantly decreased in the group treated with preventive hypervolemia. Mayer et al.[32] compared the outcome of 19 hypervolemic patients with 19 normovolemic patients using central venous pressure measurements to evaluate the state of intravascular volemia. *Hypervolemia* was defined as a central venous pressure greater than 8 mm Hg, and *normovolemia* was defined as a central venous pressure greater than 5 mm Hg. Patients in both groups received 0.9% saline solution

1,920 ml per day, as a baseline; hypervolemia was achieved by additional 5% albumin administration to increase central venous pressure as needed. Five of 19 patients in the hypervolemic group and seven of 24 patients in the normovolemic group developed symptomatic cerebral vasospasm with delayed cerebral ischemia (29% versus 26%; no significant difference). Pulmonary edema requiring treatment was observed in one patient in the hypervolemic group. The same research group published a more recent trial, using the same methodological design, randomizing 41 patients into the hypervolemic and 41 patients into the normovolemic groups.[30] The incidence of symptomatic vasospasm was 20% in both groups, and no side effects were reported from induction of hypervolemia. Solenski et al.[33] reported, however, in a large prospective observational study, that 104 of 457 (23%) treated with triple-H therapy experienced pulmonary edema. A confounding factor in the judgment of the potential complications induced by triple-H therapy may be the frequent presence of neurogenic pulmonary edema associated with SAH. In fact, Solenski et al.[33] observed an increased incidence of pulmonary edema among patients presenting in high clinical grades (WFNS IV and V), which may support the hypothesis that other factors besides induction of hypervolemia could play a role in the development of pulmonary edema. The lack of randomized controlled trials enrolling a significant number of patients (as estimated by power analysis) implies that the efficacy and safety of triple-H therapy are not well established. Guidelines, recommendations, and clinical implementation of triple-H therapy as a preventive treatment of cerebral vasospasm can therefore not be based on evidence.

## Triple-H Therapy as Treatment

Triple-H therapy as a treatment of symptomatic cerebral vasospasm consists of a more aggressive implementation of triple-H therapy in patients with established symptomatic cerebral vasospasm. A step-by-step concept of triple-H therapy (progressive from prevention to treatment) was proposed by Levy et al.[34]: First, in all patients with SAH, a hypervolemic state is induced. Second, in patients manifesting neurologic compromise, additional infusions of colloids are started to achieve a pulmonary artery wedge pressure of 14 mm Hg. Third, in patients without improvement of neurologic status over the next few hours, cardiac output (cardiac index greater than or equal to 3.5) and arterial pressure (20–30%) are increased with intravenous infusion of dobutamine, a beta-1-adrenergic receptor agonist. In a prospective observational study applying this protocol, a reversal of the delayed ischemic symptoms was obtained in 18 of 23 patients (78%). Whereas Levy et al.[34] support a hyperdynamic model to decrease delayed ischemic deficits (i.e., increase of cardiac output to increase cerebral blood flow), other authors support a hypertensive model (i.e., an increase of systemic arterial pressure). Miller et al.[35] administered phenylephrine, a selective alpha-1-adrenergic receptor agonist, to increase mean arterial pressure by 20–25% above the patient's baseline and even up to 35% above the patient's baseline, if the neurological deficit is not reversed. With such a regimen, these authors observed neurologic improvement in 21 out of 24 patients (88%). However, dobutamine and phenylephrine both increase cardiac oxygen consumption and may, therefore, induce cardiac ischemia or infarction, contributing to the increased

68    *Clinical Trials in Neurologic Practice*

risk of lung edema.[33] None of the catecholamines has proven advantageous over the others in vasospasm treatment. Safety of triple-H therapy as treatment in patients with symptomatic cerebral vasospasm after SAH is reported rarely in the literature and is never investigated systematically.[36] As already mentioned under Triple-H Therapy as Prevention, there is a lack of randomized controlled trials analyzing efficacy and safety of triple-H therapy as treatment of delayed ischemia. Furthermore, there is a lack of consensus in defining the intermediate aims of triple H-treatment (blood pressure versus cardiac output), the type and amount of fluid to administer, and the type and dose of vasoactive drugs to use.

Guidelines, recommendations, and clinical implementation of triple H-treatment cannot be based on evidence. Clinicians have to base their decisions on clinical experience and local protocols until randomized controlled trials with sufficient group sizes are available. Triple-H therapy can, however, be recommended for prevention and treatment of delayed ischemic deficits, based on the step-by-step concept of triple-H therapy as proposed by Levy et al.[34] Patients receiving triple-H therapy must be monitored closely in an intensive care setting for hemodynamic function and electrolyte balance.

## Tirilazad in Prevention of Vasospasm

The use of tirilazad mesylate, a 21-aminosteroid free-radical scavenger, in animal models of subarachnoid hemorrhage and focal cerebral ischemia has shown a reduction of cerebral vasospasm and cerebral infarct.[37,38] Several powerful randomized controlled clinical trials with a multicenter design, including more than 3,500 patients, were conducted to test efficacy and safety of this drug.[39–42] The results of these large trials have been difficult to interpret, mainly because of differences in drug effectiveness within the studies. Despite a very similar trial design, tirilazad mesylate was more effective in the cooperative study in Europe, Australia, New Zealand, and South Africa[39] than in North America.[40] In the former study, tirilazad mesylate at a dose of 6 mg/kg per day improved overall outcome and reduced mortality at 3 months, particularly in men with admission grades IV and V. These results are at odds with the cooperative study conducted in North America that showed no statistical benefit on mortality rate, functional outcome, or ischemic symptoms. The reasons for the differing results are unclear but could include differences in epidemiologic characteristics or standard care of patients. In the North American trials, there were more patients with a history of arterial hypertension (40% and 44% versus 25% and 27%), with triple-H therapy as prevention (75% and 74% versus 45% and 60%), and with triple-H therapy as treatment (30% and 34% versus 18% and 24%). Similarly, nimodipine was more often administered per os in the North American trial compared to the European, Australian, New Zealand and South African trial. Differences were also observed in the results of the control groups. Mortality among men in North America, for example, was half that among men in the European, Australian, New Zealand, and South African trial. Alternatively, the authors suggested the possibility of lower blood levels of the study drug in the North American patients as compared to the other trial, due to broader use of antiepileptic medications as well as gender difference. For these reasons, two further studies were conducted to test the safety and efficacy of higher doses of tirilazad mesylate (15 mg/kg/

day) in women experiencing aneurysmal subarachnoid hemorrhage.[41,42] This second study conducted in Europe, Australia, New Zealand, and South Africa, showed a decreased rate of symptomatic cerebral vasospasm but did not result in better patient outcomes. In the North American trial, no beneficial effect was observed in the overall group. However, sequential analysis revealed a reduction in mortality rates among patients with neurologic grades IV and V at admission. The different responses of tirilazad in patients with various degrees of neurologic impairment could not be explained by the studies' authors. In a recent meta-analysis of trials of tirilazad mesylate, NW Dorsch (invited lecture at the 7th International Conference on Cerebral Vasospasm, June 18–21, 2000) confirmed that patients presenting in WFNS grade IV and V had a better outcome if high-dose tirilazad treatment (men 6 mg/kg/day and women 15 mg/kg/day) was started within 24 hours from subarachnoid hemorrhage.

A constant result among these trials was the safety of tirilazad mesylate administration. No major side effects were observed.

Despite experimental evidence favoring a beneficial effect of tirilazad and the discrepancies of the results of the clinical trials, and in the absence of an overall benefit in patient outcome, tirilazad mesylate cannot be recommended for routine clinical use in patients with aneurysmal SAH.

## Transluminal Balloon Angioplasty

Development of endovascular techniques since 1984 has allowed transluminal balloon angioplasty[43] to be performed in cerebral vessels affected by vasospasm with or without selective injection of papaverine into the involved territories.[44,45] Despite small anecdotal series[46–58] of angiographically confirmed reversal of cerebral vasospasm and high rates of clinical improvement, no controlled investigation of the efficacy of this procedure has been conducted. As opposed to intra-arterial administration of papaverine hydrochloride alone,[44,45] balloon angioplasty demonstrates excellent angiographic results that are, in most cases, permanent. In most of the small series, clinical improvement has been observed in approximately 60% of patients treated with angioplasty.[47,51,52,58] In a recent study, Polin et al.[59] analyzed 38 patients enrolled in the North America trial of tirilazad[42] who had angioplasty for cerebral vasospasm; the authors failed to demonstrate a benefit of angioplasty over medical treatment in patients presenting with symptomatic cerebral vasospasm.

In summary, the ability of transluminal balloon angioplasty to reverse angiographic cerebral vasospasm is unquestioned. Its clinical role, however, is not proven. Future studies have to clearly define the indications for its use. First, the clinical efficacy and not only angiographic improvement must be confirmed. Second, the anatomic types of cerebral vasospasm (proximal versus distal) amenable to angioplasty must be studied. Third, the timing of the procedure with regard to symptom onset and computed tomography (CT) findings must be defined. Balloon angioplasty has gained an important role in the algorithm of vasospasm management and it can be recommended as an adjunct to triple-H therapy, but not as a replacement for careful medical management of subarachnoid hemorrhage patients in the intensive care unit. Intra-arterial papaverine injection without balloon angioplasty cannot be recommended.[60]

70    *Clinical Trials in Neurologic Practice*

## OTHER TREATMENTS FOR VASOSPASM

One of the most important and critical aspects of SAH-induced cerebral vaso-spasm is its failure to consistently respond to treatment. A large number of phar-macologic interventions have been tried in experimental models and clinical trials with only partial success. The purpose here is not to review all of the exper-imental data. Some selected clinical data are presented in the next paragraph. The efficacy of these treatment forms has not been confirmed with large random-ized controlled trials; therefore, none of the treatments described in this para-graph can be advocated in clinical practice.

### Intracisternal Fibrinolytic Treatment

Fibrinolytic substances, such as recombinant tissue plasminogen activator (rt-PA) or urokinase, can facilitate the normal clearing of blood from the subarachnoid space and, in this manner, may prevent delayed arterial spasm after SAH. Two forms of administration of rt-PA were developed and tested: (1) single intra-operative intracisternal bolus injection[61] and (2) repetitive postoperative intra-cisternal bolus injection via a cisternal catheter.[62–64]

In a randomized controlled trial, 100 patients with ruptured intracranial sac-cular aneurysms causing severe SAH were treated with a single 10-ml intraop-erative injection of vehicle buffer solution or rt-PA into the opened basal subarachnoid cisterns immediately after aneurysm clipping.[61] The rates for no or mild, moderate, and severe angiographic vasospasm were 69%, 16%, and 15% respectively, in the rt-PA–treated group versus 42%, 35%, and 23%, respec-tively, in the placebo group. There was a trend toward lesser degrees of cerebral vasospasm in the rt-PA–treated group, but this was not statistically significant ( $p =$ .07). Overall, bleeding complication rates did not differ between the two groups. The study concluded that efficacy in preventing clinical vasospasm and its ischemic complications was not demonstrated, despite a trend toward less severe cerebral vasospasm and improved outcome.

In a prospective study examining 105 patients, postoperative rt-PA was used until all of the cerebral cisterns exhibited low-density on CT scan (mean, 4–7 days).[62] Patients showing diffuse thick subarachnoid blood clots on CT with greater than 75 Hounsfield units were included in the rt-PA therapy group; those with less than 75 Hounsfield units comprised the control group. Follow-up angiography showed that 26 cases (87%) in the rt-PA group had no cerebral vasospasm, three (10%) had moderate vasospasm, and one (3%) had severe vasospasm. In contrast, there were 11 patients (15%) with delayed ischemic neu-rologic deficits in the control group. Three complications in the rt-PA group were reported: One case of SAH caused by catheter removal, one small epidural hematoma, and one subgaleal fluid accumulation. All of these complications were treated conservatively with favorable results.

Usui and colleagues[64] retrospectively compared three groups of patients. The first was comprised of patients who had simple, spontaneous cisternal drainage through a catheter left at surgery until CT scanning showed basal cisternal clot clearance (n = 29). The second group had continuous irrigation between two cis-ternal catheters using a urokinase solution, 120 IU/ml at 21 ml per hour, started after postoperative angiography confirmed complete aneurysm ablation and continued for 5–7 days (n = 60). The third group received six hourly, intermittent injections of rt-PA via a single cisternal catheter that, after clamping for several hours, was left open to drain. The patients were not randomly allocated to treatment groups, and by design, the first group had less severe SAHs. The authors concluded that postoperative fibrinolytic treatment reduced cerebral vasospasm and that rt-PA injections were easier to administer and more effective than urokinase irrigation.

The most important trial with intrathecal urokinase investigated 217 consecutive patients classified as Fisher CT Group 3.[65] After clipping the aneurysm, irrigation tubes were placed in the Sylvian fissure (inlet) unilaterally or bilaterally and in the prepontine or chiasmal cistern (outlet). Lactated Ringer's solution with urokinase (120 IU/ml) and ascorbic acid (4 mg/ml) was infused at a rate of 30 ml/hour/side for approximately 10 days. Symptomatic cerebral vasospasm was observed in six cases (2.8%), and two of these six cases (0.9%) demonstrated sequelae. Complications occurred in eight patients during irrigation therapy: Two patients experienced seizures, two patients developed meningitis, and four patients had an intracranial hemorrhage. All recovered without neurologic deficits.

Confirmation or denial of significant clinical cerebral vasospasm prevention, with less ischemic infarction and improved overall outcome, requires a larger randomized trial, as does any meaningful comparison of fibrinolytic treatment methods. Fibrinolytic treatment appears to bear acceptable bleeding risk, providing surgery is uncomplicated and aneurysm clipping complete. However, the studies have confirmed the extreme danger of fibrinolytic treatment when the aneurysm is incompletely secured.

## Intravenous Thromboxane Synthetase Inhibitor

In a large, randomized, and double-blind trial at 48 neurosurgical services in Japan, the thromboxane synthetase inhibitor OKY-046 was investigated in two different doses and compared with placebo.[66] In subjects with severe cerebral vasospasm, the incidence of delayed ischemic deficit was significantly lower, with better functional prognosis, in the low dosage (80 mg per day) of thromboxane synthetase inhibitor group than in the placebo group. Additionally, in subjects with severe grades on the Glasgow Coma Scale, Japan Coma Scale, or High Density Score, the functional prognosis at 1 month after aneurysmal rupture was significantly better although no significant differences were seen in the overall investigation. Combinations of thromboxane synthetase inhibitors and serine protease inhibitors[67] or calcium antagonists[68] were investigated without random allocation.

Further randomized controlled trials, including groups with combination therapies should be performed to confirm the efficacy of thromboxane synthetase inhibitors before definitive recommendations can be formulated.

## Endothelin Receptor Antagonists and Natrium Nitroprusside

Numerous metabolic pathways that regulate vascular tone are present in both the smooth muscle and endothelial cells.[69] An imbalance between vasoconstriction and vasodilation may play a major role in cerebral vasospasm development. The

72    *Clinical Trials in Neurologic Practice*

endothelial cell produces both endothelium-derived relaxing factors, most notably nitric oxide, and endothelium-derived constricting factors, most notably endothelin. The fine equilibrium between vasoconstriction and vasodilation can be modified by several conditions. Endothelium-dependent relaxation has been shown to be impaired after SAH. [69] Similarly, increased endothelin content in cerebrospinal fluid has been reported after SAH.[69] Oral or intravenous endothelin receptor antagonists[70,71] and intrathecal nitric oxide donors, such as sodium nitroprusside,[72] are promising drugs against cerebral vasospasm. The efficacy of these agents needs to be investigated in large clinical trials.

## CONCLUSION

Intensive care of a patient with aneurysmal subarachnoid hemorrhage should focus on treatment and prevention of the most frequent and deleterious complications of the disease: rebleeding and cerebral vasospasm. Several recent randomized trials have been conducted or are ongoing to try to improve management of patients with ruptured aneurysms.

Continuous development and technical advancement in microsurgery and endovascular surgery have opened new avenues in aneurysm treatment. The ISAT study is comparing the results of aneurysm patients treated with surgical clipping or with endovascular coiling. The results of this large study will eventually help to define the indications and limitations of each treatment option in regard to aneurysm type and location.

Acute cerebral vasospasm is still characterized by high morbidity and mortality. Thus, it is clear that more basic research and clinical studies are needed to further elucidate the underlying mechanisms and to improve outcome of SAH-induced cerebral vasospasm.

## REFERENCES

1. Yundt KD, Dacey RG Jr, Diringer MN. Hospital resource utilization in the treatment of cerebral aneurysms. J Neurosurg 1996;85:403–409.
2. Turtz A, Allen D, Koenigsberg R, Goldman HW. Nonvisualization of a large cerebral aneurysm despite high-resolution magnetic resonance angiography. Case report. 1995;82:294–295.
3. Orz Y, Osawa M, Tanaka Y, et al. Surgical outcome for multiple intracranial aneurysms. 1996;138:411–417.
4. Kassell NF, Torner JC, Jane JA, et al. The International Cooperative Study on the timing of aneurysm surgery. Part 2: surgical results. J Neurosurg 1990;73:37–47.
5. Tettenborn D, Ebara K. Prevention and treatment of delayed ischemic dysfunction in patients with aneurysmal subarachnoid hemorrhage. Stroke 1990;21:85–89.
6. Mayberg MR, Batjer HH, Dacey R, et al. Guidelines for the management of aneurysmal subarachnoid hemorrhage. A statement for healthcare professionals from a special writing group of the Stroke Council, American Heart Association. 1994;25:2315–2328.
7. Kassell NF, Torner JC, Haley EC Jr, et al. The International Cooperative Study on the timing of aneurysm surgery. Part 1: overall management results. J Neurosurg 1990;73:18–36.
8. Serbinenko FA. Balloon catheterization and occlusion of major cerebral vessels. J Neurosurg 1974;41:125–145.
9. Guglielmi G, Viñuela F, Dion J, Duckwiler G. Electrothrombosis of saccular aneurysms via endovascular approach. Part 2: preliminary clinical experience. J Neurosurg 1991;75:8–14.

## Aneurysmal Subarachnoid Hemorrhage Trials    73

10. Molyneux A, Kerr R. International Subarachnoid Aneurysm Trial. J Neurosurg 1999;91:352–353.
11. Leipzig TJ, Redelman K, Horner TG. Reducing the risk of rebleeding before early aneurysm surgery: a possible role for antifibrinolytic therapy. J Neurosurg 1997;86:220–225.
12. Roos Y. Antifibrinolytic treatment in subarachnoid hemorrhage: a randomized placebo-controlled trial. STAR Study Group. Neurology 2000;54:77–82.
13. Pickard JD, Murray GD, Illingworth R, et al. Effect of oral nimodipine on cerebral infarction and outcome after subarachnoid haemorrhage: British aneurysm nimodipine trial. BMJ 1989;298:636–642.
14. Allen GS, Ahn HS, Preziosi TJ, et al. Cerebral arterial spasm—a controlled trial of nimodipine in patients with subarachnoid hemorrhage. N Engl J Med 1983;308:619–624.
15. Philippon J, Grob R, Dagreou F, et al. Prevention of vasospasm in subarachnoid haemorrhage. A controlled study with nimodipine. Acta Neurochir 1986;82:110–114.
16. Mee E, Dorrance D, Lowe D, Neil-Dwyer G. Controlled study of nimodipine in aneurysm patients treated early after subarachnoid hemorrhage. Neurosurgery 1988;22:484–491.
17. Ohman J, Heiskanen O. Effect of nimodipine on the outcome of patients after aneurysmal subarachnoid hemorrhage and surgery. J Neurosurg 1988;69:683–686.
18. Petruk KC, West M, Mohr G, et al. Nimodipine treatment in poor-grade aneurysm patients. Results of a multicenter double-blind placebo-controlled trial. J Neurosurg 1988;68:505–517.
19. Haley EC, Jr., Kassell NF, Torner JC. A randomized controlled trial of high-dose intravenous nicardipine in aneurysmal subarachnoid hemorrhage. J Neurosurg 1993;78:537–547.
20. Jan M, Buchheit F, Tremoulet M. Therapeutic trial of intravenous nimodipine in patients with established cerebral vasospasm after rupture of intracranial aneurysms. Neurosurgery 1988;23:154–157.
21. Neil-Dwyer G, Mee E, Dorrance D, Lowe D. Early intervention with nimodipine in subarachnoid haemorrhage. Eur Heart J 1987;8:41–47.
22. Messeter K, Brandt L, Ljunggren B, et al. Prediction and prevention of delayed ischemic dysfunction after aneurysmal subarachnoid hemorrhage and early operation. Neurosurgery 1987;20:548–553.
23. Shibuya M, Suzuki Y, Sugita K, et al. Effect of AT877 on cerebral vasospasm after aneurysmal subarachnoid hemorrhage. Results of a prospective placebo-controlled double-blind trial. J Neurosurg 1992;76:571–577.
24. Mercier P, Alhayek G, Rizk T, et al. Are the calcium antagonists really useful in cerebral aneurysmal surgery? A retrospective study. Neurosurgery 1994;34:30–36;discussion 36–37.
25. Asari S, Ohmoto T. Growth and rupture of unruptured cerebral aneurysms based on the intraoperative appearance. Acta Medica Okayama 1994;48:257–262.
26. Araki Y, Kohmura E, Tsukaguchi I. A pitfall in detection of intracranial unruptured aneurysms on three-dimensional phase-contrast MR angiography. AJNR Am J Neuroradiol 1994;15:1618–1623.
27. Feigin VL, Rinkel GJ, Algra A, et al. Calcium antagonists in patients with aneurysmal subarachnoid hemorrhage: a systematic review. Neurology 1998;50:876–883.
28. Barker FG II, Ogilvy CS. Efficacy of prophylactic nimodipine for delayed ischemic deficit after subarachnoid hemorrhage: a meta-analysis. J Neurosurg 1996;84:405–414.
29. Dorsch NW. Cerebral arterial spasm—a clinical review. Br J Neurosurg 1995;9:403–412.
30. Lennihan L, Mayer SA, Fink ME, et al. Effect of hypervolemic therapy on cerebral blood flow after subarachnoid hemorrhage: a randomized controlled trial. Stroke 2000;31:383–391.
31. Rosenwasser RH, Delgado TE, Buchheit WA, Freed MH. Control of hypertension and prophylaxis against vasospasm in cases of subarachnoid hemorrhage: a preliminary report. Neurosurgery 1983;12:658–661.
32. Mayer SA, Solomon RA, Fink ME, et al. Effect of 5% albumin solution on sodium balance and blood volume after subarachnoid hemorrhage. Neurosurgery 1998;42:759–767; discussion 767–768.
33. Solenski NJ, Haley EC Jr, Kassell NF, et al. Medical complications of aneurysmal subarachnoid hemorrhage: a report of the multicenter, cooperative aneurysm study. Participants of the Multicenter Cooperative Aneurysm Study. Crit Care Med 1995;23:1007–1017.
34. Levy ML, Rabb CH, Zelman V, et al. Cardiac performance enhancement from dobutamine in patients refractory to hypervolemic therapy for cerebral vasospasm. J Neurosurg 1993;79:494–499.
35. Miller JA, Dacey RG Jr, Diringer MN. Safety of hypertensive hypervolemic therapy with phenylephrine in the treatment of delayed ischemic deficits after subarachnoid hemorrhage. Stroke 1995;26:2260–2266.
36. Solomon RA, Fink ME, Pile-Spellman J. Surgical management of unruptured intracranial aneurysms. J Neurosurg 1994;80:440–446.
37. Zuccarello M, Marsch JT, Schmitt G, et al. Effect of the 21-aminosteroid U74006F on cerebral vasospasm following subarachnoid hemorrhage. J Neurosurg 1989;71:98–104.
38. Steinke DE, Weir BK, Findlay JM, et al. A trial of the 21-aminosteroid U74006F in primate model of chronic cerebral vasospasm. Neurosurgery 1989;24:179–186.

## 74 *Clinical Trials in Neurologic Practice*

39. Kassell NF, Haley EC Jr, Apperson-Hansen C, Alves WM. Randomized, double-blind, vehicle-controlled trial of tirilazad mesylate in patients with aneurysmal subarachnoid hemorrhage: a cooperative study in Europe, Australia, and New Zealand. J Neurosurg 1996;84:221–228.
40. Haley EC Jr, Kassell NF, Apperson-Hansen C, et al. A randomized, double-blind, vehicle-controlled trial of tirilazad mesylate in patients with aneurysmal subarachnoid hemorrhage: a cooperative study in North America. J Neurosurg 1997;86:467–474.
41. Lanzino G, Kassell NF. Double-blind, randomized, vehicle-controlled study of high-dose tirilazad mesylate in women with aneurysmal subarachnoid hemorrhage. Part II. A cooperative study in North America. J Neurosurg 1999;90:1018–1024.
42. Lanzino G, Kassell NF, Dorsch NW, et al. Double-blind, randomized, vehicle-controlled study of high-dose tirilazad mesylate in women with aneurysmal subarachnoid hemorrhage. Part I. A cooperative study in Europe, Australia, New Zealand, and South Africa. J Neurosurg 1999;90:1011–1017.
43. Zubkov YN, Nikiforov BM, Shustin VA. Balloon catheter technique for dilatation of constricted cerebral arteries after aneurysmal SAH. Acta Neurochir 1984;70:65–79.
44. Elliott JP, Newell DW, Lam DJ, et al. Comparison of balloon angioplasty and papaverine infusion for the treatment of vasospasm following aneurysmal subarachnoid hemorrhage. J Neurosurg 1998;88:277–284.
45. Polin RS, Hansen CA, German P, et al. Intra-arterially administered papaverine for the treatment of symptomatic cerebral vasospasm. Neurosurgery 1998;42:1256–1264; discussion 1264–1267.
46. Barnwell SL, Higashida RT, Halbach VV, et al. Transluminal angioplasty of intracerebral vessels for cerebral arterial spasm: reversal of neurological deficits after delayed treatment. Neurosurgery 1989;25:424–429.
47. Bejjani GK, Bank WO, Olan WJ, Sekhar LN. The efficacy and safety of angioplasty for cerebral vasospasm after subarachnoid hemorrhage. Neurosurgery 1998;42:979–986; discussion 986–987.
48. Brothers MF, Holgate RC. Intracranial angioplasty for treatment of vasospasm after subarachnoid hemorrhage: technique and modifications to improve branch access. AJNR Am J Neuroradiol 1990;11:239–247.
49. Coyne TJ, Montanera WJ, Macdonald RL, Wallace MC. Percutaneous transluminal angioplasty for cerebral vasospasm after subarachnoid hemorrhage. Can J Surg 1994;37:391–396.
50. Dion JE, Duckwiler GR, Vinuela F, et al. Pre-operative micro-angioplasty of refractory vasospasm secondary to subarachnoid hemorrhage. Neuroradiology 1990;32:232–236.
51. Eskridge JM, McAuliffe W, Song JK, et al. Balloon angioplasty for the treatment of vasospasm: results of first 50 cases. Neurosurgery 1998;42:510–516; discussion 516–517.
52. Fujii Y, Takahashi A, Yoshimoto T. Effect of balloon angioplasty on high grade symptomatic vasospasm after subarachnoid hemorrhage. Neurosurg Rev 1995;18:7–13.
53. Higashida RT, Halbach VV, Dowd CF, et al. Intravascular balloon dilatation therapy for intracranial arterial vasospasm: patient selection, technique, and clinical results. Neurosurg Rev 1992;15:89–95.
54. Konishi Y, Maemura E, Shiota M, et al. Treatment of vasospasm by balloon angioplasty: experimental studies and clinical experiences. Neurol Res 1992;14:273–281.
55. Livingston K, Guterman LR, Hopkins LN. Intraarterial papaverine as an adjunct to transluminal angioplasty for vasospasm induced by subarachnoid hemorrhage [published erratum in AJNR Am J Neuroradiol 1993;14(4):1025]. AJNR Am J Neuroradiol 1993;14:346–347.
56. Newell DW, Eskridge J, Mayberg M, et al. Endovascular treatment of intracranial aneurysms and cerebral vasospasm. Clin Neurosurg 1992;39:348–360.
57. Rosenwasser RH, Armonda RA, Thomas JE, et al. Therapeutic modalities for the management of cerebral vasospasm: timing of endovascular options. Neurosurgery 1999;44:975–979;discussion 979–980.
58. Terada T, Kinoshita Y, Yokote H, et al. The effect of endovascular therapy for cerebral arterial spasm, its limitation and pitfalls. Acta Neurochir 1997;139:227–234.
59. Polin RS, Coenen VA, Hansen CA, et al. Efficacy of transluminal angioplasty for the management of symptomatic cerebral vasospasm following aneurysmal subarachnoid hemorrhage. J Neurosurg 2000;92:284–290.
60. Polin RS, Hansen CA, German P, et al. Intra-arterially administered papaverine for the treatment of symptomatic cerebral vasospasm. Neurosurg 1998;42:1256–1264.
61. Findlay JM, Kassell NF, Weir BK, et al. A randomized trial of intraoperative, intracisternal tissue plasminogen activator for the prevention of vasospasm. Neurosurgery 1995;37:168–176; discussion 177–178.
62. Mizoi K, Yoshimoto T, Takahashi A, et al. Prospective study on the prevention of cerebral vasospasm by intrathecal fibrinolytic therapy with tissue-type plasminogen activator. J Neurosurg 1993;78:430–437.
63. Sasaki T, Ohta T, Kikuchi H, et al. A phase II clinical trial of recombinant human tissue-type plasminogen activator against cerebral vasospasm after aneurysmal subarachnoid hemorrhage. Neurosurgery 1994;35:597–604; discussion 604–605.

## Aneurysmal Subarachnoid Hemorrhage Trials    75

64. Usui M, Saito N, Hoya K, Todo T. Vasospasm prevention with postoperative intrathecal thrombolytic therapy: a retrospective comparison of urokinase, tissue plasminogen activator, and cisternal drainage alone. Neurosurgery 1994;34:235–244; discussion 244–245.
65. Kodama N, Sasaki T, Kawakami M, et al. Cisternal irrigation therapy with urokinase and ascorbic acid for prevention of vasospasm after aneurysmal subarachnoid hemorrhage outcome in 217 patients. Surg Neurol 2000;53:110–117.
66. Suzuki S, Sano K, Handa H, et al. Clinical study of OKY-046, a thromboxane synthetase inhibitor, in prevention of cerebral vasospasms and delayed cerebral ischaemic symptoms after subarachnoid haemorrhage due to aneurysmal rupture: a randomized double-blind study. Neurol Res 1989;11:79–88.
67. Kaminogo M, Yonekura M, Onizuka M, et al. Combination of serine protease inhibitor FUT-175 and thromboxane synthetase inhibitor OKY-046 decreases cerebral vasospasm in patients with subarachnoid hemorrhage. Neurol Med Chir 1998;38:704–708; discussion 708–709.
68. Nakashima S, Tabuchi K, Shimokawa S, et al. Combination therapy of fasudil hydrochloride and ozagrel sodium for cerebral vasospasm following aneurysmal subarachnoid hemorrhage. Neurol Med Chir 1998;38:805–810; discussion 810–811.
69. Dietrich HH, Dacey RG. Molecular keys to the problems of cerebral vasospasm. Neurosurgery 2000;46:517–530.
70. Roux S, Breu V, Ertel SI, Clozel M. Endothelin antagonism with bosentan: a review of potential applications. J Mol Med 1999;77:364–376.
71. Roux S, Breu V, Giller T, et al. Ro 61-1790, a new hydrosoluble endothelin antagonist: general pharmacology and effects on experimental cerebral vasospasm. J Pharmacol Exp Ther 1997;283:1110–1118.
72. Thomas JE, Rosenwasser RH, Armonda RA, et al. Safety of intrathecal sodium nitroprusside for the treatment and prevention of refractory cerebral vasospasm and ischemia in humans. Stroke 1999;30:1409–1416.

# 5
# Head Injuries
Hugh J. L. Garton and Thomas G. Luerssen

Traumatic brain injury (TBI) is a major cause of disability and death. Perhaps as many as 10 million people worldwide suffer a severe head injury every year, and approximately half of the 150,000 deaths due to trauma each year in the United States are due to head injury.[1,2] Trauma is a disease generally affecting the young and healthy, exacting a particularly heavy toll on individual and societal levels. It would appear, then, that TBI would be an ideal candidate disease for randomized clinical trials (RCTs), because it is common and it poses a significant burden of illness. Although many of the standard therapies used in head injury have not been tested in the randomized controlled trial format, the 1990s have seen a burgeoning of clinical trials in head injury, most of which concentrate on pharmacologic interventions and the management of more severe head injuries. Mild and moderate head injuries have received much less scrutiny.

A recent evidence-based review of this literature by the American Association of Neurological Surgeons and the Brain Trauma Foundation made three definitive statements regarding the management of severe head injuries.[2] The standards of clinical care included the following: (1) avoidance of chronic hyperventilation in the absence of elevated intracranial pressure (ICP), (2) avoidance of glucocorticoids for improving outcomes or reducing ICP, and (3) avoidance of prophylactic anticonvulsants for the prevention of late post-traumatic seizures. A fourth point, supported almost at the level of a standard, addresses the importance of avoiding hypotension and hypoxia but is not ethically testable in an RCT.[2] Other reviewers suggest that even these conclusions may be premature.[3–6]

The goals of this chapter are to identify sources of clinical trials information in head injury, to describe critical assessment skills as they pertain to head injury trials, and to review the published randomized controlled trials relevant to head injury with an aim toward evidence-based practice for head injury.

78   *Clinical Trials in Neurologic Practice*

*Table 5.1*   Journals publishing head injury clinical trials, 1966–1999

| Journal title | Count |
| --- | --- |
| *Journal of Neurosurgery* | 24 |
| *Critical Care Medicine* | 6 |
| *Journal of Neurotrauma* | 4 |
| *Acta Neurochirurgica* | 3 |
| *Journal of Neurology, Neurosurgery and Psychiatry* | 3 |
| *Journal of Trauma* | 2 |
| *Intensive Care Medicine* | 2 |
| *New England Journal of Medicine* | 2 |
| *Neurosurgery* | 2 |
| Other | 38 |

See text for description of search methods and criteria for inclusion.

## DATA SOURCES FOR HEAD INJURY TRIALS

Head injury trials may be identified through regular perusal of the primary literature, searches through general databases of the medical literature such as MEDLINE, or through the use of clinical trial registers such as those of the Cochrane Collaboration. To provide the data for this review, we have attempted to identify all randomized clinical trials published in peer-reviewed journals pertaining to head injury. We conducted a MEDLINE search based on the key words *head injury* and *controlled trial*. We considered only human subjects trials in which there was random allocation between experimental and control groups. Similarly, we limited consideration to trials in which the study population was predominantly or exclusively head-injured patients, not considering studies of general trauma management, in which a small proportion of the patients were head injured. To supplement this, we reviewed the bibliographies of trial reports and the Cochrane Controlled Trials Register. Trials reported only in book chapters or other non-peer-reviewed formats were also excluded. Thus, we identified 86 reports, some of which are duplicate or augmented reports of trials reported elsewhere. This number does not include reports from trials that have been concluded but that have not yet been reported in a peer-reviewed format, including *N*-methyl-D-aspirate (NMDA) antagonist trials for Selfotel and Cerestat and hypothermia.[7]

Clinical trials in head injury appear in a variety of journals. Table 5.1 lists the number of human subjects head injury trials published since 1966. Approximately one-third of these trials were published in the *Journal of Neurosurgery*. *Critical Care Medicine, Journal of Neurotrauma, Journal of Neurology, Neurosurgery and Psychiatry,* and *Acta Neurochirurgica* were the only other journals with more than two trial reports. The distribution of these trials by year of publication is given in Figure 5.1. The burgeoning lit-

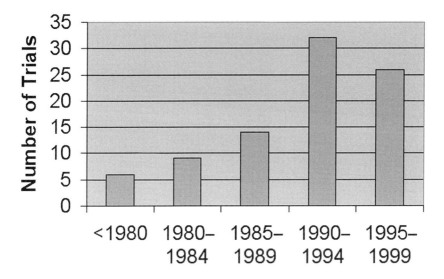

*Figure 5.1*  Clinical trial in head injury by year of publication. See text for specifics of search and inclusion criteria.

erature highlights not only the growing understanding of the importance of the clinical trial, but also the need for critical review skills on the part of the practitioner.

Searching for head injury–related trials on databases such as MEDLINE offers a more focused approach to evidence identification. The success of the search is, however, highly dependent on the search criteria. There is not currently any precise label or tag available to identify randomized controlled trials in these databases. In addition to keywords specific to the particular area of interest, phrases such as *controlled trial, randomized group, double-blinded method*, and *comparative study* can help to narrow the search results. In our identification of trials, we also noted that our MEDLINE searches were unable to detect approximately 6% of available trials because, in most cases, the journal in which they appeared was not available on MEDLINE. Similar findings have been noted in other fields.[8]

A third way to identify the relevant literature is to use a clinical trial database such as the Cochrane Controlled Trials Register. This database provides links to systematic reviews of the information provided by review groups in various fields, including head injury. Although it may be less accessible or familiar to clinicians than MEDLINE, its relative completeness and focus on clinical trials make it an ideal source for identifying primary data as well as evidence-based reviews of selected topics. Data are available in compact disc format or through the Internet and are available at many medical school libraries.

80   *Clinical Trials in Neurologic Practice*

## CRITICAL ASSESSMENT OF HEAD INJURY TRIALS

Head injury as a medical disease offers specific challenges to trial design and, therefore, interpretation and assessment. Assessment of these studies can be simplified by asking the following basic questions: *Why? How? Who? What? How many?* and *So what?*[9]

## Why?

Study reports should provide sufficient evidence to justify the plausibility or scientific rationale for the study. It is apparent in the analysis of several large, expensive, randomized trials of neuroprotective agents that the underlying logic on which the study was based was flawed. For example, to have a reasonable expectation of success, a pharmacologic agent mitigating the effects of secondary brain injury should act on a mechanism that has been clearly demonstrated to be present in the human central nervous system.[7] Experimental data from animal models must be carefully scrutinized for its relevance. Is a therapy delivered to humans in a similar fashion to its delivery when it demonstrated efficacy in the laboratory? For example, high-dose corticosteroids have been shown to limit the extent of brain injury in experimental models, but they must be administered immediately at or even before the time of injury. Clearly, this is not possible to achieve in the clinical setting. One can suggest that the positive or negative results of a trial should be considered as a probabilistic statement. If the study rationale is poor and lacks logical coherence, then the possibility that the study is reporting a false-positive must be considered.

The purpose and hypothesis of a study must be clearly stated, as they accordingly dictate the population to be studied and the parameters of interest. For example, two small clinical studies evaluated the effect of the cervical collar on ICP. The stated purpose of these studies was to investigate whether cervical collars would raise ICP in head-injured patients. However, the study populations consisted of patients having elective spinal anesthesia or lumbar puncture. None of these patients was head injured.[10,11] Improperly applied cervical collars likely do raise ICP by venous compression, but from a methodologic standpoint, these studies cannot hope to accomplish their stated purposes because no head-injured patients were actually studied.

Besides purpose and hypothesis, it must be determined whether a study addresses the efficacy or effectiveness of a given maneuver. In clinical trials parlance, a therapy is efficacious if, under ideal circumstances, the intervention results in a specific outcome. One restatement of the concept might be that in carefully selected patients with proven disease who properly comply with a therapy, the physiologic parameter monitored changes in a meaningful way. Effectiveness studies by contrast address the general question of whether the adoption of a particular therapeutic maneuver produces more good than harm. Diagnosis and treatment may be imperfect, and the outcomes of interest are generally broader than the physiologic parameters used in an efficacy setting. Both types of studies are common in the head injury literature, although they often are not labeled as such. Readers seeking evidence from an efficacy trial must assess whether the strict conditions under which the trial was conducted and the physiologic parameter improvement reported are relevant to the particular clinical question of interest.

## How?

Experimental and control groups must be selected from the participants in a truly random fashion. Nonrandomized or quasirandomized allocation of study subjects, such as alternating patients (e.g., first ten to treatment A, next ten to treatment B), is prone to significant bias and offers no real advantages. Although randomization should on average produce experimental and control groups that are similar, there is no guarantee that this will be the case. In fact, several of the phase III neuroprotectant trials experienced this phenomenon. Despite randomizing more than 1,100 patients, the European- and Australian-based phase III trial of the aminosteroid tirilazad experienced an imbalance between control and experimental groups in the occurrence of prerandomization hypotension: 16.1% of the tirilazad group was hypotensive compared to 10.5% in the control group ($p < .05$).[12] Similar imbalances existed for hypoxia as well. Previous studies have suggested that a single episode of hypotension is associated with as much as a doubling of mortality in head-injured patients.[13] Even if the differences between the groups are not statistically significant, a pronounced effect on outcome can still be seen.[14] However, ascribing additional therapeutic power to an otherwise marginal gain for the intervention when imbalances such as these occur ignores the fact that other factors, known and unknown, may also have exerted a differential effect on outcome. *Post hoc* analytical techniques are available to correct for these imbalances, but such techniques have their limitations. Stratified randomization is one solution that permits an even distribution of patients with potent prognostic characteristics between the experimental and control groups. Variables considered for stratification in head injury trials include the following: prerandomization hypotension/hypoxia, presenting Glasgow Coma Scale (GCS) score, age, admission, computed tomography (CT) scan findings, and in a multicenter trial, admitting center, to account for variations in practice patterns. In an unstratified trial, the reader must pay close attention to the assessment of baseline characteristics for these variables.

In many head injury trials, concealing the allocation of subjects is not possible. This is particularly true when the maneuver involves aspects of critical care such as hyperventilation or hypothermia. Even when the outcome measure is relatively free of bias, such as mortality, or when those assessing outcome can be separated from those providing the maneuver, the unblinded nature of the study allows substantial opportunity for co-interventions that limit or bias the study conclusions. In theory, the best protection against this is a standardized management protocol that limits variation in treatment style. Readers should carefully assess the methods section, to determine how this was achieved, and the study results, for evidence that the plan was successful.

82    *Clinical Trials in Neurologic Practice*

**Who?**

Head-injured patients are a heterogeneous group in terms of severity of injury, age, mechanism, and speed of access to definitive care. To determine whether a particular study offers relevant information, one must determine the population from which the sample is drawn, as well as the inclusion and exclusion criteria for entry into the trial, and the number of patients who were eligible for the study but did not participate or were lost to follow-up. When a large percentage of patients who were eligible did not enter the study, one must ask whether those who were not entered somehow differed from those who were. If this is the case, then the generalizability of the study may be compromised.

Most of the trials in this review focus on the severely head–injured patient. The most common definition of severity of injury uses the GCS.[15] Most investigators have accepted the general categorization into mild (GCS, 13–15), moderate (GCS, 9–12), and severe (GCS, equal to or less than 8) injuries. Typically, patients enrolled in RCTs must fall below a high and usually above a low threshold of GCS to be included in the trial. However, *severe head injury* as a phrase in context of a report may represent anything from patients with GCS 15 but with abnormal radiographs to the more typical GCS equal to or less than 8.

The timing of the intervention is also of significance. Based on the clinical examples in spinal cord injury, vasospasm in subarachnoid hemorrhage, and thrombolytic therapy for stroke, the timing at which an intervention occurs relative to the initial insult is critically linked to the likelihood of success. Readers should pay careful attention to the specifics of how far removed in both time and space the patients were from the initial insult.

Most trials to date have specifically excluded the pediatric age group from their study sample. Accordingly, there are few available data from randomized controlled trials to direct clinical practice in children with head injuries. An analysis of the relevance of the American Association of Neurological Surgeons, and Brain Trauma Foundation's *Guidelines for the Management of Severe Head Injuries* (herein after simply referred to as the *Guidelines*) for the management of pediatric head injury provides even fewer standards of care than the reference document.[16]

**What?**

The intervention under study must be identified in a manner that makes it reproducible by others. Did patients in the study successfully complete the maneuver? Were additional therapies (*co-interventions*) administered to one group of patients that might suggest alternative explanations for the results? When a study aims to assess the efficacy of a therapy, it is reasonable to exclude patients who were not compliant with the therapy if the reason for noncompliance was not directly related to the therapy itself. Thus, in a hypothermia trial it is reasonable to exclude a patient who could not be kept cold because of equipment failure, but not when hypotension in a patient necessitated rewarming. In effectiveness trials, patients who are noncompliant for any reason are generally included in the analysis.

All patients randomized must be accounted for in the trial report. Reasons why patients did not complete a study protocol are very important in assessing safety and potential biases. The proper way of handling such patients depends heavily on the study aims, but readers are encouraged to reassess the study conclusions by placing withdrawn and lost patients in the worst outcome category. A robust study should have similar results regardless of the inclusion of these patients. An alternative rule, often used in outcome assessment when several measurements are taken over time, is to use the last available measurement for the subsequent missing entries. When this is used for global outcome assessment in severely head–injured patients, treatment effects are generally underestimated because the overall trend for TBI over time is one of improvement.

The outcome measure used in a study should be clinically relevant to the study's aims. For head-injured patients, aside from mortality, the best-known and most widely used global measure of outcome is the Glasgow Outcome Scale (GOS).[17] This system categorizes patients on the following scale: 1–*dead*, 2–*vegetative*, 3–*severely disabled*, 4–*moderately disabled*, and 5–*good*. Many clinical trials assign patient outcome into favorable (GOS, 4 and 5) and unfavorable (GOS, 1–3) to give a dichotomized scale. This is done to simplify outcome reporting as well as statistical design. Furthermore, a difference in dichotomized outcomes can be clearly understood as an improvement. This outcome measure is somewhat subjective: A blinded outcome assessment is crucial to avoid bias. The GOS has come under criticism as lacking in sensitivity.[7,18,19] Indeed, the majority of patients end up at one of the extremes of the scale. This so-called U-distribution means that there are fewer patients in the intermediate grades of outcome in which greater sensitivity to improvement might be seen.

ICP, blood pressure, or cerebral perfusion pressure, as well as other physiologic parameters, are often used as surrogate end points. Each of these appears to impact outcome and their consideration, especially in smaller trials early in the assessment of a therapy, is appropriate. Nevertheless, the reader must remember that improvements in these parameters are suggestive of, but not necessarily proof of, improvements in actual neurologic or functional outcome.

## How Many?

Readers often focus on the *p* values for a study. A *p* value of less than .05 is taken to mean that the observed difference is not likely due to chance. However, in considering the results of a trial, the number of questions asked and analyses performed must be considered. A study reporting multiple outcomes has an increased likelihood of having falsely positive results. Secondary analyses— those determined after the data have been initially assessed—are more likely to represent chance variation. When multiple outcomes are assessed, the test of the study's prespecified primary hypothesis must be the focus of attention and main study result.

Many head injury trials have small sample sizes. In assessing trials that report no difference between therapies, the principal statistical question to answer is "How likely is it that a clinically meaningful difference could be detected using the sample size in the study?" This is known as the study *power*, and it is equal to $1 - \beta$ error, in which $\beta$ is the probability of a conclusion that a difference does not exist when, in reality, it does (false-negative rate). The main determinants of study power are sample size, rate of events, variability of measurement, and degree of difference to be detected. Rare events require large samples to identify change;

84   *Clinical Trials in Neurologic Practice*

the same is true detecting small differences in more common events. Determining study power requires knowledge of sample size calculations and is well described in most elementary medical statistics texts. As an example, to have an 80% chance of detecting a 25% reduction in the baseline unfavorable outcome rate of 50% for severe closed head injury by dichotomized GOS, and with a determinant of significance of $p <.05$, a trial has to enroll 520 patients. Relatively few studies in this review have such large samples. Systematic reviews attempt to address the difficulty of multiple small studies by combining data in meta-analyses, several of which exist for issues in the management of head injury.

## So What?

Are the study results applicable beyond the confines of the trial itself? In truth, the results of a study can only be generalized to the type of patients included in the study. Readers must carefully assess whether patients in their specific clinical setting are similar enough to apply the study results. In this regard, it is worth reassessing the inclusion and exclusion criteria, the institutions in which the maneuver was performed, and the degree to which the intervention can be accurately replicated. Perhaps the most important question to answer is whether the outcome being assessed really matters to the patient.

## HEAD INJURY TRIALS

For organizational purposes, we have grouped the available trials along thematic lines. Drug trials are the most common type of studies represented. Studies involving specific aspects of the routine management of severe head injury, such as hyperventilation and temperature regulation, are fewer in number. There remains a relative lack of information about many of the routine therapies that have been or are being used such as cerebrospinal fluid (CSF) drainage, cerebral perfusion pressure management, and mannitol use.[4]

### Anticonvulsants

Seizures after head trauma occur in 3–30% of patients, depending on the nature and severity of the injury. We identified seven trials of antiepileptic drug therapy involving carbamazepine (one study), phenytoin (four studies), phenobarbital (one study), and valproate (one study). The primary outcome measure in these studies is the occurrence of early or late post-traumatic seizures.

Glotzner and colleagues investigated carbamazepine begun immediately on presentation in 139 patients older than age 15 years.[19] There was a statistically significant reduction in seizure frequency in the experimental group, most of which was due to a reduction in early seizures (i.e., those occurring in the first week) as opposed to late seizures. However, patients in the treatment group had worse outcomes.[20] Studies by McQueen et al.[21] and Young et al.[22] evaluated the efficacy of phenytoin and noted no difference in seizure frequency or mortality.

Both studies had a low rate of seizures among the subjects, limiting the power of the studies to detect differences. In a higher-risk population, prophylactic phenytoin was shown to significantly reduce early seizures in the experimental group.[23] In the largest study to date, Temkim and colleagues[24] reported on 404 head-injured patients randomized to phenytoin or placebo. Only 3.6% of patients receiving the drug experienced seizures within the first 7 days, compared to 14.2% of control patients (relative risk [RR] = 0.27; 95% confidence interval [CI], 0.12–0.62). The study inclusion criteria specified that patients had to have any of the following: an intra- or extra-axial hematoma on CT, a depressed skull fracture, a clinical seizure within 24 hours of injury, a penetrating head wound, or a GCS of 10 or below. Children younger than 16 years of age were excluded. No differences in the incidence of late seizures or mortality could be found between the groups at the 1- or 2-year follow-up intervals.[24]

Manaka[25] reported on 169 head-injured patients randomized to receive phenobarbital or placebo. The study addressed only late-onset seizures, and there were no significant differences between the two groups.

In a meta-analysis of the above trials, the general trends apparent in the preceding discussion were supported—namely, the pooled RR of early seizures with treatment was 0.34 times that without treatment (95% CI, 0.21–0.54). The authors estimated that early seizures could be prevented in 10 patients for every 100 patients treated. In the combined analysis, no benefit could be seen in preventing late seizures, and no evidence supporting an improvement in overall neurologic outcome was identified.[4,5]

In a second study by Temkin and colleagues, valproate was assessed in a trial involving three arms: phenytoin for 1 week, valproate for 1 month, and valproate for 6 months.[26] A total of 379 patients were randomized. Inclusion and exclusion criteria were similar to the investigators' phenytoin trial noted above, except there was no maximum GCS for enrollment as long as the other entry criteria were met. No significant differences in early or late seizure rates were noted between the phenytoin and valproate groups. There was a nonsignificant ($p = .07$) trend toward increased mortality in the groups receiving valproate. The authors concluded that the lack of benefit, as well as the potential increased risk, argued against the use of valproate as a prophylactic agent for post-traumatic epilepsy.

## Barbiturates

Elevated ICP is a common accompaniment of brain injury that appears to have important prognostic implications.[27,28] High-dose barbiturate therapy has been shown to acutely lower ICP, probably by reducing metabolic demand and the associated coupled cerebral blood flow.[29] Trials by Ward et al.[30] and a multicenter study reported by Eisenberg et al.[31] compared pentobarbital to standard therapy. The timing and application of this therapy were different for these trials, as were the primary end points. The multicenter study showed some improvement in ICP control. In both studies, hypotension was more common in the barbiturate group. Outcomes assessed at one year by GCS were no different between the treatment groups.

A third trial compared pentobarbital to mannitol in 59 patients with a GCS of 7 or below whose ICP was 25 or greater after resuscitation and evacuation of

86    *Clinical Trials in Neurologic Practice*

mass lesions. Patients were treated with 1 g/kg bolus of mannitol with supplementation as needed to control ICP up to a serum osmolarity of 320 mOsm, or with 10 mg/kg pentobarbital bolus followed by continuous infusion to a level of 45 mg/liter. Eleven patients were excluded because of unspecified protocol violations. There was a small, nonsignificant improvement in 3-month survival for the mannitol group (RR, 1.36; 95% CI, 0.81–2.30). Mannitol was more effective as an initial agent in controlling ICP, with twice as many patients in the pentobarbital group crossing over to use mannitol rather than the reverse.[32]

In these trials, the power to detect a difference in outcome is small. A meta-analysis indicated that the pooled effect of barbiturates on outcome was negligible with the RR of death equal to 1.09 (95% CI, 0.81–1.47), whereas the chances of hypotension were significantly elevated (RR, 1.80; 95% CI, 1.05–2.92).[4,33]

## Calcium Channel Blockers

The calcium channel–blocking agents have been shown to reduce cell death by reducing the toxic influx of calcium into cells after injury. After the studies that apparently demonstrated improved outcomes in patients with aneurysmal subarachnoid hemorrhage who were treated with calcium channel–blocking agents, studies were conducted to investigate the benefit of these drugs in patients with TBI. We identified four randomized controlled trials reported in seven publications from 1990 to 1996.

An efficacy study showed that nicardipine significantly reduced elevated Doppler blood flow velocities of the intracerebral circulation (greater than or equal to 100 cm/second lasting 6 hours) compared to placebo ($p<.001$) in patients with a GCS of 8 or less. However, no differences in clinical outcomes of the patients were seen.[34]

The Head Injury Trials (HIT I–III) evaluated nimodipine in these patients. HIT I, published as three reports, enrolled 351 patients who could not obey commands (GCS motor less than 6).[35–37] Patients younger than 15 years, sustaining penetrating injury, or clinically brain dead were excluded. Despite an 80% study power to detect an increase in favorable outcome from 50% to 65%, no difference could be detected in the percentage of patients achieving this outcome (53% versus 49%: RR, 1.08; 95% CI, 0.88–1.33) or in overall survival. Hypotension was more common in the treatment group.

The HIT II trial was designed to detect a more modest effect of nimodipine (i.e., a 10% improvement in favorable outcome at 6 months). This trial accrued 852 patients. Inclusion and exclusion criteria were similar to that of the HIT I trial. As before, no overall differences in outcomes were noted. However, a planned subgroup analysis of patients with traumatic subarachnoid hemorrhage (tSAH) showed a nonsignificant trend indicating a beneficial treatment effect, which became stronger when only compliant patients were considered. As with the previous trial, hypotension was more common in the experimental group ($p=.013$).[38]

The HIT III trial focused exclusively on patients with tSAH. Patients with all injury severities were included, as long as they could begin therapy within 12 hours of the time of injury and had any amount of subarachnoid hemorrhage in any location on the initial head CT. The experimental paradigm tested placebo versus intravenous nimodipine for 7–10 days, followed by oral nimodipine for a total of 21 days. Outcome was assessed according to the dichotomized GOS at 6 months postinjury. One hundred and twenty-three patients were randomized. Seventy-five percent of patients in the nimodipine group had a favorable outcome, compared with 54% in the placebo group ($p = .02$). Hypotension was the most frequently reported complication, but its incidence was similar in the two groups. A treatment benefit was present (92% versus 72% favorable outcome) in the 31 patients who had a GCS greater than 12 at admission, but it was not significant in this small subgroup ($p = .62$).[39]

Summarizing the information from these trials, there seems to be no benefit to nimodipine given in unselected cases of TBI. There does appear to be a benefit in patients with tSAH, especially when the degree of tSAH is more significant and when nimodipine can be given within 12 hours of injury and continued for 21 days. A HIT IV trial is under way in the Far East and Australia to further assess nimodipine in tSAH.[19]

## Corticosteroids

The use of corticosteroids for the management of head injuries has been studied in a number of clinical trials. Controversy as to their true efficacy still exists. In our review, we identified 16 trial reports, of which 12 had meaningful clinical end points.[40–48] The overall results from these studies show no significant improvement in survival or neurologic outcome, although several subgroups demonstrated improved GOS scores at 6 months postinjury. For example, in the largest of these studies, Grumme and associates[48] noted that the administration of triamcinolone produced a nonsignificant 11% trend toward improved outcome compared to placebo. In a *post hoc* analysis, they further identified a subgroup of patients with an admission GCS of less than 8 and contusions on admission CT who had a significant (18%, $p < .01$) reduction in mortality in the treatment group.

The *Guidelines* cite these overall negative findings in its recommendation against the use of corticosteroids in head injury management.[2] However, a large meta-analysis concluded that there is as-yet insufficient evidence to clearly rule out a beneficial trial. None of the trials identified above had more than a 50% chance to detect a 25% improvement in outcome. In an analysis of 2,119 patients, involving these trials as well as others published in non-peer-reviewed formats, there was a 1.3% decrease in the risk of death, with a CI ranging from 5.2% less to 2.5% more. A trial to detect a 2.6% benefit would require 20,000 patients.[3,49] The Corticosteroid Randomization After Significant Head Injury trial, begun in early 1999, aims to accrue such a patient population throughout 63 centers in Europe,[50] although the need for and wisdom of this study have been questioned.[51]

## Free Radical Scavengers and Antioxidants

Among the more recently developed agents to be tested as neuroprotective agents are the free-radical scavenger polyethylene glycol conjugated superoxide dismutase (PEG-SOD), or pegorgotein, and the novel aminosteroid tirilazad. In animal studies, oxygen-mediated degradative processes figure prominently in secondary brain injury. Superoxide dismutase, an oxygen free–radical scaven-

88    *Clinical Trials in Neurologic Practice*

ger, has shown beneficial effects in laboratory models of brain injury.[52] Muize-laar and colleagues[53] published a phase II dose-escalation trial of PEG-SOD in human subjects in 1993. Entry criteria included blunt head injury with a GCS of 8 or below, inability to follow command after emergency room resuscitation, age of 16 years or older, and administration of the drug within 12 hours of injury. One hundred and four patients were randomized. Patients received placebo or a one-time administration of PEG-SOD at one of three doses: 2,000, 5,000, or 10,000 U/kg. No difference in mortality was noted between the groups. Using an adjusted analysis to control for the effects of age, GCS score, and institution, there was a significant increase in favorable outcomes at 3 months for the treatment group receiving 10,000 U/Kg. No significant adverse effects were noted. The investigators noted that ICP was less frequently elevated and easier to control in patients receiving the higher PEG-SOD dose compared to placebo.

These promising results led to a multicenter phase III trial in which 463 patients were randomized to receive placebo, 10,000 U/kg, or 20,000 U/kg of PEG-SOD.[54] Entry criteria were similar to the phase II trial, except that the drug had to be administered within 8 hours of injury. Outcome was assessed by the GOS at 3 months and grouped into good (GOS, 5,4), fair (GOS, 3), and poor (GOS, 2,1). An 8% absolute improvement in 3-month trichotomized GOS was noted at the 10,000 U/kg dose, but this was not significant ($p = .15$); the agent is not available for clinical use for head-injured patients.

The use of tirilazad, a free-radical scavenger that inhibits lipid peroxidation has been studied in two large clinical trials, one of which has been reported to date. The European/Australian tirilazad trial enrolled 1,120 patients to receive placebo or 10 mg/kg of tirilazad mesylate every 6 hours for 5 days by intravenous infusion.[55] Inclusion criteria included patients between 15 and 65 years of age, GCS less than 13, abnormal CT scan, and initiation of treatment within 4 hours of injury. The study was powered to have an 80% chance of detecting a 10% improvement in the severely head–injured group. No significant effect of tirilazad was seen in the study population as a whole or in the moderate and severe subgroups. In a preplanned analysis of patients with tSAH, an improvement in mortality (43% versus 34%), but not good outcome, was seen for severely injured men only. The authors raise appropriate cautions about the interpretation of such subgroup assessments, but note that a similar finding of male-specific protection was seen in trials of tirilazad in patients with aneurysmal subarachnoid hemorrhage. Despite the large sample size, imbalances existed in the important baseline characteristics of hypotension and hypoxia and the presence of an epidural hematoma. An adjusted outcome assessment was not presented. Both the PEG-SOD and tirilazad trials have been criticized on grounds that the drug target—free radicals— have not been demonstrated to be produced in human traumatic brain injury.[7]

## Hyperventilation

The use of hyperventilation has been a widely practiced and long-standing therapy for head injury in the United States.[56] This therapy clearly reduces elevated ICP, presumably by causing cerebral vasoconstriction. Concern has been raised that this induced vasoconstriction could reduce cerebral blood flow to the point of ischemia, at least in some regions of the injured brain, thereby actually contributing to injury and worsening the neurologic outcome. Despite the long history of this therapy and the real potential for critical evaluation through RCTs, few studies have been conducted. One trial has compared "normal" ventilation ($PaCO_2$, 30–35 mm Hg) to hyperventilation ($PaCO_2$, 24–28 mm Hg), with a third group receiving both hyperventilation and the buffering agent tromethamine (THAM) to act as an additional bicarbonate buffer in the central nervous system.[53,57] One hundred and thirteen patients were randomized. The study included patients aged 3 years and over who had GCS of 8 or below after resuscitation. Treatment was maintained for 5 days. Fourteen percent of patients had elevated ICP at admission. Outcome was measured at 3, 6, and 12 months by a single unblinded evaluator. Although the hyperventilation group as a whole demonstrated worse 3- and 6-month outcomes by dichotomized GOS, this difference was not significant ($p = .08$). An adjusted analysis accounting for differences in age and admission motor GCS showed that the subset of patients with the best motor scores (GCS, 4 or 5) faired significantly worse in the hyperventilation group at 3 and 6, but not 12, months. Patients receiving THAM had outcomes similar to the control group. The authors concluded that the routine use of prolonged hyperventilation retarded recovery from severe closed head injury. The *Guideline* used this study as justification for its recommendation against the use of prophylactic chronic hyperventilation.[2] However, Roberts and colleagues[4,6] reviewed this trial and calculated the RR of death or severe disability using the 1-year outcome without regard to subgroupings. They noted that the 95% CI for the RR of hyperventilation ranged from a 20% reduction to a 50% increase in poor outcome. Because of the small sample size and the lack of a significant difference in overall outcome, they concluded that there is insufficient evidence to determine the best practice with regard to hyperventilation.

In a second study focusing on the effects of THAM in patients experiencing hyperventilation to a milder degree ($PaCO_2$, 32–35 mm Hg), no significant differences were seen in GOS scores. Fewer patients in the THAM group had ICP elevations over 20 mm Hg, and fewer measures, such as the use of barbiturates, were required for ICP control.[58]

## Hypothermia

We identified seven reports outlining the trial protocols or reporting results from three randomized trials of hypothermia.[59–65] Shiozaki and colleagues[59] studied mild hypothermia in 33 patients older than 10 years of age who had GCS of 8 or below and could be treated within 2 hours of injury. Patients with refractory ICP despite therapy that included barbiturates, but not mannitol or steroids, were eligible. Patients randomized to hypothermia were cooled actively to 34°C and rewarmed slowly, as long as ICP remained stable. At 6 months, mortality and death or severe disability was significantly lower in the patients treated with hypothermia. The treatment was associated with lower cerebral blood flow and cerebral metabolic rates.

Clifton and colleagues investigated the efficacy of moderate hypothermia (32°–33°C), randomizing 46 patients to standard therapy or systemic cooling begun within 6 hours of injury.[61] Patients with hypoxia or hypotension were excluded. Patients in the treatment group were maintained for 48 hours after reaching the target temperature of 33°C, and then rewarmed at a prescribed rate

90    *Clinical Trials in Neurologic Practice*

of 1°C every 4 hours. There was a 16% reduction in the rate of poor outcome in the treatment group, although this was not statistically significant. There was a nonsignificant increase in sepsis in the hypothermic group.

Marion and colleagues[64] reported results from a similar trial of 82 patients, aged 16–75 years, with closed head injuries and GCS less than 8. An abnormal CT scan was required, as was the initiation of treatment within 6 hours of injury. Patients with prerandomization hypotension or hypoxia were excluded. The study was of similar design to that of Clifton et al.,[61] except that hypothermia was maintained for 24 hours. A 14% reduction in death and severe disability was seen for the treatment group, which was not statistically significant. Using a logistic regression model to adjust for GCS and CT classification of injury,[66] the risk reduction attributable to the hypothermia was 0.5 (95% CI, 0.2–1.2). Most of the benefit was seen in patients with admission GCS greater than 4. Statistically significant differences seen in the first 36 hours for the hypothermic patients as a group included lower ICP, higher cerebral perfusion pressure, and lower cerebral blood flow. There was no overall increase in the complication rate for the cooled patients.

These promising but inconclusive trials led to a larger multicenter phase III trial investigating the efficacy of induced hypothermia in adult patients with severe closed head injury. The trial was halted prematurely in 1998. The report from this trial has not yet been published, but preliminary information indicates that there was no overall benefit seen for hypothermia (G. Clifton, personal communication, 1999). As with the trial performed and reported by Marion et al., some degree of efficacy was seen in certain subgroups of patients, specifically those younger than 45 years of age and those with higher GCS scores. At present, hypothermia is best regarded as an unproven therapy.

## Mannitol and Hypertonic Saline

We have previously noted the trial titled *The University of Toronto Head Injury Treatment Study*, which compared mannitol to pentobarbital for patients with refractory ICP.[32] Smith and colleagues[67] compared 80 patients with severe head injuries treated with mannitol boluses in response to ICP elevations or on a routine schedule of mannitol (0.25 g/kg every 2 hours), as long as the serum osmolality was less than 310 mOsm/kg. For clinical deterioration, the scheduled group was given an additional dose of 0.75 g/kg and head CT in search of a treatable cause. The RR of death or severe disability at 1 year using ICP-directed therapy was 0.88 times (95% CI, 0.55–1.38) that of scheduled therapy. Although this was not significant, the sample size offered only a 20% chance of detecting a true reduction in poor outcomes of 25%.

Prophylactic mannitol administered before patient arrival at the hospital has been assessed in 44 head-injured patients who were older than age 18, had GCS less than 12, required intubation, and were seen by flight transport teams within 6 hours of injury. Patients were randomized to receive placebo or a one-time dose of mannitol (1 g/kg). The primary study end point was systolic blood pressure measured every 15 minutes for 2 hours and was similar between the groups. Mortality, apparently measured at 2 hours after enrollment, was 25% in the mannitol group and 14% in placebo group ($p = .38$).[68]

Two trials that assessed the use of hypertonic saline for resuscitation of head trauma victims provide conflicting results. In the first of these, 32 children, age

## Head Injuries    91

younger than 16 years with GCS less than 8, were randomized to receive lactated Ringer's solution or hypertonic saline over a 3-day period. ICP and cerebral perfusion pressure were similar between the groups, but more interventions were required in the placebo group to keep ICP under 15 mm Hg ($p$ <.01). The authors concluded that the use of hypertonic saline made ICP management easier in the first 3 days after injury.[69] In a similar trial, Shackford and colleagues[70] compared lactated Ringer's solution to 1.6% hypertonic saline in 41 adult patients with blunt head trauma and GCS of 13 or below who had an abnormal head CT and required ICP monitoring. Baseline GCS and ICP were worse in the hypertonic saline group. Significantly more interventions were required to control ICP in the hypertonic saline group. Average ICP and GOS at discharge were similar between the groups, although seven patients (17%) who died during the first 48 hours were not considered in the outcome data. Neither of these two studies provides sufficient outcome data to make any assessment of the effectiveness of the therapy.

### Nutrition

Body energy requirements after head injury are typically elevated, and patients are prone to catabolism and nitrogen wasting.[71–73] Head-injured patients typically require 130–140% of usual daily caloric needs. Rapp and colleagues studied the timing of supplemental nutrition in head-injured patients.[74] Thirty-eight patients with intracranial hematomas or neurologic deficits were randomized to receive total parenteral nutrition (TPN) within 48 hours of admission or enteral feedings via nasogastric (NG) tube as soon as bowel sounds were present and NG output was less than 100 ml/hr. Patients in the NG group were fed much less because of gastrointestinal intolerance. Therefore, this study has been generally considered to compare early versus late feeding. At 1 year follow-up, mortality in the TPN group was 15%, compared to 55% in the NG feeding group ($p$ = .02). Other studies with more aggressive NG feeding regimens have shown better outcomes.[75,76] In addition, TPN and enteral feeding have been shown to have similar impacts on ICP in head-injured patients.[77]

Jejunal feeding has been considered as an alternative to gastric feedings. Grahm compared 32 patients with GCS lower than 10 allocated to nasojejunal (NJ) feeds begun within 36 hours of admission or NG feeds begun after 3 days.[78] Caloric and nitrogen intake, as well as nitrogen balance, were all significantly better in the NJ feeding group. In addition, patients in the NJ group experienced fewer infectious complications ($p$ <.05). Neurologic outcomes were not reported. This study suffers from methodologic limitations, in that the patients were allocated to their groups on the basis of day of admission, and at least four patients in each group were assigned to their groups directly. Substantial variability in metabolic and nitrogen needs over the course of recovery occurred, and repeated assessments with indirect calorimetry and urea nitrogen measurements were recommended.[79] The *Guidelines* recommend that nutritional replacement begin within 72 hours of injury to allow for full replacement of caloric expenditure by 1 week.[2] They suggest that there is some evidence that NJ feeding is preferable to NG feeding and equivalent to TPN.

92   *Clinical Trials in Neurologic Practice*

What patients should be fed has been investigated on a number of fronts. Nitrogen wasting is dramatic after head injury, and head-injured patients derive more than 20% of their caloric needs from protein.[80] Several studies address whether increasing the level of nitrogen replacement could improve nitrogen retention and avoid visceral protein losses. Clifton et al.[81] compared a diet with 14% caloric protein to one with 22% caloric protein in 20 patients with random allocation to the groups. A nonsignificant trend of improved nitrogen balance was seen in the group fed 22% caloric protein. In concordance with this, recommendations are that the diet should contain more than 15% protein calories.[2] One trial suggests that supplemental branched chain amino acids may lower rates of nitrogen excretion and improve nitrogen balance.[82]

Hyperglycemia appears to have a deleterious effect on head injury.[83] Two small trials studying glucose- and carbohydrate-free diets have shown that patients fed these diets have increased ketogenesis, reduced CSF lactate, and improved nitrogen balance. Neurologic outcomes were not reported.[84,85]

The administration of insulin-like growth factor 1 (IGF-1), which may play an intermediary role in anabolic processes, has been studied in 33 patients aged 18–59 years with GCS of 4–10. Patients randomized to the experimental group received IGF-1 at 0.01 mg/kg for 14 days. Neurologic outcome was improved in a subset of patients with admission GCS of 5–7, but not for the cohort as a whole. Nitrogen balances were better in the treated patients compared to controls in the first week after the injury, but both groups had similar negative nitrogen balances in the second week. The authors noted a trend toward improved outcomes in patients with higher levels of IGF-1.[86] IGF-1 may also play a role in limiting T-cell immunosuppression seen in head-injured patients.[87]

Because of its role in NMDA channel control, protein synthesis and a wide spectrum of central nervous system biochemistry, the neuroprotective effect of zinc in the diets of severely head–injured patients has also been investigated. In a small randomized trial, 68 patients were fed enriched zinc (12 mg elemental zinc) or standard zinc (2.5 mg elemental zinc) TPN, followed by enteral zinc supplements (22 mg elemental zinc) or placebo for 3 months after injury.[88] The mortality at 1 month after injury was 12% in the supplemented group compared to 26% in the control group ($p = .09$), and there was a trend toward improved GCS scores. A larger follow-up study has not yet been reported.

## Infection Control, Immune Response, and Gastric Protection

The role of prophylactic antibiotics in the management of head-injured patients remains unclear. Penicillin prophylaxis for CSF otorrhea did not alter rates of meningitis, but the sample size limited study power.[89] In a trial of 100 intubated patients, the majority of whom were head injured, prophylactic cefuroxime (two doses of 1,500 mg given 12 hours apart) significantly reduced the incidence of clinically suspected and microbiologically confirmed pneumonia, as well as intensive care unit and hospital lengths of stay.[90]

Immune system dysfunction in head-injured patients can be demonstrated as altered $CD_4/CD_8$ ratios[90] and abnormal humoral immune responses.[91] Gooding and colleagues[92] assessed whether intravenous immunoglobulin prophylaxis could decrease secondary infection and found trends toward lower rates of pneumonia and proven sepsis.

Ranitidine has been compared to placebo for the prevention of stress-induced gastric ulcers in head-injured patients. Metz and colleagues[93] reported a 19% rate of gastrointestinal bleeding in the control group compared to a 3% rate in the experimental group, which received 6.25 mg/hr continuous ranitidine infusion over a 5-day period beginning within 24 hours of injury ($p = .002$).

## Sedation

Sedatives, analgesics, and paralytic agents are used to ameliorate agitation and improve mechanical ventilation and, as such, are significant aids to the management of elevated ICP. There is limited evidence that identifies the optimal agents or methods for applying these agents. In a small study of 15 patients randomized to propofol or morphine and midazolam, patients receiving propofol had a smaller arteriovenous difference in oxygen concentration early after injury, implying reduced cerebral metabolism.[94] In a larger, randomized, phase II trial, a 5-day course of propofol (10–200 μg/kg/min) was compared to morphine sulfate (0.25–5.00 mg/kg/min) as the primary sedative.[95] Among 42 randomized adult patients, ICP, cerebral perfusion pressure, and therapy intensity were similar, and 6-month outcome and mortality were (nonsignificantly) better in the propofol group, despite greater degrees of hypoxia and hypotension and more patients with GCS between 3 and 5 at admission and with compressed basal cisterns on CT scan in the propofol control group. However, serious complications have been reported with its use for more than 48 hours in children.[96]

## PREVENTION

Bicycle accidents are a common source of head injuries in children, and helmet use should reduce the rate of injury in them.[97] Two studies by Cushman and colleagues[98,99] attest to the difficulty of achieving this goal in head injury prevention. The first of these compared the use of a specific instructional program promoting helmet use, provided in the ambulatory setting, to cyclists 5–18 years old. No noticeable impact on the rate of helmet purchase was noted (7.2% versus 7.0%), despite the fact that only one in four of the families owned bike helmets at the onset of the study.[98] In a separate study, even when the sample consisted exclusively of the families of children presenting to the emergency room after a bicycle accident, helmet promotion was equally ineffective in generating helmet purchase.[99]

## NEUROPSYCHOLOGICAL AND OTHER INTERVENTIONS

The role of methylphenidate in ameliorating the neurobehavioral deficits occurring after traumatic brain injury has been assessed in three trials. Two of these

94    *Clinical Trials in Neurologic Practice*

(44 total patients) show no effect on cognitive outcome,[100,101] whereas the study by Plenger and colleagues[102] noted some improvement in the rate but not the final extent of recovery.

The use of early follow-up, such as counseling and neuropsychological and behavioral therapy, has been assessed in a large trial of 1,156 head-injured patients, 76% of whom were not admitted and 59% of whom were lost at 6-month follow-up. A subset of patients who were admitted or who had more than 1 hour of post-traumatic amnesia did have significantly better quality of life scores in the early intervention group (i.e., those seen within 7–10 days, compared to the control group seen at 6 months).[103]

Trials have been conducted to assess the optimal method of endotracheal tube suctioning for intubated head-injured patients[104] and the effect of hyperbaric oxygen[105] and the use of kinetic beds to prevent pulmonary complications in head-injured patients.[106] None of these studies demonstrated improved neurologic outcome in experimental compared to control patients.

## REFERENCES

1. Alexander E Jr. Global Spine and Head Injury Prevention Project (SHIP) [editorial]. Surg Neurol 1992;38(6):478–479.
2. Bullock R, Chestnut R, Clifton G, et al. Guidelines for the management of severe head injury: Brain Trauma Foundation, American Association of Neurological Surgeons, Joint Section on Neurotrauma and Critical Care. J Neurotrauma 1996;13:643–734.
3. Alderson P, Roberts I (eds). Corticosteroids for Acute Traumatic Brain Injury. The Cochrane Library. Oxford: Update Software, 1999.
4. Roberts I, Schierhout G, Alderson P. Absence of evidence for the effectiveness of five interventions routinely used in the intensive care management of severe head injury: a systematic review. J Neurol Neurosurg Psychiatry 1998;65:729–733.
5. Schierhout G, Roberts I (eds). Anti-epileptic Drugs for Preventing Seizures Following Acute Traumatic Brain Injury. The Cochrane Library. Oxford: Update Software, 1999.
6. Schierhout G, Roberts I (eds). Hyperventilation Therapy for Acute Traumatic Brain Injury. The Cochrane Library. Oxford: Update Software, 1999.
7. Bullock MR, Lyeth BG, Muizelaar JP. Current status of neuroprotection trials for traumatic brain injury: lessons from animal models and clinical studies. Neurosurgery 1999;45:207–217.
8. Dickersin K, Scherer R, Lefebvre C. Identifying relevant studies for systematic reviews. BMJ 1994;309:1286–1291.
9. Schechter MT, LeBlanc FE, Lawrence VA. Appraising New Information. In H Tyroidl, MF McNealy, DS Mulder, et al. Surgical Research. New York: Springer-Verlag, 1998.
10. Kolb JC, Summers RL, Galli RL. Cervical collar-induced changes in intracranial pressure. Am J Emerg Med 1999;17:135–137.
11. Raphael JH, Chotai R. Effects of the cervical collar on cerebrospinal fluid pressure. Anaesthesia 1994;49:437–439.
12. Marshall LF, Maas AI, Marshall SB, et al. A multicenter trial on the efficacy of using tirilazad mesylate in cases of head injury. J Neurosurg 1998;23:560–567.
13. Chesnut RM, Marshall LF, Klauber MR, et al. The role of secondary brain injury in determining outcome from severe head injury. J Trauma 1993;34:216–222.
14. Altman DG. Comparability of randomised groups. The Statistician 1985;34:125–136.
15. Teasdale G, Jennett B. Assessment of coma and impaired consciousness. A practical scale. Lancet 1974;2:81–84.
16. Luerssen TGL. Neurological injuries in infants and children. An overview of current management strategies. Clin Neurosurg 2000;46:170–184.
17. Jennett B, Bond M. Assessment of outcome after severe brain damage. Lancet 1975;1:480–487.
18. Scheuler ML, Pedley TA. The evaluation and treatment of seizures. N Engl J Med 1990;323:1468–1474.

*Head Injuries* 95

19. Maas AI, Steyerberg EW, Murray GD, et al. Why have recent trials of neuroprotective agents in head injury failed to show convincing efficacy? A pragmatic analysis and theoretical considerations. Neurosurgery 1999;44:1286–1298.
20. Glotzner FL, Haubitz I, Miltner F, et al. Seizure prevention using carbamazepine following severe brain injuries. Neurochirurgia (Stuttg) 1983;26:66–79.
21. McQueen JK, Blackwood DH, Harris P, et al. Low risk of late post-traumatic seizures following severe head injury: implications for clinical trials of prophylaxis. J Neurol Neurosurg Psychiatry 1983;46:899–904.
22. Young B, Rapp RP, Norton JA, et al. Failure of prophylactically administered phenytoin to prevent late posttraumatic seizures. J Neurosurg 1983;58:236–241.
23. Lauxerois M, Pechadre J, Colnet G, et al. Prevention des crises d'epilepsie posttraumatiques precoces par les hydantoines (Hydantoins in the prevention of early posttraumatic epileptic crises). Epilepsies 1990;2:5–10.
24. Temkin NR, Dikmen SS, Wilensky AJ, et al. A randomized, double-blind study of phenytoin for the prevention of post-traumatic seizures. N Engl J Med 1990;323:497–502.
25. Manaka S. Cooperative prospective study on posttraumatic epilepsy: risk factors and the effect of prophylactic anticonvulsant. Jpn J Psychiatry Neurol 1992;46:311–315.
26. Temlain NR, Dikenen SS, Anderson GD, et al. Valproate theraphy for prevention of post traumatic seizures: a randomized trial. J Neurosurg 1999;91:593–600.
27. Miller JD, Becker DP, Ward JD, et al. Significance of intracranial hypertension in severe head injury. J Neurosurg 1977;47:503–516.
28. Narayan RK, Kishore PR, Becker DP, et al. Intracranial pressure: to monitor or not to monitor? A review of our experience with severe head injury. J Neurosurg 1982;56:650–659.
29. Kassell NF, Hitchon PW, Gerk MK, et al. Alterations in cerebral blood flow, oxygen metabolism, and electrical activity produced by high dose sodium thiopental. Neurosurgery 1980;7:598–603.
30. Ward JD, Becker DP, Miller JD, et al. Failure of prophylactic barbiturate coma in the treatment of severe head injury. J Neurosurg 1985;62:383–388.
31. Eisenberg HM, Frankowski RF, Contant CF, et al. High-dose barbiturate control of elevated intracranial pressure in patients with severe head injury. J Neurosurg 1988;69:15–23.
32. Schwartz ML, Tator CH, Rowed DW, et al. The University of Toronto head injury treatment study: a prospective, randomized comparison of pentobarbital and mannitol. Can J Neurol Sci 1984;11:434–440.
33. Roberts I (ed). Barbiturates for Acute Traumatic Brain Injury. The Cochrane Library. Oxford: Update Software, 1999.
34. Compton JS, Lee T, Jones NR, et al. A double blind placebo controlled trial of the calcium entry blocking drug, nicardipine, in the treatment of vasospasm following severe head injury. Br J Neurosurg 1990;4:9–15.
35. Bailey I, Bell A, Gray J, et al. A trial of the effect of nimodipine on outcome after head injury. Acta Neurochir 1991;110:97–105.
36. Teasdale G, Bailey I, Bell A, et al. A randomized trial of nimodipine in severe head injury: HIT I. British/Finnish Co-operative Head Injury Trial Group. J Neurotrauma 1992;9(Suppl 2):S545-S550.
37. Teasdale GM, Pettigrew LE, Wilson JT, et al. Analyzing outcome of treatment of severe head injury: a review and update on advancing the use of the Glasgow Outcome Scale. J Neurotrauma 1998;15:587–597.
38. A multicenter trial of the efficacy of nimodipine on outcome after severe head injury. The European Study Group on Nimodipine in Severe Head Injury. J Neurosurg 1994;80:797–804.
39. Harders A, Kakarieka A, Braakman R. Traumatic subarachnoid hemorrhage and its treatment with nimodipine. German tSAH Study Group. J Neurosurg 1996;85:82–89.
40. Alexander E, Jr. Medical management of closed head injuries. Clin Neurosurg 1972;19:240–250.
41. Saul TG, Ducker TB, Salcman M, et al. Steroids in severe head injury: a prospective randomized clinical trial. J Neurosurg 1981;54:596–600.
42. Cooper PR, Moody S, Clark WK, et al. Dexamethasone and severe head injury. A prospective double-blind study. J Neurosurg 1979;51:307–316.
43. Braakman R, Schouten HJ, Blaauw-van Dishoeck M, et al. Megadose steroids in severe head injury. Results of a prospective double-blind clinical trial. J Neurosurg 1983;58:326–330.
44. Giannotta SL, Weiss MH, Apuzzo ML, et al. High dose glucocorticoids in the management of severe head injury. Neurosurgery 1984;15:497–501.
45. Dearden NM, Gibson JS, McDowall DG, et al. Effect of high-dose dexamethasone on outcome from severe head injury. J Neurosurg 1986;64:81–88.
46. Chacon L. Edema cerebral en traumatismo craneoencefalico severo en niños tratados con y sin dexametasona. Med Crit Venez 1987;2:75–79.

## 96  Clinical Trials in Neurologic Practice

47. Zagara G, Scaravilli P, Bellucci MC, et al. Effect of dexamethasone on nitrogen metabolism in brain-injured patients. J Neurosurg Sci 1987;31:207–212.
48. Grumme T, Baethmann A, Kolodziejczyk D, et al. Treatment of patients with severe head injury by triamcinolone: a prospective, controlled multicenter clinical trial of 396 cases. Res Exp Med 1995;195:217–229.
49. Alderson P, Roberts I. Corticosteroids in acute traumatic brain injury: systematic review of randomised controlled trials. BMJ 1997;314:1855–1859.
50. Kmietowicz Z. Trial of steroids for treating head injury begins. BMJ 1999;318:1441.
51. Gregson B, Todd NV, Crawford D, et al. CRASH trial is based on problematic meta-analysis. BMJ 1999;319:578.
52. Kontos H. Oxygen Radicals in Experimental Brain Injury. In J Hoff, A Betz (eds), Intracranial Pressure VII. Berlin: Springer-Verlag, 1989;787–798.
53. Muizelaar JP, Marmarou A, Young HF, et al. Improving the outcome of severe head injury with the oxygen radical scavenger polyethylene glycol-conjugated superoxide dismutase: a phase II trial. J Neurosurg 1993;78:375–382.
54. Young B, Runge JW, Waxman KS, et al. Effects of pegorgotein on neurologic outcome of patients with severe head injury. A multicenter, randomized controlled trial. JAMA 1996;276:538–543.
55. Marshall LF, Maas AI, Marshall SB, et al. A multicenter trial on the efficacy of using tirilazad mesylate in cases of head injury. J Neurosurg 1998;89:519–525.
56. Ghajar J, Hariri RJ, Narayan RK, et al. Survey of critical care management of comatose, head-injured patients in the United States. Crit Care Med 1995;23:560–567.
57. Marmarou A, Holdaway R, Ward JD, et al. Traumatic brain tissue acidosis: experimental and clinical studies. Acta Neurochir Suppl 1993;57:160–164.
58. Wolf AL, Levi L, Marmarou A, et al. Effect of THAM upon outcome in severe head injury: a randomized prospective clinical trial. J Neurosurg 1993;78:54–59.
59. Shiozaki T, Sugimoto H, Taneda M, et al. Effect of mild hypothermia on uncontrollable intracranial hypertension after severe head injury. J Neurosurg 1993;79:363–368.
60. Clark RS, Kochanek PM, Obrist WD, et al. Cerebrospinal fluid and plasma nitrite and nitrate concentrations after head injury in humans. Crit Care Med 1996;24:1243–1251.
61. Clifton GL, Allen S, Barrodale P, et al. A phase II study of moderate hypothermia in severe brain injury. J Neurotrauma 1993;10:263–271.
62. Clifton GL. Hypothermia and hyperbaric oxygen as treatment modalities for severe head injury. New Horiz 1995;3:474–478.
63. Marion DW, Obrist WD, Carlier PM, et al. The use of moderate therapeutic hypothermia for patients with severe head injuries: a preliminary report. J Neurosurg 1993;79:354–362.
64. Marion DW, Penrod LE, Kelsey SF, et al. Treatment of traumatic brain injury with moderate hypothermia. N Engl J Med 1997;336:540–546.
65. Resnick DK, Marion DW, Darby JM. The effect of hypothermia on the incidence of delayed traumatic intracerebral hemorrhage. Neurosurgery 1994;34:252–255.
66. Marshall LF, Marshall SB, Klauber MR, et al. A new classification of head injury based on computerized tomography. J Neurosurg 1991;75:S14–S20.
67. Smith HP, Kelly DL, Jr., McWhorter JM, et al. Comparison of mannitol regimens in patients with severe head injury undergoing intracranial monitoring. J Neurosurg 1986;65:820–824.
68. Sayre MR, Daily SW, Stern SA, et al. Out-of-hospital administration of mannitol to head-injured patients does not change systolic blood pressure. Acad Emerg Med 1996;3:840–848.
69. Simma B, Burger R, Falk M, et al. A prospective, randomized, and controlled study of fluid management in children with severe head injury: lactated Ringer's solution versus hypertonic saline. Crit Care Med 1998;26:1265–1270.
70. Shackford SR, Bourguignon PR, Wald SL, et al. Hypertonic saline resuscitation of patients with head injury: a prospective, randomized clinical trial. J Trauma 1998;44:50–58.
71. Clifton GL, Robertson CS, Grossman RG, et al. The metabolic response to severe head injury. J Neurosurg 1984;60:687–696.
72. Deutschman CS, Konstantinides FN, Raup S, et al. Physiological and metabolic response to isolated closed-head injury. Part 1: Basal metabolic state: correlations of metabolic and physiological parameters with fasting and stressed controls. J Neurosurg 1986;64:89–98.
73. Bruder N, Dumont JC, Francois G. Evolution of energy expenditure and nitrogen excretion in severe head-injured patients. Crit Care Med 1991;19:43–48.
74. Rapp RP, Young B, Twyman D, et al. The favorable effect of early parenteral feeding on survival in head-injured patients. J Neurosurg 1983;58:906–912.

*Head Injuries* 97

75. Hadley MN, Grahm TW, Harrington T, et al. Nutritional support and neurotrauma: a critical review of early nutrition in forty-five acute head injury patients. Neurosurgery 1986;19:367–373.

76. Young B, Ott L, Twyman D, et al. The effect of nutritional support on outcome from severe head injury. J Neurosurg 1987;67:668–676.

77. Young B, Ott L, Haack D, et al. Effect of total parenteral nutrition upon intracranial pressure in severe head injury. J Neurosurg 1987;67:76–80.

78. Grahm TW, Zadrozny DB, Harrington T. The benefits of early jejunal hyperalimentation in the head-injured patient. Neurosurgery 1989;25:729–735.

79. Borzotta AP, Pennings J, Papasadero B, et al. Enteral versus parenteral nutrition after severe closed head injury. J Trauma 1994;37:459–468.

80. Duke JH Jr, Jorgensen SB, Broell JR, et al. Contribution of protein to caloric expenditure following injury. Surgery 1970;68(1):168–174.

81. Clifton GL, Robertson CS, Contant CF. Enteral hyperalimentation in head injury. J Neurosurg 1985;62:186–193.

82. Ott LG, Schmidt JJ, Young AB, et al. Comparison of administration of two standard intravenous amino acid formulas to severely brain-injured patients. Drug Intell Clin Pharm 1988;22:763–768.

83. Merguerian PA, Perel A, Wald U, et al. Persistent nonketotic hyperglycemia as a grave prognostic sign in head-injured patients. Crit Care Med 1981;9:838–840.

84. Robertson CS, Goodman JC, Narayan RK, et al. The effect of glucose administration on carbohydrate metabolism after head injury. J Neurosurg 1991;74:43–50.

85. Ritter AM, Robertson CS, Goodman JC, et al. Evaluation of a carbohydrate-free diet for patients with severe head injury. J Neurotrauma 1996;13:473–485.

86. Hatton J, Rapp RP, Kudsk KA, et al. Intravenous insulin-like growth factor-I (IGF-I) in moderate-to-severe head injury: a phase II safety and efficacy trial. J Neurosurg 1997;86:779–786.

87. Kudsk KA, Mowatt-Larssen C, Bukar J, et al. Effect of recombinant human insulin-like growth factor I and early total parenteral nutrition on immune depression following severe head injury. Arch Surg 1994;129:66–70.

88. Young B, Ott L, Kasarskis E, et al. Zinc supplementation is associated with improved neurologic recovery rate and visceral protein levels of patients with severe closed head injury. J Neurotrauma 1996;13:25–34.

89. Klastersky J, Sadeghi M, Brihaye J. Antimicrobial prophylaxis in patients with rhinorrhea or otorrhea: a double-blind study. Surg Neurol 1976;6:111–114.

90. Rixen D, Livingston DH, Loder P, et al. Ranitidine improves lymphocyte function after severe head injury: results of a randomized, double-blind study. Crit Care Med 1996;24:1787–1792.

91. Wilson NW, Ochs HD, Peterson B, et al. Abnormal primary antibody responses in pediatric trauma patients. J Pediatr 1989;115:424–427.

92. Gooding AM, Bastian JF, Peterson BM, et al. Safety and efficacy of intravenous immunoglobulin prophylaxis in pediatric head trauma patients: a double-blind controlled trial. J Crit Care 1993;8:212–216.

93. Metz CA, Livingston DH, Smith JS, et al. Impact of multiple risk factors and ranitidine prophylaxis on the development of stress-related upper gastrointestinal bleeding: a prospective, multicenter, double-blind, randomized trial. The Ranitidine Head Injury Study Group. Crit Care Med 1993;21:1844–1849.

94. Stewart L, Bullock R, Rafferty C, et al. Propofol sedation in severe head injury fails to control high ICP, but reduces brain metabolism. Acta Neurochir 1994;60(Suppl):544–546.

95. Kelly DF, Goodale DB, Williams J, et al. Propofol in the treatment of moderate and severe head injury: a randomized, prospective double-blinded pilot trial. J Neurosurg 1999;90:1042–1052.

96. Bray RJ. Propofol infusion syndrome in children. Paediatr Anaesth 1998;8:491–499.

97. Thompson RS, Rivara FP, Thompson DC. A case-control study of the effectiveness of bicycle safety helmets. N Engl J Med 1989;320:1361–1367.

98. Cushman R, James W, Waclawik H. Physicians promoting bicycle helmets for children: a randomized trial. Am J Public Health 1991;81:1044–1046.

99. Cushman R, Down J, MacMillan N, et al. Helmet promotion in the emergency room following a bicycle injury: a randomized trial. Pediatrics 1991;88:43–47.

100. Bohnen NI, Twijnstra A, Jolles J. A controlled trial with vasopressin analogue (DGAVP) on cognitive recovery immediately after head trauma. Neurology 1993;43:103–106.

101. Speech TJ, Rao SM, Osmon DC, et al. A double-blind controlled study of methylphenidate treatment in closed head injury. Brain Inj 1993;7:333–338.

102. Plenger PM, Dixon CE, Castillo RM, et al. Subacute methylphenidate treatment for moderate to moderately severe traumatic brain injury: a preliminary double-blind placebo-controlled study. Arch Phys Med Rehabil 1996;77:536–540.
103. Wade DT, Crawford S, Wenden FJ, et al. Does routine follow up after head injury help? A randomised controlled trial. J Neurol Neurosurg Psychiatry 1997;62:478–484.
104. Rudy EB, Turner BS, Baun M, et al. Endotracheal suctioning in adults with head injury. Heart Lung 1991;20:667–674.
105. Rockswold GL, Ford SE, Anderson DC, et al. Results of a prospective randomized trial for treatment of severely brain-injured patients with hyperbaric oxygen. J Neurosurg 1992;76:929–934.
106. Clemmer TP, Green S, Ziegler B, et al. Effectiveness of the kinetic treatment table for preventing and treating pulmonary complications in severely head-injured patients. Crit Care Med 1990; 18:614–617.

# 6
# Clinical Trials in Spinal Cord Injury
Charles H. Tator and Michael G. Fehlings

An average incidence of 11,000 cases per year makes spinal cord injury (SCI) a serious cause of morbidity and mortality in North America.[1,2] The pharmacotherapy trials with methylprednisolone (MP) by the National Acute Spinal Cord Injury Studies (NASCIS-2 and NASCIS-3)[3,4] have shown improved neurologic recovery in patients with SCI. The improvement was modest with only slight functional benefit. Recent advances in the safety and efficacy of surgical decompression of the spinal cord also offer some potential for improving neurologic recovery after SCI.[5–7] However, the appropriate timing (early or late) and clinical indications (e.g., complete or incomplete injuries) for pharmacotherapy or surgery are not clear because of the paucity of prospective, randomized controlled trials. This chapter reviews the clinical evidence for the value of pharmacotherapy and other measures, such as surgical decompression for the treatment of patients with SCI. The emphasis is on randomized controlled trials in the acute phase of the condition, although trials in the chronic phase are also discussed. The chapter concentrates on trials aimed at improvement of neurologic function and omits those designed to reduce such complication rates as those for deep venous thrombosis.

## IMPORTANCE OF SPINAL CORD INJURY

Traffic accidents, sports and recreational activities, accidents at work, falls in the home, and violence are the main causes of SCI in North America.[1,2] Many of the injuries occur in young people: 70% of the patients in the NASCIS-2 trial were younger than 35 years of age.[3] The lack of effective treatments for restoring neurologic function below the level of the injury means that the vast majority of SCI victims faces many years of lost independence and continued medical expenses. The financial cost of care for acute SCI is enormous. In 1975, Kraus et al.[1] estimated an "annual cost to the United States for support and treatment of all persons with a spinal cord injury of two billion dollars," and in

100　*Clinical Trials in Neurologic Practice*

*Table 6.1*　Primary and secondary mechanisms of injury in acute spinal cord injury

**Primary injury mechanisms**
Acute compression
Impact
Distraction
Laceration
Sheer
Missile
**Secondary injury mechanisms**
Systemic events
　Systemic shock
　Spinal shock
　Hypoxia
　Hyperthermia
　Injudicious movement of the unstable spine leading to worsening compression
Extracellular factors
　Microcirculatory vascular damage leading to ischemia or hemorrhage
　Tissue swelling
　Inflammation
Intracellular factors
　Ischemic cascade
　Ionic shifts
　Neurotransmitter excess
　Excitotoxicity
　Lipid peroxidation
　Free radical injury
　Loss of energy metabolism
　Apoptosis
　Edema
　Cytokine excess
　Loss of neurotrophic factor support

1990, Stripling[8] estimated that this figure had risen to four billion dollars annually. Acute care hospitalization is a considerable component of the total cost, and complications such as pneumonia, pressure sores, and urinary tract infections are a major factor.[9,10]

## BIOLOGICAL RATIONALE FOR EARLY TREATMENT OF ACUTE SPINAL CORD INJURY

The spinal cord behaves as a linear elastic model under small strains[11] and exhibits nonlinear elastic characteristics under larger strains.[12] The pathophysiology of experimental SCI and the prospects for clinical recovery vary with several primary and secondary injury mechanisms (Table 6.1), including force of compres-

*Clinical Trials in Spinal Cord Injury*   101

sion, duration of compression, displacement, impulse, and kinetic energy.[13–21] For example, persisting compression of the spinal cord appears to cause secondary injury mechanisms that are potentially reversible.[13,14] In the majority of humans with SCI, the primary mechanisms of injury to the spinal cord include acute compression, impact, distraction, laceration, shear, and missile injury[22] (see Table 6.1). These primary events initiate a secondary injury, usually involving several additional damaging processes. The concept of secondary injury was first postulated in 1911 by Allen, who found that surgical myelotomy and removal of the post-traumatic hematomyelia resulted in improvement of neurologic function in dogs subjected to experimental acute SCI.[23] Pathologic evidence for sequential change includes progressive hemorrhage, edema, and axonal and neuronal necrosis, followed by infarction, demyelination, and cyst formation.[24–28] As outlined in Table 6.1, numerous pathophysiologic mechanisms and autodestructive biochemical processes have been postulated to explain the progressive post-traumatic destruction of the spinal cord.[29–31] There is evidence that the following secondary injury mechanisms are important in acute SCI: (1) vascular changes, including reduction in blood flow, loss of autoregulation, neurogenic shock, hemorrhage, loss of microcirculation, vasospasm, and thrombosis (see references 32, 33 for reviews); (2) electrolyte shifts, including increased intracellular calcium, increased extracellular potassium, and increased sodium permeability[34]; (3) neurotransmitter accumulation, such as serotonin or catecholamines[35] and extracellular glutamate, the latter producing excitotoxicity[36]; (4) arachidonic acid release; free radical production, especially oxygen free radicals[37]; and eicosanoid production, especially prostaglandins and lipid peroxidation[11]; (5) endogenous opioids[38,39]; (6) edema formation[40]; (7) inflammation[41]; and (8) loss of energy metabolism, especially decreased adenosine triphosphate (ATP) production.[42] These theories of secondary injury have been the subject of several reviews.[21,43–45]

The evolution of these pathophysiologic processes that lead to progressive pathologic changes during the first few hours after injury is important with respect to pharmacotherapy and surgical treatment of SCI. The improved understanding of the pathophysiology of acute SCI has led to improved pharmacologic strategies to attenuate the effects of the secondary injury. The NASCIS-2 study demonstrated a beneficial effect of high-dose MP if given within 8 hours of injury in patients with complete and incomplete spinal cord injuries[3]; this emphasizes the importance of the timing of treatment. Also, the NASCIS-3 study gave some evidence that treatment within 3 hours may have been superior to treatment begun 3–8 hours after injury.[4] The severity of the pathologic changes and the degree of recovery are directly related to the duration of acute compression, as demonstrated by experimental studies in which longer compression times produced less clinical recovery.[13,14,46–49] The clinical evidence of the relationships between duration of compression, timing of treatment, recovery of spinal cord function, and complication rates are not well established and depend largely on anecdotal accounts of improved recovery after rapid decompression by traction or surgery.[50–53] There is only one prospective randomized controlled trial of the timing of surgical decompression, and in this study early decompression (less than 72 hours after injury) did not produce significantly improved neurologic recovery as compared with late decompression (5 days or longer after injury).[54]

102    *Clinical Trials in Neurologic Practice*

*Table 6.2*    Current optimal treatment of acute spinal cord injury

First hour
1.  Manage any airway, breathing, and circulation (ABC) problems.
2.  Immobilize the spine.
3.  Restore any systemic hypotension to normotension.
4.  Give methylprednisolone.
5.  Treat in appropriate facility with multidisciplinary team.

Later
1.  Treat the whole patient.
2.  Obtain detailed imaging to detect persisting compression of the cord.
3.  Detect and relieve persisting compression of the cord in selected patients.
4.  Achieve spinal stability.
5.  Mobilize the patient.
6.  Actively avoid complications.

## OPTIMAL TREATMENT FOR THE MANAGEMENT OF SPINAL CORD INJURY

The initial management of patients with SCI (Table 6.2) has improved considerably in most countries. There is better training and deployment of first aid personnel, and many citizens have received special training or are otherwise aware of the necessity for swift, judicious management. There is also greater awareness of the importance for the prevention of hypoxia and hypotension, and early attention is given to the establishment of optimal airway, breathing, and circulation (i.e., the "ABCs" of trauma management). There is improved knowledge among emergency personnel and the general public about the necessity for early immobilization of the spine and for avoidance of injudicious movement of the spine. In most countries, there is also acknowledgment of the advantages of regionalization of the acute management of SCI patients in organized units with specialized equipment and trained personnel, and that referral to these units within the first 2–3 hours of trauma is advantageous.[10] All these measures have the potential for neuroprotection of the injured cord by preventing or treating the systemic secondary mechanisms of injury, especially the hypotension associated with spinal or systemic shock, and hypoxia associated with compromised respiration secondary to airway obstruction or paralysis of diaphragmatic or intercostal muscles.

Hypotension frequently occurs after SCI, due to systemic or spinal shock.[55] Restoration of any systemic hypotension to normotension is a principle of first aid management in SCI. This is based on the recognition that there is vascular compromise of the injured cord by local microcirculatory events, including vasospasm and small-vessel thrombosis,[56,57] which would be made worse by hypotension. Indeed, some investigators have recently advocated *aggressive* medical management of SCI patients: this includes invasive monitoring and the administration of vasopressors as required.[58,59] Invasive monitoring consists of an arterial line to maintain mean systemic arterial pressure at 85 mm Hg, a central venous line to maintain central venous pressure at 5–10 mm Hg, and a pulmonary artery catheter to maintain a pulmonary artery capillary wedge pressure of 18 mm Hg or higher. In most cases, these parameters can be achieved with the liberal use of crystalloid and colloid solutions, but vasopressors such as dopamine (or dobutamine) at 2.5–5.0 µg/kg per minute or norepinephrine (Levophed) at 0.01–0.2 µg/kg per minute[59] are advocated if necessary to restore adequate hemodynamic homeostasis. Invasive monitoring combined with frequent clinical observation by trained personnel in an intensive care setting prevents fluid overload and minimizes the risk of pulmonary edema. These measures are designed to ensure optimal conditions for spinal cord recovery, but in the absence of a randomized trial it is not known whether such aggressive medical management improves neurologic recovery.

The autonomic hemodynamic manifestations of spinal shock and reflex loss may last for several days or weeks after injury. In contrast, the somatic motor and sensory deficits of spinal shock usually terminate within an hour of injury. Thus, structural damage to the cord is usually the cause of motor and sensory neurologic deficits persisting for more than 1 hour after SCI rather than spinal shock.

The principles of early management also include the concept of *treating the whole patient*, which requires attention to prevention of gastric dilatation and vomiting, with its attendant risk of aspiration, prevention of bladder distension, pressure sores, and deep venous thrombosis. These protective measures against the known complications of SCI are essential for trials of neuroprotection to enhance cord recovery, because the recovery potential of the injured cord is adversely affected by any hypoxic, hypotensive, inflammatory, or infectious complications of SCI.


## NATURAL HISTORY OF NEUROLOGIC RECOVERY AFTER ACUTE SPINAL CORD INJURY

To assess the results of current clinical trials in SCI, it is essential to be aware of the natural history of neurologic recovery from SCI in the absence of major attempts to alter the prognosis. The majority of SCI patients experience some neurologic recovery,[60] although the potential is much greater in those who have incomplete injuries (as defined below). Neurologic recovery includes recovery of nerve root function at the level of the injury or caudally and cord recovery at the level of the injury or caudally. The biological basis for such recovery includes the following: resolution of acute injury events, such as hypoxia or ischemia; resolution of secondary injury events, such as ionic, neurotransmitter, or vascular changes; and recovery by long-term process, such as axonal regeneration or remyelination. The National Spinal Cord Injury Database, reported by Stover et al.,[61] is a source of information about neurologic recovery in almost 10,000 SCI patients that was compiled by the Model Spinal Cord Injury System Program at 19 centers in the United States from 1973 to 1985. The Frankel system of grading was used and showed that even a small number of neurologically complete cases can recover some caudal neurological function indicative of cord recovery.[62] Hansebout[63] conducted a review of the neurologic recovery of complete cases and found that approximately 1% of complete cases recovered the

104 *Clinical Trials in Neurologic Practice*

ability to ambulate. Stover et al.[61] found the best recovery in the B and C categories of the Frankel grading system of incomplete injuries, in which 30–50% of patients improved 1 Frankel grade. Sixty percent of patients with SCI have incomplete injuries[64]; thus, these high rates of natural recovery, especially among incomplete patients who received the standard of care existent during the era before the development of formal clinical trials, make it mandatory to use rigorous study methodology and accurate outcome measures in clinical trials of patients with SCI.

## METHODOLOGY OF OUTCOME STUDIES AND OUTCOME MEASURES USED IN CLINICAL TRIALS IN SPINAL CORD INJURY

A variety of outcome study methodologies and outcome measures have been used in clinical trials in acute SCI (Table 6.3). Although much has been learned from retrospective analyses of large case series, such as the natural history of recovery noted in the previous section, many previous therapeutic studies failed because of faulty study design. Individual case series using retrospectively collected data provide minimal opportunity to establish new treatments. Meta-analysis of groups of retrospective studies might improve the quality of the analysis and the validity of the results in some instances. The optimal method for studying a new treatment in SCI is the prospective randomized control trial, in which a statistically sound design is used during a reasonably practical period of time, such as 3–5 years. There have been only 10 such studies (described below) due to the costs involved and the reluctance of some investigators to participate. Prospective data collection has improved the quality of the data collected in some nonrandomized SCI trials,[6] and a double-blind crossover trial design has been used to study pharmacotherapy in the chronic phase of SCI.[65]

The most important outcome measures in clinical trials of acute SCI are neurologic recovery and functional improvement. Other useful outcome variables include the following: mortality rate, morbidity rates in terms of specific complications of SCI, length of acute and rehabilitation hospital stay, incidence of intractable pain, return to work, and patient satisfaction. Radiologic outcome variables such as adequacy of decompression and confirmation of restoration of spinal alignment and stability are also useful. It is unfortunate that neurophysiologic tests have not been included as outcome measures in any of the published trials, although tests such as the recording of somatosensory-evoked potentials have been shown to be of prognostic value[66] and are often used for monitoring SCI patients who are having surgical treatment.[67] Electrophysiology measures and patient satisfaction surveys have been used in clinical trials in the chronic phase of SCI.

With respect to clinical trials, the American Spinal Injury Association (ASIA), with the collaboration of the International Medical Society of Paraplegia (IMSOP), has developed scales for the neurologic grading and assessment of neurologic recovery of patients with acute SCI.[68] In most countries, the ASIA/IMSOP system has replaced other systems, such as the Frankel[62] and Sunnybrook[69] systems, for grading neurologic function and assessing neuro-

*Clinical Trials in Spinal Cord Injury*   105

*Table 6.3*   Outcome measures for clinical trials in acute spinal cord injury

| Outcome measure | Method | Comment |
|---|---|---|
| Clinical neurologic examination<br>Frankel grade<br>ASIA/IMSOP grade<br>Sunnybrook grade<br>Benzel grade<br>ASIA/IMSOP motor score<br>ASIA/IMSOP sensory score | Compare the numbers of patients who change one or two grades, or the changes between baseline and follow-up in mean motor or sensory scores (use raw data or % of baseline, or % of potential recovery). | ASIA/IMSOP is more useful than the others, but there is a ceiling effect for grade D and uncommon improvement from grade A to B. |
| Functional assessment<br>FIM<br>Functional MRI | Compare the mean raw scores of clinical ability. | Functional Independence Measures (FIM) has only been applied to two randomized prospective controlled trials in acute SCI. |
| Neurophysiologic studies<br>SSEP<br>Motor-evoked potential | Measures of sensory or motor conduction in the cord. Compare mean latencies or amplitudes or presence/absence. | Somatosensory-evoked potential (SSEP) has been used to predict prognosis, but has not been used in a controlled trial. |
| Imaging features<br>Relief of compression<br>Restoration of alignment<br>Assessment of stability | MRI best for spinal cord and nerve roots.<br>Computed tomography best for spine. | MRI has not yet been used as an outcome measure for cord recovery in a clinical trial. |
| Mortality/ morbidity | Compare complication rates such as sepsis between treatment groups, centers, or both. | Frequently used and provides important data about side effects of drugs and performance of centers. |

ASIA/IMSOP = American Spinal Injury Association/International Medical Society of Paraplegia; MRI = magnetic resonance imaging.

logic recovery in SCI patients, because it is more precise and comprehensive. For these reasons, the ASIA/IMSOP method has been used in most recent clinical trials in SCI. Comparisons between treatment groups can be made on the basis of the numbers of patients who show a change in neurologic grade or on the basis of change in motor or sensory scores, which are obtained by adding the individual values given for muscle strength and dermatome sensitivity, respectively. It is not essential for all clinical trials to use the same outcome measures, as long as the measures used have been verified on the basis of inter-rater reliability and other measures of consistency.

However, it should be noted that the ASIA/IMSOP system still has significant shortcomings, such as the "ceiling" effect noted for Grade D patients, who may recover near-normal neurologic function but would have to recover fully and achieve a normal neurologic examination to improve to Grade E. Other classifications, such as the Benzel method and the Sunnybrook Scale,[69] include a larger number of categories (Benzel has seven; Sunnybrook has 10) especially for incomplete injuries, but these scales have been used much less often,[70] and there is no definite proof that they are superior to the ASIA system for avoiding the ceiling effect.

The methods used to compute the results of clinical trials should be clearly stated, and the statistical tests to assess the significance of the results should be reliable and appropriate. However, some investigators have used difficult mathematical formulas to compute neurologic recovery and have used statistical tests not easily understood by the practitioners. These difficulties have led to controversy about the results of some trials, especially the NASCIS-2 trial.[71] In an attempt to deal with the differing baseline neurologic status of patients in the trial, some studies have computed other outcome parameters, such as the percent increase in the potential recovery, instead of clearly stating the exact percent increase in motor score. Such manipulations serve to equalize the opportunities for recovery from injuries at different levels and of varying severity. For example, a cervical incomplete injury has the potential to recover more muscle groups than a lumbar incomplete injury. To prevent confusion and uncertainty, reports of clinical trials must contain all the raw and derived data for each outcome measure of recovery.

Clinical trials in SCI should also include outcome measures of the functional significance of the neurologic recovery. Only recently have functional outcome measures been included in the design of clinical trials in SCI. The functional measure recently used in SCI clinical trials is the test of Functional Independent Measures (FIM).[72] However, its value in this field has not yet been established. A major shortcoming of the FIM is the inability to apply it at the time of initial assessment.

## Eligibility and Stratification

All 10 clinical trials in acute SCI with a randomized, prospective controlled methodology have included men and women (men comprise 80–85% of all acute SCIs). Most trials have had age restrictions of 16–75 years of age. The younger age groups have been excluded, usually because of the difficulties of obtaining informed consent, and the older age groups have been excluded because of the high mortality of SCI in those older than 75 years of age,[73] especially those with complete injuries. All trials have excluded gunshot wounds because of their poor prognosis for recovery. Other common exclusions are patients with pre-existing neurologic diseases, previous SCI, and major medical conditions, such as heart failure or multiple trauma, which may be life-threatening or cause hemodynamic instability. This exclusion underlines the importance of prevention of secondary injury caused by such factors (discussed in the section Optimal Treatment for the Management of Spinal Cord Injury). It is of interest that one clinical trial specifically excluded patients who were hypotensive for a defined period of time.[74] All trials have excluded patients who had been drinking or who had head injuries sufficiently severe to prevent reliable scoring of neurologic function at the initial assessment.

Due to the importance of the severity of neurologic injury to the potential for recovery,[22] most studies have used stratification into complete and incom-

*Clinical Trials in Spinal Cord Injury*    107

plete injuries to ensure equal numbers of similarly injured patients in each treatment group. Some studies have also stratified for level of injury, with cervical being separated from thoracic only, or with thoracic and lumbar combined. Indeed, there is some evidence that neurologic recovery is related to level of injury.[22] Due to the slowness of neurologic recovery after acute SCI, most trials have required a 1-year follow-up examination and based the primary outcome measure on a comparison of the initial and 12-month neurologic examinations. Accordingly, most trials have excluded patients with uncertain follow-up, such as travelers and convicts.

## TEN RANDOMIZED, PROSPECTIVE CONTROL TRIALS IN ACUTE SPINAL CORD INJURY

There have been 10 randomized, prospective control trials in acute SCI (Table 6.4). Four examined the role of MP; two studied GM-1 ganglioside (GM-1); and one each examined thyrotropin-releasing hormone (TRH), gacyclidine (an *N*-methyl-D-aspartate [NMDA] receptor antagonist), and nimodipine (a calcium channel blocker). The remaining trial assessed early versus late decompression surgery.

Three of the four MP trials were conducted by the NASCIS group led by Dr. Michael Bracken, which comprised a large number of centers; all of the centers were in the United States, except for two in Toronto, Canada. Not all centers participated in all three NASCIS trials. The NASCIS trials were well organized, involved large numbers of patients and sophisticated methodology, and were supported by the National Institutes of Health in the United States and by the Upjohn Company (Kalamazoo, Michigan), which supplied the agents. Indeed, the NASCIS group performed the first multicenter, randomized, prospective control trial of any treatment modality in the field of acute SCI. The NASCIS-1 trial assessed the value of two doses of MP: The low dose was 100 mg per day intravenously (IV) for 10 days, and the high dose was 1,000 mg per day IV for 10 days. This trial involved 330 patients in nine centers and found no difference in neurologic recovery based on a novel system of classification of motor and sensory dysfunction.[75,76] There was no placebo group, because many investigators had been using MP in their practices based on favorable reports of experimental studies and had concerns about the ethical implication of withholding the drug. There was a significant increased rate of wound infections in the high-dose group. Thus, when NASCIS-2 was planned, there was less concern about including a placebo group; this was a key component of the NASCIS-2 trial that resulted in MP's producing improved neurologic recovery compared to both the placebo group and a second treatment group that received the drug naloxone, which had also been selected for study based on favorable experimental results.[3] MP was administered in very high doses, but only for 24 hours. The initial dose was 30 mg/kg IV followed by 5.4 mg/kg per hour IV for the next 23 hours. There were 487 patients randomized in 16 centers. The improvement was evident in both complete and incomplete cases, but only in patients to whom the drug was administered within the first 8 hours of injury. Furthermore, subsequent detailed analysis of the type of neurologic recovery gave strong evidence that there was

## 108   *Clinical Trials in Neurologic Practice*

*Table 6.4*   Randomized, prospective, control trials in acute spinal cord injury in humans

| Name of study and authors | Year results reported | Agent | Placebo | Neurologic result |
|---|---|---|---|---|
| NASCIS-1, Bracken et al.[75,76] | 1984 | Methylprednisolone (MP), low versus high dose | No. | No difference. |
| NASCIS-2, Bracken et al.[3] | 1990 | MP, naloxone, or placebo | Yes. | MP improved neurologic recovery. |
| NASCIS-3, Bracken et al.[4] | 1997 | MP ± tirilazad | No. | MP improved neurologic recovery. |
| Japanese MP, Otani et al.[108] | 1994 | MP or placebo | Yes. | MP improved neurologic recovery. |
| GM-1 No. 1, Geisler et al.[78] | 1991 | GM-1 ganglioside | Yes. All patients received MP at lower than NASCIS-2 dose. | GM-1 improved neurologic recovery. |
| GM-1 No. 2, Geisler et al.[79] | 1998, preliminary | GM-1 ganglioside | Yes. All patients received MP at NASCIS-2 dose. | Not available yet. |
| TRH, Pitts et al.[70] | 1995 | TRH or placebo | Yes. | No difference. |
| GK-11, Tadie et al.[80] | In progress | GK-11 or placebo | Yes. MP not given. | Not available yet. |
| Nimodipine, Petitjean et al.[81] | 1998 | Nimodipine, MP, both, or placebo | Yes. | No difference. |
| Decompression, Vaccaro et al.[54] | 1997 | Decompression <72 hrs versus >5 days | No. All patients received MP at NASCIS-2 dose. | No difference; 20 patients in trial lost to follow up. |

ASIA = American Spinal Injury Association; FIM = Functional Independent Measures; ICU = intensive care unit; NASCIS = National Acute Spinal Cord Injury Studies; TRH = thyrotropin-releasing hormone.

significant recovery at both the level of cord injury and at lower cord levels, indicating long tract recovery.[77]

For a number of reasons, some investigators and practitioners have questioned the results.[71] For example, it was surprising to note that one of the placebo groups attained the highest neurologic recovery at 1 year (the incomplete group treated after 8 hours of injury).[77] Furthermore, it has been questioned whether the division of patients into those treated in less than 8 hours and those treated in more than 8 hours was statistically valid, because this stratification was not contained in the primary question. However, the subsequent multicenter trial of MP in Japan, which included 117 patients, confirmed that MP given within 8 hours of injury produced increased neurologic recovery as compared to a placebo, and thus adds weight to the validity of the result of the NASCIS-2 trial. Since these trials were completed,

| No. of patients | No. of centers | Outcome measures | Follow-up duration | Other results |
|---|---|---|---|---|
| 306 | 9 | "Dysfunction" scores: motor and sensory, complication rates | 1 yr | Increased wound infectious in high dose group. |
| 487 | 10 | "Expanded" motor and sensory scores, complication rates | 1 yr | — |
| 499 | 16 | ASIA grade, ASIA motor scores, FIM | 1 yr | Duration of MP varies with duration of delay; MP better than tirilazad; more sepsis and pneumonia in 48 hour group. |
| 177 | 42 | "Expanded" motor score, sensory score, complication rates | 6 mos | — |
| 34 | 1 | Frankel grade, ASIA motor score | 1 yr | — |
| 800 approximately | 28 | ASIA grade, Benzel grade, ASIA scores, FIM | 1 yr | Comparison of Benzel versus ASIA systems. |
| 20 | 1 | Sunnybrook scale | 1 yr | — |
| 280 planned | 26 | ASIA grade, ASIA motor and sensory scores | 1 yr | — |
| 100 | 1 | ASIA grade, ASIA motor and sensory scores | 1 yr | More infections in MP groups; early surgery not better. |
| 62 | 1 | ASIA grade, Frankel grade, ASIA motor | 1 yr (average) | No change in stay in ICU or rehabilitation. |

the majority of patients with SCI in North America has received MP according to the NASCIS-2 recommendations. Indeed, the MP studies have had two other significant effects. First, investigators in subsequent prospective randomized control trials in SCI in North America have felt compelled to include MP in all treatment groups. Second, the 8-hour therapeutic window has been established as a benchmark for other trials, even those not involving drugs. This time window may or may not be appropriate for other treatment strategies, such as surgical decompression.

NASCIS-3 examined a number of issues, including the duration of administration of MP (24-hour versus 48-hour), and the effectiveness of a new agent, tirilazad mesylate, an antioxidant designed to prevent free radical–induced lipid peroxidation.[4] In this multicenter trial in 400 patients, MP produced more recovery than tirilazad. With MP, if administration began within 3 hours of injury, there was no additional benefit from prolonging the treatment to 48 hours from 24 hours. Fur-

110　*Clinical Trials in Neurologic Practice*

thermore, patients receiving MP for 48 hours had a higher incidence of severe sepsis and pneumonia than those treated for 24 hours. However, if MP was delayed to the 3–8 hour postinjury interval, then neurologic recovery was improved by continuing MP for 48 hours rather than 24 hours. The NASCIS-3 study is also noteworthy because it is the first randomized trial in patients with acute SCI to include a functional outcome measure (FIM). This additional outcome measure was useful for confirming the results.

GM-1 is a complex acidic bovine glycolipid that, in experimental studies, enhanced neuronal sprouting and regeneration and counteracted some secondary injury processes, such as glutamate-induced excitotoxicity. The first GM-1 study in SCI patients was a single-center randomized prospective control trial in only 34 patients, and it included a placebo group.[78] The patients received GM-1 at 100 mg IV daily for a mean of 26 days, with the first dose given at a mean of 48 hours after injury. All patients also received MP, but at much lower doses than in NASCIS-2. There was a remarkable improvement in neurologic recovery, including several patients who improved by two Frankel grades, and although the number of patients was small, a statistically significant result was achieved. The outcome measures included Frankel grade changes and ASIA motor scores. The second GM-1 trial was a multicenter trial that included 28 centers and approximately 800 patients with grading on the basis of ASIA and Benzel grades. As noted above, the latter system divides the incomplete injuries into a larger number of categories in an attempt to overcome the ceiling effect. The final report of this study had not been published at the time of submission of this chapter, but the preliminary results were announced in 1998 and showed no significant overall difference between the treatment and placebo groups at 26 weeks, although there was better recovery in the GM-1 patients at 8 and 16 weeks after injury. There was also a trend toward better recovery in the ASIA B patients who received the drug compared with the ASIA B patients who received only the placebo.[79]

The clinical trial with TRH, an antagonist of endogenous opioids, was a single-center trial comprised of only 20 patients.[70] The patients began treatment within 12 hours of injury and received TRH IV, 0.2 mg/kg bolus, and 0.2 mg/kg per hour for 6 hours. The study included a placebo group, and the primary neurologic outcome measure was the Sunnybrook scale developed by the senior author in 1970,[69] which, as noted above, contains an expanded number of grades of incomplete SCI. Pitts et al.[70] found no significant difference in neurologic recovery between the patients treated with TRH and the placebo group.

Gacyclidine is an NMDA antagonist that is being investigated in patients with acute SCI in a multicenter, randomized prospective controlled trial in France.[80] The inclusion criteria for this study are very strict and exclude many ASIA grade D patients with minimal neurologic deficits and those with significant systemic hypotension. This trial is noteworthy because the first dose of the drug was administered within 2 hours of injury, and the protocol thus required the cooperation of all the emergency retrieval and first aid groups in a large portion of France. The ASIA/IMSOP grading system was taught to these groups, and they were often responsible for administering the first dose of the drug or placebo. It is also noteworthy that MP was not included in the protocol. Three different doses of gacyclidine are being examined, and a total of 280 patients are being studied. The final results had not been reported at the time of submission of this chapter.

Nimodipine, a calcium channel blocker, was examined in 100 patients with acute SCI in a single-center randomized prospective trial in France.[74,81] Four

Clinical Trials in Spinal Cord Injury    111

groups of patients were studied: nimodipine alone, nimodipine plus MP, MP alone, and placebo. Nimodipine was given IV at 0.015 mg/kg per hour for 2 hours, followed by 0.03 mg/kg per hour for 7 days, and MP was given at the same dose rate as in NASCIS-2 (30 mg/kg bolus over 1 hour, followed by 5.4 mg/kg per hour for 23 hours). The onset of treatment was within 6 hours of injury in all cases, with the average interval being approximately 3.5 hours. Patients with persistent hypotension were excluded. There was no significant difference between the four treatment groups. With only 100 patients among the four treatment groups, this trial is at high risk of a type 2 error and would have been improved by the inclusion of more patients. The authors also examined the results based on the timing of surgical treatment for stabilization of the spine or decompression of the spinal cord and found no relationship between improved neurologic function and the timing of surgery. However, it should be noted that there was no randomization of patients on the basis of the timing of surgery.

Vaccaro et al.[54] have performed the only randomized prospective controlled trial reported of the timing of surgical decompression in patients with SCI. The subject of the timing of surgical decompression in clinical and experimental SCI was reviewed by the present authors.[82] The surgical trial by Vaccaro et al.[54] was a single center trial in which 62 patients were randomized to early or late surgery. The early surgery group was defined as surgical treatment in less than 72 hours from the time of trauma and had a mean time of decompression of 1.8 days. The late surgery group was defined as surgical treatment more than 5 days after trauma and had a mean time of decompression of 16.8 days. There was no difference in ASIA motor score or ASIA grade at follow-up, approximately one year after injury, and there was no difference between the groups in the length of stay in the intensive care unit or in in-patient rehabilitation time. It should be noted that 20 of the 62 patients enrolled in the trial were lost to follow-up and that the statistical power of this trial was low.

## NONRANDOMIZED STUDIES IN ACUTE SPINAL CORD INJURY

Although this chapter has emphasized the importance of the 10 randomized, prospective controlled trials in acute SCI, information has also been obtained from other trials. For example, knowledge about the treatment of hypotension was obtained from the nonrandomized, prospective study by Vale et al.,[59] in which 77 patients with acute SCI were resuscitated according to a standard protocol to maintain mean arterial pressure above 85 mm Hg and were recommended to have early surgical decompression as soon after medical resuscitation as possible. They prospectively recorded the data in a consistent fashion using standard outcome measures, including the Frankel and ASIA grades, and found improved neurologic recovery compared with a selected series of patients identified by a search of the literature. Although Vale et al. successfully resuscitated the patients without a randomized prospective control methodology, they did not prove the value of their approach involving aggressive medical and surgical management.

Evidence for the effectiveness of surgery in patients with SCI is fragmentary. Pioneers in the management of patients with SCI held markedly different views about surgical intervention. Richard Schneider was one of the most experienced spinal neurosurgeons and advocated early surgery for some patients, such as

## 112    Clinical Trials in Neurologic Practice

those with the acute anterior cervical cord syndrome who had total paralysis with preservation of some posterior column function—essentially, ASIA B patients.[83] Conversely, he strongly argued against early surgery, or indeed any surgery on other groups of patients, such as the patients with immediate complete SCI without a spinal canal block (based on the jugular vein compression test of Queckenstedt) or those with acute central cord syndrome.[84,85] In the 1940s to 1970s, when Schneider practiced, early surgery was generally performed within the first week of injury and almost never on the day of injury. Several reports up to the 1960s from experienced clinicians, including Comarr and Kaufman,[86] Guttman,[87,88] and Bedbrook[89] and colleagues, documented a higher incidence of neurologic deterioration and impaired recovery after attempted surgical decompression, mainly by laminectomy alone. It is now well recognized that laminectomy as the sole surgical technique is contraindicated in most cases of acute SCI, because it usually fails to produce adequate decompression of the cord and often causes spinal instability, which itself can lead to neurologic deterioration. There are still many centers, especially outside North America, that advocate conservative, nonoperative treatment for spinal cord injury, even incomplete cervical injury.[90] Improved imaging by computed tomography and magnetic resonance imaging has shown that, in most cases, compression occurs from an anterior direction and cannot be adequately relieved by posterior approaches such as laminectomy. Also, spine surgeons now have an array of devices and instruments to stabilize the spine and ensure postdecompression stability.

However, even in the presence of precise imaging and accurately performed decompression and surgical techniques, which ensure postdecompression stability, it is unknown whether decompression improves neurologic recovery. There have been several studies, almost all retrospective, of the value of surgical decompression in nonrandomized patients that have attempted to compare decompressed and nondecompressed groups; they have used historical controls or patient groups treated by different surgeons in the same hospital who have followed surgical or nonsurgical protocols on the basis of personal preference or other biases (Table 6.5).[6,21,58,59,91–100] The value of surgical decompression cannot be determined from these nonrandomized studies. The prospective study of surgical decompression reported in 1987 by one of the present authors (C. H. T.) is characteristic of these studies.[6] In that case-control study, there was no improved benefit to surgical decompression in 118 patients who had surgery performed at various times after acute SCI compared to a concurrent control group of 92 patients who did not undergo surgery. However, this study showed that surgery can be performed on acute SCI patients without causing changes in mortality rate or in the rates of most of the common complications sustained by patients with acute SCI. As shown in Table 6.5, almost all the other studies were retrospective and nonrandomized and attempted to compare early and late surgery with no convincing results. In almost all of these studies, except that of Wagner and Chehrazi,[97] the early surgery group received surgery 24 hours or more after injury.

As shown in Table 6.5 and noted in the previous section, the only prospective randomized trial of the timing of decompression was reported by Vaccaro et al. in 1997.[54] In this trial of 62 patients with cervical cord injury, 34 were randomized to early decompression within 72 hours of injury (m = 1.8 days), and 28 were randomized to late decompression, defined as longer than 5 days after injury (m = 16.8 days). There was no significant difference in neurologic recovery between the two groups.

## TRIALS IN CHRONIC SPINAL CORD INJURY

Several reports showed high recovery rates among patients who have had late decompression weeks or months after acute SCI (Table 6.6). Although these results are impressive and support the concept that persisting compression should be treated, they do not provide evidence about the relative merits of early versus late decompression. Furthermore, all these studies of late decompression were retrospective.[95,101–104]

There have been few pharmacotherapy trials to enhance neurologic function in chronic SCI patients. However, 4-aminopyridine, an agent found to improve conduction in the damaged but incompletely interrupted spinal cord, has received considerable attention. Randomized double-blind crossover trials by Hansebout et al.[105] and Potter et al.[65] showed temporary improvement in neurologic function after IV[105] or oral administration.[65]

Trials of antispasticity pharmacotherapy with agents such as baclofen have proven the feasibility of prolonged intrathecal administration of agents in patients with chronic SCI.[106] It can be expected that there will be future trials using this route for agents designed to improve recovery and regeneration of the spinal cord, such as neurotrophic factors.[107]

## CONCLUSIONS

In addition to the major improvement in our understanding of the pathophysiology of acute SCI through experimental studies that have elucidated the primary and secondary injury mechanisms, there have been major advances in the diagnosis and management of patients with acute SCI. These advances include improved first aid, especially through the rapid deployment of trained personnel skilled in recognition and judicious early management. Improvement has also been derived from the development of regional multidisciplinary units with the necessary personnel and equipment for managing acute SCI patients. Improved medical management has come from techniques to monitor, prevent, or treat early hypotension and hypoxia, which can worsen any remaining neurologic function and reduce the potential for neurologic recovery. Diagnostic regimens now include highly accurate and noninvasive techniques to image the injured spinal cord and nerve roots by magnetic resonance and to image the injured spinal column by computed tomography.

Improved surgical techniques allow decompression of the spinal cord through a variety of surgical approaches, and stabilization of the spinal column with various new techniques involving instrumentation, which can be performed with increased precision and lower morbidity. Finally, the advances include much more accurate methods of grading and scoring the clinical neurologic examination and the functional outcome of SCI patients, especially the ASIA system, which have improved the precision and validity of clinical trials. These advances have prompted clinical investigators to conduct many outstanding, well-designed clinical trials of neuroprotection and other treatment modalities, such as surgical decompression in patients with SCI. The methodology used in the trials has also been refined in terms of patient numbers, duration of follow-up, and the inclusion of functional outcome measures.

114   *Clinical Trials in Neurologic Practice*

*Table 6.5*   Trials of spinal surgery and recovery of neurologic function in patients with acute spinal cord injury

| Authors, yr | No. of patients | Timing of surgery |
|---|---|---|
| Larson et al.,[95] 1976 | 44<br>First wk, 8<br>>1 wk, 36 | Early, <1 wk<br>Late, >1 wk |
| Maynard et al.,[96] 1979 | 123; 43% early surgery | Within 4 wks |
| Wagner, Chehrazi,[97] 1982 | 22 OP<br>20 non-OP | Early, <8 hrs<br>Late, 9–48 hrs |
| Benzel, Larson,[92] 1986 | 35, all complete<br>25 anterior OP<br>10 posterior OP | 1–4 wks |
| Benzel, Larson,[91] 1987 | 99, all cervical | Mean, 29 days |
| Donovan et al.,[93] 1987 | 17 OP<br>43 non-OP | Within 3 wks |
| Tator et al.,[6] 1987 | 116 OP<br>75 decompressed or reduced<br>41 fusion<br>92 non-OP | Within 4 weeks |
| Wiberg, Hauge,[100] 1988 | 30 | Early, <24 hours; n = 8; m = 12 days |
| Weinshel et al.,[99] 1990 | 90 OP | m = 13 days |
| Levi et al.,[58] 1991 | Early, 45<br>Late, 58 | <24 hrs<br>>24 hrs |
| Duh et al.,[94] 1994 | 303 OP | Mean, 200 hrs<br>38 in <25 hrs |
| Waters et al.,[98] 1996 | 184 non-OP<br>269 | Mean, >14 days, up to 3.5 mos |
| Vale et al.,[59] 1997 | 77, mostly OP | <24 hrs in 11 of 64 with follow-up |
| Vaccaro et al.,[54] 1997 | 34<br>28 | <72 hrs; m = 1.80 days<br>>5 days; m = 16.8 days |

OP = operation.

The most reliable and useful information from the clinical trials in SCI has been obtained from the randomized, prospective control trials, although some useful information has also come from other study formats. MP has been proven to improve neurologic function if administered within 8 hours of injury. In turn, the MP studies show that there is a therapeutic window after trauma that allows time

| Type of study | Questions | Results |
|---|---|---|
| Retrospective | Does early surgery improve neurologic recovery? | No difference in neurologic recovery between early and late, preferable to wait. |
| Retrospective | Does early surgery improve neurologic recovery? | Surgery within 4 wks does not improve neurologic recovery. |
| Retrospective | Does early or late surgery improve neurologic recovery? | Surgery does not improve recovery (early, <8 hrs, not better than late, 9–48 hrs). |
| Retrospective | Does nerve root decompression improve root recovery? | Anterior decompression improves root recovery. |
| Retrospective | Is there a relationship between trauma to time of decompression and neurologic recovery? | No relationship between time to decompression and neurologic recovery. |
| Retrospective | Does surgical fusion improve neurologic recovery? | Fusion did not improve neurologic recovery. Many complete cases recovered in both groups. |
| Prospective, nonrandom | Does surgical decompression reduce or fusion improve neurologic recovery? | Surgery did not improve neurologic recovery. No change in length of stay. |
| Retrospective | Does OP improve neurologic recovery? | Decompression improves neurologic recovery, especially in incompletes. |
| Retrospective | Does surgical decompression improve neurologic recovery? | Surgical decompression improved neurologic recovery more than fusion alone. |
| Retrospective | Does early surgery improve neurologic recovery? | Early is preferred, but no significant difference in neurologic recovery. |
| Prospective, randomized but not on basis of surgery | Does early or late surgery improve neurologic recovery? | Surgery does not improve neurologic recovery (early, <25 hrs, or late, >200 hrs, may be better). |
| Prospective, nonrandom | Does surgery improve neurologic recovery from a baseline of 30 days? | Surgery did not improve neurologic recovery. |
| Prospective, nonrandom | Does early surgery improve neurologic recovery? | Timing of surgery had no effect on neurologic recovery. |
| Prospective, randomized | Does early surgery improve neurologic recovery in cervical cord injury? | No difference in neurologic outcome. |

for treatment to be administered to interrupt secondary injury processes. There is a need for further, well-designed clinical trials of neuroprotection afforded by pharmacotherapy, surgery, and other means in acute SCI.

The duration of the time window of opportunity for early treatment to reverse or prevent the damaging pathophysiologic processes is unknown. In animal studies,

116　*Clinical Trials in Neurologic Practice*

*Table 6.6*　Late surgical decompression and recovery of neurologic function
in patients with spinal cord injury

| Authors, yr | No. of patients | Timing | Type of study | Results |
|---|---|---|---|---|
| Bohlman, Freehafer,[102] 1975 | 27 | Average, 22 mos | Retrospective | Improved neurologic recovery in eight incompletes |
| Larson et al.,[95] 1976 | 44 | <1 wk to several yrs | Retrospective | Improved neurologic recovery in completes and incompletes |
| Bohlman,[101] 1979 | 100 | Average, 12 mos | Retrospective | Improved neurologic recovery in many |
| Brodkey et al.,[103] 1980 | 8 | 3 wks to 4 yrs | Retrospective | Improved neurologic recovery in incompletes |
| Maiman et al.,[104] 1984 | 20 | 1 mo to 5 yrs | Retrospective | Improved neurologic recovery in most |
| Anderson, Bohlman,[109] 1992 | 51 | 1 mo to 8 yrs (m = 15 mos) | Retrospective | Improved neurologic recovery in 25 completes (one or two levels, caudal cord in only one patient) |
| Bohlman, Anderson,[37] 1992 | 58 | 1 mo to 9 yrs (m = 13 mos) | Retrospective | Improved neurologic recovery in 46 incompletes (cord recovery) |

the treatment window for decompression appears to extend for several hours from
the time of onset of compression. With respect to decompression in patients, it has
not yet been possible to accurately determine the time window. Guidance about the
duration of the therapeutic window in human SCI may be gained from the acute
pharmacotherapy treatment trials. Both the North American and Japanese trials with
high-dose MP have shown that this agent was successful in improving neurologic
recovery if given within the first 8 hours of injury.[3,4,108] However, in the GM-1 trial,
which showed improved neurologic recovery, the therapeutic window in humans
with SCI extended for at least 48 hours after SCI, because the first dose of this agent
was not given until an average of 48 hours after injury.[78] It should be noted that the
biological properties of this agent include reversal of acute injury events and longer-
term repair by promotion of regeneration. In summary, the available evidence in
human SCI shows that there is uncertainty about the length of the time window for
treatment. Intuitively, the duration probably relates to a number of factors, including
the severity of the injury, patient age, and the effectiveness of the treatment.

## Acknowledgments

The authors wish to acknowledge the assistance of Ms. Sandi Amaral in the
preparation of this manuscript and the financial assistance of the Joint Sections
of Neurotrauma and Critical Care and Disorders of the Spine and Peripheral
Nerves of the AANS/CNS, which have encouraged the development of clinical
trials in acute SCI. Dr. Fehlings is supported by a Career Scientist Award from
the Ontario Ministry of Health.

## REFERENCES

1. Kraus JF, Franti CE, Riggins RS, et al. Incidence of traumatic spinal cord lesions. J Chron Dis 1975;28:471–492.
2. Tator CH. Epidemiology and General Characteristics of the Spinal Cord Injury Patient. In EC Benzel, CH Tator (eds), Contemporary Management of Spinal Cord Injury. Park Ridge, IL: American Association Neurological Surgery, 1995;9–13.
3. Bracken MB, Shepard MJ, Collins WF, et al. A randomized clinical trial of methylprednisolone and naloxone used in the initial treatment of acute spinal cord injury: results of the second National Acute Spinal Cord Injury Study. N Engl J Med 1990;322:1405–1411.
4. Bracken MB, Shepard MJ, Holford TR, et al. Administration of methylprednisolone for 24 or 48 hours or tirilazad mesylate for 48 hours in the treatment of acute spinal cord injury. Results of the third national acute spinal cord injury randomized controlled trial. JAMA 1997;277:1597–1604.
5. Papadopoulos SM. Cervical spine instability: Instrumentation and other methods of management. Presented at American Association of Neurological Surgeons. Practical Clinic, 1994.
6. Tator CH, Duncan EG, Edmonds VE, et al. Comparison of surgical and conservative management in 208 patients with acute spinal cord injury. Can J Neurol Sci 1987;14:60–69.
7. Wilberger J. Diagnosis and management of spinal cord trauma. J Neurotrauma 1991;(Suppl 1):S21–S30.
8. Stripling TE. The cost of economic consequences of traumatic spinal cord injury. Paraplegia News. August, 1990;50–54.
9. Tator CH, Duncan EG, Edmonds VE, et al. Complications and costs of management of acute spinal cord injury. Paraplegia 1993;31:700–714.
10. Tator CH, Duncan EG, Edmonds VE, et al. Neurological recovery, mortality and length of stay after acute spinal cord injury associated with changes in management. Paraplegia 1995;33:254–262.
11. Hung TK, Albin MS, Brown TD, et al. Biomechanical responses to open experimental spinal cord injury. Surg Neurol 1981;15:471–476.
12. Somerson SK, Stokes BT. Functional analysis of an electromechanical spinal cord injury device. Exp Neurol 1987;96:82–96.
13. Dolan EJ, Tator, CH, Endrenyi L. The value of decompression for acute experimental spinal cord compression injury. J Neurosurg 1980;53:749–755.
14. Guha A, Tator CH, Endrenyi L, Piper I. Decompression of the spinal cord improves recovery after acute experimental spinal cord compression injury. Paraplegia 1987;25:324–339.
15. Hung TK, Chang GL, Chang JL, Albin MS. Stress-strain relationship and neurological sequelae of uniaxial elongation of the spinal cord of cats. Surg Neurol 1975;15:471–476.
16. Noyes DH, Bresnahan JC. Correlation between spinal cord lesion volume and impact parameters. Proc Biophys Soc 1981;33:H12.
17. Panjabi MM. Experimental spinal cord trauma. A biomechanical viewpoint. Paraplegia 1987; 25:217–220.
18. Rivlin AS, Tator CH. Effect of duration of acute spinal cord compression in a new acute cord injury model in the rat. Surg Neurol 1978;10:39–43.
19. Tarlov IM. Spinal cord injuries—early treatment. Surg Clin North Am 1955;35:591–607.
20. Tator CH. Experimental and clinical studies of the pathophysiology and management of acute spinal cord injury. J Spinal Cord Med 1996;19:206–214.
21. Tator CH, Fehlings MG. Review of the secondary injury theory of acute spinal cord trauma with emphasis on vascular mechanisms. J Neurosurg 1991;75:15–26.
22. Tator CH. Spine-spinal cord relationships in spinal cord trauma. Clin Neurosurg 1983;30:479–494.
23. Allen AR. Surgery of experimental lesion of spinal cord equivalent to crush injury of fracture dislocation of spinal column. A preliminary report. JAMA 1911;57:878–880.
24. Blight AR. Cellular morphology of chronic spinal cord injury in the cat: analysis of myelinated axons by line-sampling. Neuroscience 1983;10:521–543.
25. Bresnahan JC, King JS, Martin GF, et al. A neuroanatomical analysis of spinal cord injury in the Rhesus monkey (Macaca Mulatta). J Neurol Sci 1976;28:521–542.
26. Bunge RP, Puckett WR, Becerra JL, et al. Observations on the pathology of human spinal cord injury. Adv Neurol 1993;59:75–89.
27. Kakulas BA. Pathology of spinal injuries. Cent Nerv Syst Trauma 1984;1:117–129.
28. Wallace MC, Tator CH, Lewis AJ. Chronic regenerative changes in the spinal cord after cord compression injury in rats. Surg Neurol 1987;27:209–219.
29. Collins WF. A review and update of experimental and clinical studies of spinal cord injury. Paraplegia 1983;21:204–219.

## 118   Clinical Trials in Neurologic Practice

30. Hall ED, Yonkers PA, Horan KL, Braughler JM. Correlation between attenuation of posttraumatic spinal cord ischemia and preservation of tissue vitamin E by the 21-aminosteroid U74006F: evidence for an in vivo antioxidant mechanism. J Neurotrauma 1989;6:169–176.
31. Young W. Secondary CNS injury. J Neurotrauma 1988;5:219–221.
32. Tator CH. Ischemia as a Secondary Neuronal Injury. In SK Salzman, AI Faden (eds), Neurobiology of Central Nervous System Trauma. New York: Oxford University Press, 1994;209–215.
33. Tator CH. Review of experimental spinal cord injury with emphasis on the local and systemic circulatory effects. Neurochirurgie 1991;37:291–302.
34. Young W, Koreh I. Potassium and calcium changes in injured spinal cords. Brain Res 1986;365:42–53.
35. Osterholm JL, Mathews GJ. Altered norepinephrine metabolism following experimental spinal cord injury. Part I: relationship to hemorrhagic necrosis and post-wounding neurological deficits. J Neurosurg 1972;36:386–394.
36. Faden AI, Simon RP. A potential role for excitotoxins in the pathophysiology of spinal cord injury. Ann Neurol 1988;23:623–626.
37. Demopoulos HB, Flamm ES, Pietronigro DD, et al. The free radical pathology and the microcirculation in the major central nervous system disorders. Acta Physiol Scand 1980;492(Suppl 111):91–119.
38. Faden AI, Jacobs TP, Holaday JW. Comparison of early and late naloxone treatment in experimental spinal injury. Neurology 1982;32:677–681.
39. Faden AI, Jacobs TP, Smith MT: Evaluation of the calcium channel antagonist nimodipine in experimental spinal cord ischemia. J Neurosurg 1984;60:796–799.
40. Wagner FC Jr, Stewart WB. Effect of trauma dose on spinal cord edema. J Neurosurg 1981;54:802–806.
41. Xu J, Hsu CY, Junker H, et al. Kininogen and Kinin in experimental spinal cord injury. J Neurochem 1991;57:975–980.
42. Anderson DK, Means ED, Waters TR. Spinal cord energy metabolism in normal and postlaminectomy cats. J Neurosurg 1980;52:387–391.
43. Anderson DK, Hall ED. Pathophysiology of spinal cord trauma. Ann Emerg Med 1993;22:987–992.
44. Faden AI. Experimental neurobiology of central nervous system trauma. Crit Rev Neurobiol 1993;7:175–186.
45. Young W, Huang PP, Kume-Kick J. Cellular, Ionic and Biomolecular Mechanisms of the Injury Process. In EC Benzel, CH Tator (eds), Contemporary Management of Spinal Cord Injury. Park Ridge, IL: American Association of Neurological Surgeons, 1995;27–42.
46. Carlson GD, Warden KE, Barbeau JM, et al. Viscoelastic relaxation and regional blood flow response to spinal cord compression and decompression. Spine 1997;22:1285–1291.
47. Delamarter RB, Sherman J, Carr JB. Pathophysiology of spinal cord injury: Recovery after immediate and delayed decompression. J Bone Joint Surg 1995;77-A:1042–1049.
48. Nystrom B, Berglund JE. Spinal cord restitution following compression injuries in rats. Acta Neurol Scand 1988;78:467–472.
49. Tarlov IM. Spinal Cord Compression: Mechanisms of Paralysis and Treatment. Springfield, IL: Charles C Thomas, 1957.
50. Gillingham J. Letter to the editor. Early management of spinal cord trauma. J Neurosurg. 1976;44:766–767.
51. Hadley M, Fitzpatrick B, Sonntag V, Browner C. Facet fracture-dislocation injuries of the cervical spine. Neurosurg 1992;30:661–666.
52. Sussman BJ. Letter to the editor. Early management of spinal cord trauma. J Neurosurg 1976;44:766.
53. Wolf A, Levi L, et al. Operative management of bilateral facet dislocation. J Neurosurg 1991;75:883–890.
54. Vaccaro AR, Daugherty RJ, Sheehan TP, et al. Neurologic outcome of early versus late surgery for cervical spinal cord injury. Spine 1997;22:2609–2613.
55. Kiss ZHT, Tator CH. Neurogenic Shock. In ER Geller (ed), Shock and Resuscitation. New York: McGraw-Hill, 1993;421–440.
56. Anthes DL, Theriault E, Tator CH. Ultrastructural evidence for arteriolar vasospasm after spinal cord trauma. Neurosurgery 1996;39:804–814.
57. Koyanagi I, Tator CH, Lea PJ. Three-dimensional analysis of vascular system in the rat spinal cord with scanning electron microscopy of vascular corrosion casts. Part 2: acute spinal cord injury. Neurosurgery 1993;33:285–292.
58. Levi L, Wolf A, Belzberg H. Hemodynamic parameters in patients with acute cervical cord trauma: description, intervention, and prediction of outcome. Neurosurgery 1993;33:1007–1017.

59. Vale FL, Burns J, Jackson AB, Hadley MN. Combined medical and surgical treatment after acute spinal cord injury: results of a prospective pilot study to assess the merits of aggressive medical resuscitation and blood pressure management. J Neurosurg 1997;87:239–246.
60. Tator CH. Biology of neurological recovery and functional restoration after spinal cord injury. Neurosurgery 1998;42:696–708.
61. Stover SL, DeLisa JA, Whiteneck GG. Spinal Cord Injury. Clinical Outcomes from the Model Systems. Gaithersburg, MD: Aspen Publications, 1995.
62. Frankel H, Hancock D, Hyslop G, et al. The value of postural reduction in the initial management of closed injuries of the spine with paraplegia and tetraplegia part 1. Paraplegia 1969;7:179–192.
63. Hansebout RR. A Comprehensive Review of Methods of Improving Cord Recovery after Acute Spinal Cord Injury. In CH Tator (ed), Early Management of Acute Spinal Cord Injury. New York: Raven Press, 1982;181–196.
64. Tator CH. Clinical Manifestations of Acute Spinal Cord Injury. In EC Benzel, CH Tator (eds), Contemporary Management of Spinal Cord Injury. Park Ridge, IL: American Association of Neurological Surgeons, 1995;15–26.
65. Potter PJ, Hayes KC, Segal JL, et al. Randomized double-blind crossover trial of Fampridine-SR (sustained release 4-aminopyridine) in patients with incomplete spinal cord injury. J Neurotrauma 1998;15:837–849.
66. Rowed DW. Value of Somatosensory Evoked Potentials for Prognosis in Partial Cord Injuries. In CH Tator (ed), Early Management of Acute Spinal Cord Injury. New York: Raven Press, 1982;167–180.
67. Li S, Tator CH. Spinal Cord Blood Flow and Evoked Potentials as Outcome Measures for Experimental Spinal Cord Injury. In E Stalberg, HS Sharma, Y Olsson (eds), Spinal Cord Monitoring. Basic and Clinical Aspects. New York: Springer Verlag, 1998;365–392.
68. American Spinal Injury Association. Standards for Neurological and Functional Classification of Spinal Cord Injury. Revised Edition. Chicago, Il: American Spinal Injury Association, 1992.
69. Tator CH, Rowed DW, Schwartz ML. Sunnybrook Cord Injury Scales for Assessing Neurological Injury and Neurological Recovery. In CH Tator (ed), Early Management of Acute Spinal Cord Injury. New York: Raven Press, 1982;7–24.
70. Pitts LH, Ross A, Chase GA, Faden AI. Treatment with thyrotropin-releasing hormone (TRH) in patients with traumatic spinal cord injuries. J Neurotrauma 1995;12(3):235–243.
71. Nesathurai S. Steroids and spinal cord injury: revisiting the NASCIS 2 and NASCIS 3 trials. J Trauma 1998;45:1088–1093.
72. Keith RA, Granger CV, Hamilton BB, Sherwin FS. The functional independence measure: a new tool for rehabilitation. Adv Clin Rehab 1987;1:6–18.
73. Tator CH, Duncan EG, Edmonds VE, et al. Changes in epidemiology of acute spinal cord injury from 1947 to 1981. Surg Neurol 1993;40:207–215.
74. Petitjean ME, Pointillart V, Dixmerias F, et al. Traitement medicamenteux de la lesion medullaire traumatique au stade aigu. Ann Fr Anesth Reanim 1998;17:114–122.
75. Bracken MB, Collins WF, Freeman DF, et al. Efficacy of methylprednisolone in acute spinal cord injury. JAMA 1984;251:45–52.
76. Bracken MB, Shepard MJ, Hellenbrand KG, et al. Methylprednisolone and neurological function 1 year after spinal cord injury. Results of the National Acute Spinal Cord Injury Study. J Neurosurgery 1985;63:704–713.
77. Bracken MB, Holford TR. Effects of timing of methylprednisolone or naloxone administration and recovery of segmental and long tract neurological function in NASCIS II. J Neurosurg 1993;79:500–507.
78. Geisler FH, Dorsey FC, Coleman WP. Recovery of motor function after spinal cord injury—a randomized placebo-controlled trial with GM-1 ganglioside. N Engl J Med 1991;324:1829–1939.
79. Geisler FH, Dorsey FC, Patarnello F, et al. Sygen acute spinal cord injury study. J Neurotrauma 1998;15:868.
80. Tadie M, Jin O, Lui S, Privat A. Experimental and clinical study of an inhibitor of NMDA receptors in the early treatment of spinal cord injuries. J Neurotrauma 1995;12:349.
81. Petitjean ME, Pointillart V, Daverat P, et al. Administration of methylprednisolone or nimodipine or both versus placebo at the acute phase of spinal cord injury. J Neurotrauma 1995;12:456.
82. Fehlings MG, Tator CH. An evidence-based review of surgical decompression for acute spinal cord injury: Rationale, indications and timing based on experimental and clinical studies. J Neurosurg 1999;91(Suppl 1):1–11.
83. Schneider RC. A syndrome in acute cervical spine injuries for which early operation is indicated. J Neurosurgery 1951;8:360–367.

## 120 *Clinical Trials in Neurologic Practice*

84. Schneider RC, Crosby EC, Russo RH, Gosch HH. Traumatic spinal cord syndromes and their management. Clin Neurosurg 1973;20:424–492.
85. Schneider RC, Thompson JM, Bebin J. The syndrome of the acute central cervical spinal cord injury. J Neurol Neurosurg Psychiatry 1958;21:216–227.
86. Comarr AE, Kaufman AA. A survey of the neurological results of 858 spinal cord injuries. A comparison of patients treated with and without laminectomy. J Neurosurg 1956;13:95–106.
87. Guttmann L. Initial Treatment of Traumatic Paraplegia and Tetraplegia. In P Harris (ed), Spinal Injuries Symposium. Edinburgh, UK: Morrison & Gibb, Ltd., Royal College of Surgeons, 1963;80–92.
88. Guttmann L. Spinal Cord Injuries. Comprehensive Management and Research (2nd ed). Oxford: Blackwell, 1976.
89. Bedbrook GM, Sakae T. A review of cervical spine injuries with neurological dysfunction. Paraplegia 1980;20:321–333.
90. Katoh S, El Masry WS, Jaffray D, et al. Neurologic outcome in conservatively treated patients with incomplete closed traumatic cervical spinal cord injuries. Spine 1996;21(20):2345–2351.
91. Benzel EC, Larson SJ. Functional recovery after decompressive spine operation for cervical spine fractures. Neurosurgery 1987;20:742–746.
92. Benzel EC, Larson SJ. Recovery of nerve root function after complete quadriplegia from cervical spinal fractures. Neurosurgery 1986;19:809–812.
93. Donovan WH, Kopaniky D, Stolzmann E, Carter RE. The neurological and skeletal outcome in patients with closed cervical cord injury. J Neurosurg 1987;66:690–694.
94. Duh M, Shepard MJ, Wilberger JE, Bracken MB. The effectiveness of surgery on the treatment of acute spinal cord injury and its relation to pharmacological treatment. Neurosurgery 1994;35:240–249.
95. Larson SJ, Holst RA, Hemmy DC, Sances A Jr. Lateral extracavitary approach to traumatic lesions of the thoracic and lumbar spine. J Neurosurg 1976;45:628–637.
96. Maynard F, Reynolds G, Fountain S, et al. Neurological prognosis after traumatic quadriplegia. Three year experience of California Regional Spinal Cord Injury Care System. J Neurosurg 1979;50:611–616.
97. Wagner FC Jr, Chehrazi B. Early decompression and neurological outcome in acute cervical spinal cord injuries. J Neurosurg 1982;56:699–705.
98. Waters RL, Adkins RH, Yakura JS, Sie I. Effect of surgery on motor recovery following traumatic spinal cord injury. Spinal Cord 1996;34:188–192.
99. Weinshel SS, Maiman DJ, Baek P, Scales L. Neurologic recovery in quadriplegia following operative treatment. J Spinal Disord 1990;3:244–249.
100. Wiberg J, Hauge HN. Neurological outcome after surgery for thoracic and lumbar spine injuries. Acta Neurochir 1988;91:106–112.
101. Bohlman HH. Acute fractures and dislocations of the cervical spine. An analysis of three hundred hospitalized patients and review of the literature. J Bone Joint Surg 1979;61A:1119–1142.
102. Bohlman HH, Freehafer A. Late anterior decompression of spinal cord injuries. J Bone Joint Surg Am 1975;57:1025.
103. Brodkey JS, Miller CF Jr, Harmody RM. The syndrome of acute central cervical spinal cord injury revisited. Surg Neurol 1980;14:251–257.
104. Maiman DJ, Larson SJ, Benzel EC. Neurological improvement associated with late decompression of the thoracolumbar spinal cord. Neurosurgery 1984;14:302–307.
105. Hansebout RR, Blight AR, Fawcett S, Reddy K. 4-Aminopyridine in chronic spinal cord injury: a controlled, double-blind, crossover study in eight patients. J Neurotrauma 1993;10:1–8.
106. Penn RD, Savoy SM, Corcos D, et al. Intrathecal baclofen for severe spinal spasticity. N Engl J Med 1989;321:1517–1521.
107. Penn RD, Kroin JS, York MM, Cedarbaum JM. Intrathecal ciliary neurotrophic factor delivery for treatment of amyotrophic lateral sclerosis (Phase 1 Trial). Neurosurgery 1997;40:94–100.
108. Otani K, Abe H, Kadoya S, et al. Beneficial effect of methylprednisolone sodium succinate in the treatment of acute spinal cord injury. Sekitsui Sekizui J 1994;7:633–647.
109. Anderson PA, Bohlman HH. Anterior decompression and arthrodesis of the cervical spine: long-term motor improvement. Part II. Improvement in complete traumatic quadriplegia. J Bone Joint Surg 1992;74A:683–692.

# 7
# Clinical Trials in Epilepsy

Pierre Loiseau and Pierre Jallon

Almost all forms of seizure disorders should be treated because of the deleterious consequences of recurrent seizures. Approximately 50% of previously untreated patients with epilepsy achieve a permanent remission by the first prescription of a marketed antiepileptic drug (AED), and an additional 10–20% are controlled by dosage adjustment of this drug or alternative monotherapy. Thus, medical treatment remains unsatisfactory for 20–30% of patients with epilepsy. Furthermore, it has been estimated that approximately 30% of patients treated with available AEDs experience moderate to severe adverse effects.[1] Therefore, the need remains for new agents with higher efficacy or lesser toxicity.[2]

In 1857, Sir Charles Locock reported a clear reduction in seizures among women given potassium bromide; this simple report resulted in widespread use of this substance. In 1912, Hauptmann reported the antiepileptic properties of phenobarbital prescribed as a sedative. For a long period, showing acceptable therapeutic value was enough. Phenytoin, carbamazepine, and valproic acid, at least in Europe, were approved early after their discovery after open clinical trials only. However, as such trials may lead to overoptimistic results, more detailed information is currently required before a drug is approved for general use in patients.

At present, efficacy must be shown beyond any statistical doubt, as well as safety. The current basis for the development of all novel AEDs has been a set of guidelines offered in 1989 by the International League Against Epilepsy.[3] Pilot studies are necessary for an adequate development plan. However, the essential aspect of development is double-blind randomized clinical trials in which the new drug is compared to control treatment.

Antiepileptic drug trials are difficult to perform; no single trial design will be appropriate for all drugs or for all patients affected with epilepsy.[4] A standard approach is the classical crossover or parallel-group add-on randomized controlled trial, in which the new drug or a comparator is added to unchanged pre-existing therapy. In response-conditional crossover trials, only patients with an insufficient response to treatment cross over to alterna-

121

122    *Clinical Trials in Neurologic Practice*

tive treatment. Response-dependent (enrichment) designs begin with an open titration period, to a determined dosage or the maximum tolerated dose in an individual patient, followed by an open fixed-dose period. Only improved patients enter a double-blind crossover or parallel-group phase. Drug interactions, difficulties in analyzing individual drug action, and the fact that monotherapy is chosen in a majority of patients with epilepsy resulted in innovative trial designs.[5] Finally, to obtain an indication for monotherapy, the new drug should have demonstrated value in a monotherapy trial. In classical active-control monotherapy trials, an investigational drug is compared with a conventional drug given at its usual dosage, but if such a comparison demonstrates only equivalence, and no difference in outcome, this could mean that neither drug was effective.[6] For this reason, new designs aim to show only indisputable antiseizure activity of the investigational compounds and do not need to show drug equivalency or superiority to a usual dose of a marketed drug. These studies are named therapeutic failure design trials, in which outcome is assessed in terms of failure or completers. Failure means that patients meet some protocol-determined escape criterion before the planned duration of the trial (e.g., worsening of epilepsy or intolerance to study medication). Completers are those patients who can complete the trial without a significant increase in seizure frequency. Attenuated active-control designs are randomized, double-blind, parallel-group trials, in which patients in one treatment arm receive an estimated therapeutic dose of the investigational drug, and in the other arm they receive a pseudoplacebo—that is, a minimally effective dose of the investigational drug, or a low dose of an established drug. Presurgical withdrawal designs are another form of monotherapy trials. A monotherapy, placebo-controlled trial may be performed during presurgical evaluation of refractory patients with partial epilepsy, taking advantage of the fact that many of these subjects have all medication discontinued during presurgical evaluation. Patients are randomized to the drug or to the placebo. Both time to exit and absolute percentage of completers are analyzed as trial outcomes.

## CONTROLLED TRIALS OF ANTIEPILEPTIC DRUGS

Only double-blind randomized controlled trials (RCTs) are summarized.

### Conventional Antiepileptic Drugs

Phenobarbital

*Summary*

Phenobarbital was introduced in clinical practice in 1912. When compared to chlorazepate, a trend to improve seizure control was found with phenobarbital, but chlorazepate had less toxicity.[7] Phenobarbital was also compared with phenytoin, primidone, and carbamazepine in the treatment of 622 untreated or undertreated adults with simple or complex partial seizures (n = 265) or secondarily generalized seizures (n = 357).[1] The study protocol was designed to conform as closely as possible to standards of optimal clinical practice, except that treatment was double-blind. Patients were randomly assigned to receive one of the four drugs and were followed up for 2 years, or until the drug failed to control seizures or caused unacceptable side effects. Sample size was calculated so that important clinical differences in outcome could be detected with a power of at least 0.8 and a significance level of 0.05. Treatment failure and time to first seizure were analyzed with an actuarial lifetime method. As for overall efficacy, phenobarbital was statistically equal to the other drugs. Complete control of generalized tonic-clonic seizures was similar (phenobarbital, 43%; phenytoin, 43%; carbamazepine, 48%; primidone, 45%). Fewer patients with partial seizures were controlled with phenobarbital than with carbamazepine. Unacceptable side effects led to phenobarbital withdrawal in 19% of treated patients.

## Comments

These two comparative trials are in keeping with a long-lasting clinical practice. Phenobarbital is an effective medication in chronic, as well as in newly diagnosed epilepsies. It is as effective as phenytoin and primidone in primary or secondarily generalized tonic-clonic seizures, but probably less effective in patients with partial seizures. Its dose-related toxicity remains a practical problem.

## Phenytoin

### Summary

Phenytoin was introduced for the treatment of epilepsy in 1938 in the United States and soon after World War II in Europe. To the best of our knowledge, no double-blind, placebo-controlled trial was ever performed. Conversely, as its efficacy and safety have been made evident, newer drugs have been compared against phenytoin. Phenytoin was one of the four drugs compared for efficiency as monotherapy in the multicenter, double-blind trial conducted by the Veterans Administration.[1] Phenytoin's overall efficacy was statistically equal to the other drugs. It was slightly better tolerated than phenobarbital, with toxicity leading to drug withdrawal in 16% of treated patients.

## Comments

The Veterans Administration study highlights the main problems with phenytoin. Its efficacy is unquestionable, but its tolerability is not. Apart from infrequent idiosyncratic reactions, it has a dose-related neurotoxicity and long-term cosmetic side effects, resulting in an efficiency (efficacy and toxicity) that is lower than that of more recent compounds.

124    *Clinical Trials in Neurologic Practice*

Carbamazepine

*Summary*

Carbamazepine was marketed in Europe in 1964. The U.S. Food and Drug Administration (FDA) approved carbamazepine in 1974 as an anticonvulsant for adults, in 1978 for children older than 6 years, and in 1987 without age limitations. A number of placebo-controlled and active-control trials have been published.

An early trial was done in 46 mentally impaired adult inpatients with uncontrolled generalized seizures when treated with phenobarbital, phenytoin, or primidone alone or in combination.[8] Half of each treatment group remained unchanged, whereas the other half was gradually tapered off its anticonvulsant medication and had carbamazepine gradually introduced over a 3-week period. The efficacy of carbamazepine was considered equivalent to that of phenobarbital, phenytoin, and primidone, and tolerability was good. In a psychiatric hospital, the effect of carbamazepine and a placebo as add-on therapy was compared in 22 patients with partial or generalized seizures.[9] The maximum daily dose of carbamazepine was 600 mg, maintained for 8 weeks. No significant differences between carbamazepine and placebo were found. Conversely, when patients were on carbamazepine in another placebo-controlled add-on trial in 37 hospitalized adult patients, secondarily generalized seizures were reduced by 55% and complex partial seizures by 83%.[10] Carbamazepine or placebo was added for 3-week periods to a baseline therapy of phenobarbital and phenytoin. A fourth trial was performed in 23 outpatients, aged 4–49 years, with refractory partial epilepsy.[11] During the 6.5-month duration of this study, pre-existing medications were unchanged, and carbamazepine or placebo was added for 3 months each. Carbamazepine dosage was increased, according to tolerance, up to a maximum of 1,200 mg per day. A greater than 50% reduction in seizure frequency occurred in 12 patients. The behavioral and anticonvulsant effects of carbamazepine versus phenobarbital were also evaluated in 21 chronically hospitalized patients.[12] In addition to half dosage of anticonvulsant and antipsychotic medication for 2 or 4 months, each patient received both carbamazepine (400–1,200 mg/day) and phenobarbital. Psychotropic effects were shown, but neither the number of patients having seizures nor seizure frequency was different.

A comparison of carbamazepine, 600 mg per day, with phenytoin, 300 mg per day, was subsequently done in 24 institutionalized adult patients with behavior disorders.[13] They successively received the two drugs as the exclusive medications for a total of 6 months, without demonstrable difference in their effectiveness. Another comparative study of carbamazepine versus phenytoin was done in 38 patients older than 12 years of age with complex partial seizures; these patients received carbamazepine or phenytoin as sole medications for a total of 16 weeks.[14] No significant differences in efficacy were found. Side effects were mild and encountered as often with carbamazepine as with phenytoin, with a trend in favor of carbamazepine (i.e., fewer side effects, not reaching statistical significance). A drawback of this study was the mix of naive and refractory patients. However, the authors stressed that some patients responded better to carbamazepine or phenytoin.

*Clinical Trials in Epilepsy* 125

Another comparison of carbamazepine and phenytoin prescribed as sole medication was performed.[15] Carbamazepine and phenytoin were given in two successive 4-month study blocks to 47 adult outpatients with moderately severe epilepsy. Both drugs were equally effective, but significantly fewer patients had objective side effects when on carbamazepine. Another study was conducted in 45 institutionalized adult patients with uncontrolled partial seizures.[16] During each of the three 21-day treatment periods, one-third of patients were assigned to receive phenytoin (300 mg/day), phenobarbital (300 mg/day), or carbamazepine (1,200 mg/day). In this population, carbamazepine was equal in efficacy to phenobarbital or phenytoin. Carbamazepine was compared with phenytoin in a crossover trial in 19 adult patients with partial seizures and nine with generalized tonic-clonic seizures.[17] Each treatment period lasted 10 weeks. All medications, except phenobarbital and primidone, were discontinued gradually, whereas carbamazepine or phenytoin doses were increased. Doses were adjusted according to plasma levels. No differences in efficacy were found among drugs when plasma levels were within optimum ranges. The authors stressed the efficacy of carbamazepine in partial seizures and generalized seizures (whether primary generalized or secondarily generalized).

Carbamazepine was also compared to phenytoin as initial monotherapy.[18] Thirty-five untreated adult patients with two or more seizures, or one seizure and an EEG with paroxysmal features, were treated for 6 months with each drug. Carbamazepine was as effective as phenytoin in the control of partial and generalized seizures. Complete control (81.5% versus 85.8%) was similar in both groups. Major and minor side effects were likewise similar for both drugs.

Carbamazepine was also compared to clonazepam in patients with untreated complex partial seizures.[19] Patients aged 6–72 years were allocated to 6 months of treatment with clonazepam (n = 17) or carbamazepine (n = 19). There were no significant differences between the two treatments regarding efficacy, side effects, or withdrawals.

## Comments

These RCTs share several flaws, including the following: rather unsophisticated designs, add-on trials, small number of patients, and short evaluation periods. However, they document the results of open studies and observations of daily practice. In the Veterans Administration comparative study,[1] overall and generalized seizure control was not better with carbamazepine than with the other three drugs, but carbamazepine provided significantly better control of partial seizures.

## Sodium Valproate

### Summary

Sodium valproate was marketed in France in 1967 and a decade later in the United Kingdom. The FDA approved it in 1978 for use as sole or adjunctive ther-

126  *Clinical Trials in Neurologic Practice*

apy in the treatment of absence seizures, and many years later for use in more frequent types of epilepsies.

In 1977, 39 refractory inpatients, aged 8–63 years, were entered in the first controlled valproate trial. Other medications were maintained at a constant dosage, or, when possible, at a constant plasma level. The number of seizures was significantly lower on valproate than on placebo (*p* <.01). The interaction between phenobarbital and valproate was documented.[20] A dose-ranging study in 13 adult inpatients was published 2 years later.[21] Again, concomitant treatment was maintained throughout the study with adjustment of plasma levels. The difference between the number of seizures at three different levels of valproate was statistically significant.

Valproic acid and ethosuximide were then compared in a response-conditional trial.[22] Patients aged 3–18 years with absence seizures (untreated, n = 16; refractory, n = 29) were randomly assigned to one of two treatment sequences: (1) a 6-week period with valproate followed by a 6-week period with ethosuximide, or (2) a 6-week period with ethosuximide followed by a 6-week period with valproate. Only nonresponders, or those who had serious adverse reactions, were crossed over to the alternative treatment. Efficacy was judged by the result of a 12-hour telemetry electroencephalogram. Both drugs were similarly effective and tolerated.

A large, multicenter study compared valproate with carbamazepine.[23] The study design was similar to that of the previous Veterans Administration study. Untreated or undertreated adult patients with complex partial seizures (n = 206) or secondarily generalized tonic-clonic seizures (n = 274) were followed up for 1–5 years or until there was proven inefficacy, unacceptable adverse effects, or a combination. Sodium valproate and carbamazepine, used in monotherapy, had a similar efficacy for the control of secondarily generalized seizures. For complex partial seizures, four of five outcome measures favored carbamazepine. Effectiveness (combining efficacy and toxicity) was also superior with carbamazepine. Both drugs caused minimal cognitive or affective impairment. The authors concluded that phenytoin and carbamazepine remained drugs of first choice in partial epilepsies, but that valproate should be considered as a useful alternative drug if phenytoin or carbamazepine lacked efficacy or was not tolerated. Another smaller (33 patients) study comparing valproate and carbamazepine was published in the same year.[24] Because 64% of patients were seizure-free in both groups during a 24-week maintenance period, it was concluded that valproate monotherapy was as effective as carbamazepine monotherapy. The conclusion of the Veterans Administration study was also challenged.[25,26]

*Comments*

Years after its marketing, many European physicians considered valproate as a weak drug for two reasons:(1) low dosages were prescribed, and (2) valproate was added to enzyme-inducing agents, resulting in subtherapeutic plasma concentrations. Gram and collaborators' first trial[20] was visionary because of the monitoring of valproate plasma levels; their second trial[21] demonstrated an

*Clinical Trials in Epilepsy*    127

indisputable dose-activity relationship. The well-conducted comparison of valproate versus ethosuximide[22] was fruitful, and neither the small number of patients nor the short duration of the study was a drawback. RCTs contributed to define valproate's broad spectrum of activity.

## Recent Antiepileptic Drugs

This review covers preliminary results of pivotal studies and selected abstracts without clear efficacy and safety data.

Felbamate

*Summary*

Felbamate was approved in the United States in 1993, and worldwide 1 year later, after a clinical development program that used classical and novel study design.

The first pivotal trial was a placebo-controlled, add-on crossover study with phenytoin or carbamazepine among adult patients with uncontrolled seizures.[27] Fifty-six patients completed the study. Mean seizure frequencies during the 8-week analysis were 34.9 during the felbamate period and 40.2 during the placebo period ($p = .007$).

A three-period crossover study of felbamate in inpatients with refractory complex partial seizures was also performed.[28] Patients were on carbamazepine as the only drug, and they continued taking it throughout the study. There was no significant difference in seizure frequency between the placebo and felbamate periods, but when a correction was made for the interaction-related lower carbamazepine level noted during felbamate periods, the data suggested a clear efficacy of felbamate 3,000 mg per day. Felbamate was well tolerated by all patients who completed the study; only mild adverse effects were noted.

Likewise, a presurgical trial of 64 adult patients with partial seizures was performed.[29] When presurgical evaluation was completed, most had the major part of their therapy discontinued, and felbamate or placebo was added after randomization. The efficacy variable (time to the fourth seizure) was statistically in favor of felbamate.

Using an attenuated active-control design, felbamate monotherapy was evaluated in 44 patients with refractory partial seizures.[30] Patients were randomized to felbamate (3,600 mg/day) or to valproate (15 mg/kg/day, considered a subtherapeutic level). Previous drugs were tapered and then discontinued. Nineteen patients on valproate and three on felbamate met escape criteria ($p < .001$), and when compared with baseline, the felbamate group had a 50–65% reduction in seizure frequency. In another multicenter study using a similar design, 111 patients were included.[31] Thirty-seven patients on valproate and 18 patients on felbamate met escape criteria ($p < .001$). Adverse events were mild or moderate in severity and less frequent than in the add-on studies.

128   *Clinical Trials in Neurologic Practice*

The efficacy of felbamate in the Lennox-Gastaut syndrome was studied in 73 patients aged 4–36 years.[32] In the treatment phase, felbamate or placebo was added to current medications for 70 days, with a 14-day titration period and a 56-day maintenance period. Dosage of felbamate was titrated to a maximum of 45 mg/kg per day or 3,600 mg per day, whichever was less. Felbamate-treated patients experienced a 19% decrease in the total frequency of seizures, as compared to a 4% increase in the placebo group ($p = .002$) and a 34% decrease in the frequency of atonic seizures, as compared to a 9% decrease in the placebo ($p = .01$).

Most frequently encountered adverse events recorded during the clinical trials were gastrointestinal (nausea, anorexia, vomiting, weight loss), and common neurotoxic symptoms (headache, dizziness, somnolence, insomnia). Many were shown to be dose-related, and a slow initial titration reduced them.

*Comments*

In postmarketing experience, higher doses of felbamate were needed for better response in very refractory partial epilepsies; dosages of up to 7,000 mg have been used in adults and 100 mg/kg in children.[33] RCTs were performed in symptomatic and cryptogenic partial and generalized epilepsies, and none in idiopathic generalized epilepsies (approximately 30% of the epilepsy population). The RCTs also missed the critical point of felbamate-associated aplastic anemia.

Gabapentin

*Summary*

Gabapentin was licensed as add-on therapy for partial epilepsy in patients older than 11 years in the United Kingdom in 1993 and in the United States in 1994, and is presently licensed worldwide. It has been approved in France as monotherapy for both drug-resistant and naive patients.

The first trial was a crossover, three-way, add-on study comparing gabapentin 300, 600, and 900 mg per day in 25 adult patients with refractory partial (n = 18) or generalized epilepsies.[34] The median frequency of all seizures was significantly reduced on gabapentin 900 mg per day compared to baseline, whereas doses of 300 and 600 mg did not reach significance. A second study included 43 adult patients with refractory partial epilepsy randomly allocated to receive a placebo or gabapentin 900 or 1,200 mg per day for 3 months.[35] A significant decrease in seizure frequency was noted only among patients receiving gabapentin 1,200 mg.

Based on these initial dose-ranging studies, three subsequent pivotal, placebo-controlled, parallel-group, add-on trials were conducted with a similar design. Baseline and double-blind treatment periods were 3 months each. Efficacy variables included responder rate, percentage change in seizure frequency, and a response ratio. In the United Kingdom trial, 127 adult patients received gabapentin 1,200 mg per day or placebo.[36] A greater percentage of patients responded to gabapentin than placebo (25% versus 9.8%). The median reduction in partial seizure frequency was also favorable, 29% versus 12%. In the United States trial,

*Clinical Trials in Epilepsy* 129

adult patients were randomly assigned to receive gabapentin 600, 1,200, or 1,800 mg per day or placebo.[37] Responder rates were 18.4%, 17.6%, and 26.4%, respectively, in the gabapentin-treated groups and 8.4% in the placebo group. For patients in each gabapentin treatment group, the mean response ratio was significantly better than that of the placebo group. An international study involving 272 patients older than 12 years of age compared gabapentin 900 and 1,200 mg/day to placebo.[38] Responder rates were 22.9% in the 900-mg group and 10.1% in the placebo group, a significant difference. There was also a slightly greater improvement for those on 1,200 mg than for those on 900 mg per day.

The efficacy of gabapentin in refractory generalized seizures was evaluated in a study that included 129 patients (age, 12–67 years).[39] Patients were randomized to receive gabapentin 1,200 mg per day or placebo added on to their standard therapy. During a 14-week evaluation period, the responder rate for generalized tonic-clonic seizures was higher among patients in the gabapentin group (27.5% versus 17.5%)—a clear but not significant trend. Absence and myoclonic seizures failed to respond to gabapentin therapy. Gabapentin was well tolerated.

Trials were also performed in children; two of these studies demonstrated no effect of gabapentin compared with placebo in children with newly diagnosed absence seizures.[40] Conversely, gabapentin was effective as add-on therapy in the treatment of refractory partial seizures in 128 children younger than 12 years.[41] Patients were randomized to receive gabapentin 23–35 mg/kg per day or placebo added on to their unchanged therapy in a 12-week treatment period.

Two parallel-group studies evaluated gabapentin monotherapy in patients over 11 years of age with refractory partial epilepsy. The first was a presurgical 8-day trial.[42] Dosages of gabapentin 300 and 3,600 mg per day were compared in 82 hospitalized patients. Time to exit was significantly longer ($p = .0001$), and completion rate was significantly higher (53% versus 17%; $p = .002$) for patients receiving gabapentin 3,600 mg per day. The second study was a study of conversion from marketed-drugs therapy to gabapentin monotherapy in three parallel groups.[43] After 2 weeks of gabapentin add-on therapy and 8 weeks of conventional drugs tapered withdrawal, gabapentin monotherapy continued for 16 weeks or until premature withdrawal due to a treatment-failure event. A total of 275 outpatients were randomized to treatment with gabapentin 600, 1,200 or 2,400 mg per day. Outcome measures, including time to exit, completion rate, and mean time on monotherapy, showed no significant differences among the dosage groups; overall, only 20% of patients completed the study.

A monotherapy trial for newly diagnosed partial seizures was conducted with a 24-week evaluation phase.[44] A total of 292 patients over 12 years of age were randomized to receive, in a blind fashion, gabapentin 300, 900, or 1,800 mg per day or open-label carbamazepine (600 mg/day). Low-dose gabapentin was chosen as the comparator rather than placebo, for ethical reasons. The chosen carbamazepine 600 mg per day was considered as appropriate initial dosage for newly diagnosed epilepsy. Time to protocol-specified exit event was significantly longer for patients on gabapentin 900 or 1,800 mg per day than for 300 mg per day. The most clinically relevant measure of retention on treatment (exit event plus adverse event withdrawal rate) was similar for carbamazepine and gabapentin 1,800 mg per day but was lower for gabapentin 900 mg per day. Adverse events were more frequent among carbamazepine-treated patients (84%) than in gabapentin-treated patients (60%).

130   *Clinical Trials in Neurologic Practice*

All studies describe excellent tolerability with the use of gabapentin. The most common complaints were somnolence (15%), fatigue (13%), dizziness (7%), and weight gain (4%).[36] Few patients withdrew for adverse events.[38] In the presurgical trial,[42] no patient exited the study due to adverse events, despite rapid initial titration of full dose within 24 hours.

Another trial addressed the effect of different doses of gabapentin on cognitive function in adult patients with refractory partial seizures.[45] Each treatment phase lasted 3 months, during which the dose of gabapentin or matched placebo was increased stepwise at 4-week intervals: 1,200, 1,800 and 2,400 mg per day. Among the 21 patients completing the study, among whom only nine were responders, the drug had no measurable effect on cognition but produced sedation at the highest dose. No interactions were observed between gabapentin and other standard drugs.

## Comments

RCTs provide unequivocal proof of efficacy for gabapentin in the treatment of partial epilepsies as a co-medication or as a sole drug. They also show a low potential for dose-related toxicity or drug hypersensitivity reactions. Studies support a dose-related antiepileptic effect: Gabapentin doses between 600 and 1,800 mg per day resulted in an overall responder rate of 25%. In open studies, gabapentin has been prescribed at doses up to 4,800 and 6,000 mg per day,[46,47] with better efficacy and without limiting side effects. Open-label extension studies failed to show tolerance up to 2 years.[48]

## Lamotrigine

### Summary

Lamotrigine was approved for adjunct treatment of partial seizures in the United Kingdom in 1991, in the United States in 1994, and in France in 1995. At present, it is approved for monotherapy in several countries.

Eight add-on, crossover controlled trials of lamotrigine in 304 patients with refractory partial seizures have been completed.[49-56] All studies had a similar design, admission criteria, and assessments. Because plasma elimination half-life is substantially prolonged with coadministration with valproate and reduced with coadministration with liver enzyme–inducing drugs, lamotrigine dosages were tailored to background therapy. Target lamotrigine dose was 300 or 400 mg per day when used with phenobarbital, phenytoin, or carbamazepine, and 150 or 200 mg per day when used with valproate. Dose was titrated according to clinical response. Treatment phases ranged from 8 to 16 weeks, and the washout period ranged from 4 to 6 weeks. Seven of the eight studies showed a statistically significant effect of lamotrigine in reducing total seizure counts. Responder rates were 67%, 7%, 11%, 30%, 22%, 18%, 29%, and 20%, respectively (mean, 22%). Adverse effects were generally minor and transient, and most frequently were neurotoxic symptoms. Withdrawal due to skin rash occurred in two studies.[54,56] Subsequently, another add-on, crossover trial evaluated 38 adult patients with refractory partial seizures.[57] Lamotrigine (75–400 mg/day), as compared to placebo, caused a significant reduction in seizure frequency for total number of seizures, complex partial and secondarily generalized.

In another multicenter, parallel-group study of 216 patients with refractory partial seizures, lamotrigine 300 and 500 mg per day were compared.[58] During 6 months of treatment, median seizure frequency decreased by 8% with placebo, 20% with lamotrigine 300 mg, and 36% with lamotrigine 500 mg. Reduction in seizure frequency was significant for those receiving 500 mg, but not for those receiving 300 mg. Responders were 20% for the 300-mg group and 34% for the 500-mg group. The trial demonstrated that the addition of lamotrigine to an ongoing regimen of standard drugs produced dose-related reductions in seizure frequency that were maintained over a 6-month treatment period.

Adverse events were generally mild or moderate in intensity and resolved over time. They were dose-related and resulted in drug withdrawal in only 9% of patients. Patients concurrently on carbamazepine had a greater frequency of neurotoxicity. Another small, short-term study was then conducted to evaluate lamotrigine high-dose tolerability and pharmacokinetic profile at a dose of 500 mg per day.[59] Lamotrigine doses of 700 mg per day can be tolerated in patients receiving concomitant enzyme-inducing AEDs, and kinetics remain linear over the range of 500–700 mg per day.

Monotherapy trials also compared lamotrigine with phenytoin and carbamazepine. In a parallel-group, double-blind, 48-week study, 181 patients (86 lamotrigine, 95 phenytoin) aged 14–75 years who had experienced more than one seizure (partial, secondary, primary generalized seizures) in the previous 6 months were entered.[60] The daily dose was lamotrigine 150 mg per day or phenytoin 300 mg per day. There were no significant differences between lamotrigine and phenytoin for any of the efficacy analyses. Neurotoxic symptoms were reported more frequently among the phenytoin-treated group. Adverse events led to withdrawal in 15% of the lamotrigine-treated patients and in 19% of the phenytoin-treated patients. Another trial compared lamotrigine and carbamazepine in newly diagnosed epilepsy.[61] After a 4-week escalation phase, the drug dosage was blindly adjusted according to efficacy and adverse experiences. No significant differences in efficacy were found between these two drugs. Overall, 15% of lamotrigine-treated patients withdrew due to adverse events, compared to 27% of carbamazepine-treated patients. The most common reason for withdrawal with both drugs was a skin rash (lamotrigine, 9%; carbamazepine, 13%).

Another trial used an attenuated active-control design.[62] Adult patients with refractory partial seizures were randomized to lamotrigine 500 mg per day (n = 50) or a low dose of valproate (1,000 mg/day) (n = 64). Study medication was added to carbamazepine or phenytoin monotherapy over a 4-week period, and then carbamazepine or phenytoin was withdrawn over the next 4 weeks. Fifty-six percent of lamotrigine patients versus 20% of valproate patients successfully completed the 12-week monotherapy phase ($p<.001$), and the time to escape was significantly longer in the lamotrigine group ($p<.001$).

Although a number of uncontrolled studies and case reports indicated that lamotrigine was effective in both idiopathic and symptomatic generalized epilepsies, the first double-blind, placebo-controlled, add-on, crossover trial in drug-resistant generalized epilepsy was published only in 1998.[63] The study consisted of two 8-week treatment periods; depending on their concomitant ther-

132    *Clinical Trials in Neurologic Practice*

apy, patients received lamotrigine 75 or 150 mg per day. Twenty-two patients aged 15–50 years, with generalized epilepsy with absence, myoclonic, or generalized tonic-clonic seizures (symptomatic epilepsies were theoretically excluded), completed the study. Half of those with generalized tonic-clonic seizures, and a third of patients with absence seizures, had a greater than 50% reduction in seizure frequency with lamotrigine compared to placebo.

Lamotrigine as add-on therapy for treatment of children and adolescents with refractory partial seizures was assessed in another study.[64] After 8-week baseline, 202 patients aged 2–16 years were entered in an 18-week treatment phase (with 6 weeks of dose increase) and were randomized to lamotrigine (1–15 mg/kg/day, depending on concurrent medication) or placebo. The lamotrigine-treated group had a significant reduction in the frequency of all seizures. There were no significant differences in the number of adverse events between lamotrigine and placebo-treated patients.

Another trial was conducted in patients aged 3–25 years with the Lennox-Gastaut syndrome, randomly assigned to a 16-week treatment with lamotrigine (n = 79) or placebo (n = 90).[65] A significant decrease in the median frequency of atonic and generalized tonic-clonic seizures was observed. Responder rates were 33% in the lamotrigine group and 16% in the placebo group ($p = .01$).

The aim of another small study was to demonstrate a synergy between two drugs with presumed complementary modes of action.[66] A dose-ranging study of additional lamotrigine was performed in patients with refractory complex partial seizures treated with an anticonvulsant regimen containing vigabatrin. Fourteen of the 20 patients who completed the study improved: Three patients were responders (with a greater than 50% seizure reduction) with lamotrigine 50 mg per day, 7 with lamotrigine 100 mg per day, and 9 with 200 mg per day. This is an interesting study, demonstrating dose-related efficacy of lamotrigine and a possible benefit of polytherapy in some refractory patients.

## Comments

Lamotrigine-pivotal RCTs addressed adults with refractory partial epilepsy, a selected population of epileptic patients. Even if these studies demonstrated the value of lamotrigine in this subgroup of patients, they failed to prove efficacy in cases of generalized idiopathic and symptomatic epilepsies. Because of anecdotal reports and uncontrolled studies indicating effectiveness of lamotrigine in refractory generalized epilepsies, two controlled trials have been performed; they demonstrated efficacy in the Lennox-Gastaut syndrome and in both tonic-clonic and absence seizures of idiopathic generalized epilepsies.

## Oxcarbazepine

### Summary

Oxcarbazepine has been registered and to date is marketed in many countries, including the United States.

*Clinical Trials in Epilepsy* 133

Phenytoin monotherapy among adult patients with mixed seizure types and unsatisfactory control or disturbing adverse effects was gradually replaced by oxcarbazepine or carbamazepine.[67] Only 34 patients completed this trial. Dosages were titrated according to clinical effect; oxcarbazepine ranged from 600 to 900 mg per day, and carbamazepine ranged from 400 to 800 mg per day. Both drugs were considered more active than phenytoin. No differences in efficacy between these two drugs were detected (31% oxcarbazepine responders, 39% carbamazepine responders); tolerability favored oxcarbazepine. A crossover design on 48 adult patients with refractory partial seizures used carbamazepine or oxcarbazepine in addition to unchanged concomitant treatment.[68] Doses were individually titrated to achieve optimum seizure control, resulting in higher mean dosages for oxcarbazepine (2,628 mg/day) than carbamazepine (1,302 mg/day). A nonstatistically significant trend toward better overall seizure control was observed with oxcarbazepine. Likewise, a significant reduction in seizures was noted among the oxcarbazepine-treated group, only for patients with tonic-clonic seizures. No differences were apparent regarding the incidence or nature of side effects.

A large parallel-group study compared oxcarbazepine to carbamazepine in adults with newly diagnosed, previously untreated epilepsy.[69] A total of 235 patients with partial seizures entered the study. Drugs were titrated according to clinical effect; final mean dosages were carbamazepine 684 mg per day and oxcarbazepine 1,040 mg per day. Mean trial duration was 336 days. Efficacy was not significantly different; more than 80% of patients had a greater than 50% reduction in seizure frequency. Complete control was achieved in 52% of oxcarbazepine-treated patients and in 60% of carbamazepine-treated patients. Side effects, such as allergic reactions, that led to drug discontinuation favored oxcarbazepine.

Three comparative trials, with similar aims and designs, were conducted. Patients had partial or primarily generalized seizures. During a flexible 8-week titration period, treatment was adjusted based on clinical response and was continued during the subsequent 48-week maintenance period, with further dose adjustment if necessary. Oxcarbazepine was compared with phenytoin in 287 patients aged 16–65 years with untreated partial or generalized seizures.[70] In the efficacy analysis, no significant differences were found between treatment groups. The number of premature discontinuations due to adverse experiences showed a significant difference in favor of oxcarbazepine. Even though patients were a nonrefractory population, 59.3% for oxcarbazepine and 58% for phenytoin became seizure-free. One hundred seventeen patients dropped out, a proportion common in naive patients. In the second study, a total of 193 patients aged 5–18 years were randomized to oxcarbazepine or phenytoin.[71] Efficacy and safety results were similar to those of the adult study. The third trial compared oxcarbazepine and valproate.[72] In the efficacy analysis comprising 212 patients aged 15–65 years, no statistically significant difference was found between treatment groups. Complete seizure control was achieved in 56.6% of oxcarbazepine-treated patients and 53.8% of valproate-treated patients. Premature discontinuation due to adverse events occurred in 15 oxcarbazepine-treated patients and in 10 valproate-treated patients.

A presurgical trial compared oxcarbazepine with a placebo and concluded that oxcarbazepine appears to be an effective monotherapy treatment of refractory

134    *Clinical Trials in Neurologic Practice*

partial epilepsy.[73] An attenuated active-control trial comparing oxcarbazepine as monotherapy at 2,400 mg per day to 300 mg per day was performed in drug-resistant patients with partial epilepsy.[74] The double-blind treatment phase consisted of a 42-day conversion period to monotherapy and an 84-day maintenance period on monotherapy. The percentage of patients meeting one of the exit criteria was significantly lower for the 2,400 mg per day group compared with the oxcarbazepine 300 mg per day group ($p < .0001$).

A problem with oxcarbazepine, as well as with carbamazepine, is its rather short elimination half-life. This issue was addressed in a study of 157 adult patients with epilepsy who were treated with flexible, individually titrated doses of oxcarbazepine monotherapy and then randomized to once- and twice-daily regimens.[75] The lack of significant differences between the two groups at 60 weeks demonstrated that once-a-day administration was possible.

### Comments

In RCTs, oxcarbazepine has been shown to have similar efficacy, similar spectrum of activity, and better tolerability than carbamazepine. The tolerability and safety of oxcarbazepine were satisfactorily assessed.

## Tiagabine

### Summary

Five placebo-controlled trials led to tiagabine approval as adjunctive therapy for adults with epilepsy in Europe and the United States.

Tiagabine was evaluated in two pilot add-on studies with a similar response-dependent (enrichment) design.[76,77] During an open individualized screening phase, tiagabine was added to existing drug therapy and then increased until clinical efficacy or tolerance was achieved. Only improved patients were randomized into the double-blind crossover phase. In the first study, tiagabine was more effective than placebo in reducing the median seizure rate ($p = .05$).[76] A 50% reduction compared to placebo was noted for complex partial seizures in 26% of patients and in 63% of patients with secondarily generalized seizures. The other study had similar results.[77]

Three pivotal, multicenter, double-blind, parallel-group, placebo-controlled, add-on trials were done in patients with complex partial seizures. The studies had similar designs, and their aims were complementary. One was a dose-ranging study, with fixed administration of 16, 32, or 56 mg per day of tiagabine in four divided doses. A total of 297 patients ranging in age from 12–77 years were randomized to the double-blind phase, and 293 patients were evaluated in the intent-to-treat analysis.[78] The two other trials were dose-frequency studies with tiagabine, 10 mg three times daily, or placebo added to existing AEDs.[79] A total of 77 patients aged 16–75 years were randomized in each arm. The other study compared tiagabine among 318 patients at a fixed dose of 32 mg per day with twice- or four-times-daily dosing with placebo.[80]

Results of integrated analysis of efficacy for the two crossover studies and the three parallel-group studies were very similar,[81] despite their different designs, allowing a global analysis with 1,032 patients enrolled (182 in the crossover studies and 850 in the parallel-group studies).[82] Tiagabine was more effective than placebo for all seizure types combined with respect to median reduction in seizure rates (25% versus 0.1%; $p = .0001$). The proportion of responders to tiagabine was 23% for all seizure types combined and 27% for complex partial seizures, compared to 9% and 13%, respectively, for the placebo group. In the parallel-group trials, responders for complex partial seizures were as follows: 35% when tiagabine ranged from 48 to 64 mg per day; 26% when dose ranged from 24 to 48 mg per day; and 15% when it was under 24 mg per day. The minimum effective dose was considered to be 32 mg per day. Despite tiagabine's short half-life, studies showed similar efficacy between once-, twice-, and four-times-daily administration.

Safety and tolerability of tiagabine were evaluated in an integrated analysis of the five add-on trials.[83] Adverse events were mostly mild to moderate in severity and often transient, occurring mainly during dose titration. Most of them were characterized by dizziness, fatigue, somnolence, headache, tremor, difficulty concentrating, nervousness, and depressed mood; these were reported by more patients receiving tiagabine than placebo. No significant adverse effects on cognitive functions with tiagabine use were found in patients included in the double-blind studies.[84–86] Tiagabine was well tolerated in patients with psychiatric history.[87] Adjunctive tiagabine therapy resulted in no consistent weight change.[88]

Another trial aimed to determine whether combinations of AEDs with different mechanisms of action was superior to combinations of drugs with a similar mechanism of action.[89] The addition of tiagabine, a γ-aminobutyric acid (GABA)–ergic agent, was better tolerated when added to sodium-channel modulators, such as carbamazepine or phenytoin, than another sodium-channel modulator, with similar efficacy.

Two double-blind trials were also conducted to assess tiagabine monotherapy in patients with partial seizures.[90] A small presurgical trial was performed; previous therapy was completely discontinued, and patients were randomized (seven tiagabine, four placebo) to receive tiagabine or placebo. For both treatment groups, the 24-hour incidence of seizures increased during the double-blind period relative to baseline. However, placebo-treated patients experienced more seizures than tiagabine-treated patients. Likewise, an attenuated active-control design was used to assess tiagabine monotherapy for patients with uncontrolled partial seizures with a single conventional drug. Ninety-six patients were randomized to a high-dose group and were titrated to tiagabine 36 mg per day, whereas 102 patients were randomized to a low-dose group and received 6 mg per day of tiagabine. Only 57 patients (29%) completed the study; 141 patients discontinued their participation prematurely. For both groups, the median rate for complex partial seizures decreased significantly between the baseline and fixed-dosage period in patients who completed the study. In the intent-to-treat analysis, the percentage of responders was 31% in the high-dose group and 18% in the low-dose group ($p = .04$). Adverse events and tolerability-related withdrawals were also greater in the high-dose group.

136    *Clinical Trials in Neurologic Practice*

## Comments

Tiagabine has been approved after a relatively short premarketing trial period. However, data on tiagabine safety and efficacy in children are scarce,[91,92] and controlled trials are still in progress. RCTs answered a number of questions regarding the short half-life of this compound. A twice-daily administration is likely to be sufficient. Efficacy and tolerability were dose-dependent. Adverse events were similar in the RCTs, and no new types of adverse events developed during long-term therapy.[93] As tiagabine is a potent and specific inhibitor of GABA uptake, melanin binding in the eye is possible. No systematic monitoring for relevant ophthalmologic changes during clinical development was requested. However, there is no evidence of retinal or optic nerve lesions in animal toxicologic studies, and a retrospective search in data from all phase II and III clinical trials (n = 2,531) failed to find any tiagabine-related fixed visual field defects.[94]

## Topiramate

### Summary

Topiramate is a new agent that has become available for use as an adjunctive for partial seizures in many countries since 1995. Pivotal trials consisted of four phases, including screening, a baseline phase of 8–12 weeks' duration, a double-blind treatment phase with a 2- to 6-week titration and an 8–12 week maintenance period, and tapering phases. Some trials compared a single-target daily dosage with placebo: 400 mg per day,[95] 600 mg per day,[96] or 800 mg per day,[97] whereas others were dose-ranging studies, with a low-dose trial of 200, 400, and 600 mg per day[98] and a high-dose trial of 600, 800 and 1,000 mg per day.[99] To qualify for entry into the double-blind phase of the study, patients aged 18–65 years had to have four or more monthly refractory partial seizures. Pooled data analysis was performed, because it allowed evaluation of efficacy end points and treatment response for a number of study subgroups otherwise not statistically valuable in individual studies.[100] The five trials included 534 patients, 360 receiving topiramate and 174 receiving placebo. Topiramate was significantly superior to placebo in reducing total seizures by 75% or by 100% ($p = .01$). Of topiramate-treated patients, 41% had a greater than 50% reduction in seizures, versus only 10% in the placebo-treated group. Topiramate reduced the frequency of simple partial, complex partial, and secondarily generalized seizures. Response according to topiramate dose was as follows: topiramate 400 mg, 35%; topiramate 600 mg, 47%; and topiramate 800 mg, 69%. Protocol-specified target dosages for topiramate-treated patients were reached in 84% of patients in the 400-mg group, 61% of patients in the 600-mg group, and 44% of patients in the 800-mg group. Withdrawals due to adverse effects occurred in 21% of patients in the 800-mg group, most of them during the rapid-titration phase. The most frequent adverse events were mild to moderate and included the following: somnolence, dizziness, headache, fatigue, cognitive impairment, depression, nausea, and confusion, all of which were related to dose and rate of titration and usually transient. No clinically significant abnormalities of liver function, renal function, hematologic parameters, or allergic reactions were noted.

A pediatric trial was also performed among children aged 2–17 years with refractory partial seizures randomized to topiramate (n = 41) or placebo (n = 45).[101] Efficacy and tolerability were similar to those seen in adults.

The efficacy and safety of topiramate as adjunctive therapy in primary generalized seizures were also evaluated. Patients aged 3–59 years with three or more generalized tonic-clonic seizures during an 8-week baseline period while receiving one to two standard AEDs were entered.[102] Thirty-nine patients were randomized to topiramate and 41 to placebo. After a 56-day titration period, placebo or topiramate treatment was continued for 12 weeks. Among topiramate-treated patients, seizure frequency was significantly reduced (57% versus 9%; $p$ = .02); more patients had 50% seizure reduction (generalized tonic-clonic seizures, 56% versus 20%; $p$ = .001) or were seizure-free (generalized tonic-clonic seizures, 13% versus 5%) compared with placebo.

Another trial evaluated topiramate as an adjunctive therapy in patients (2–42 years of age) with the Lennox-Gastaut syndrome.[103] Patients were randomized to topiramate (n = 48) or placebo (n = 50). Falls were significantly reduced among those receiving topiramate compared to placebo, and global seizure severity was also significantly improved (53% versus 28%; $p$ = .04).

Topiramate monotherapy was also evaluated in a therapeutic failure trial; 48 patients with refractory partial seizures were randomized to receive topiramate 100 mg per day or topiramate 1,000 mg per day.[104] During a 5-week conversion phase, baseline drug(s) were gradually discontinued, whereas topiramate 100 mg per day was continued or topiramate dosage was titrated to a dose of 500 mg twice daily. An 11-week maintenance monotherapy phase followed. Time until exit was longer ($p$ = .002), and success frequency (study completion) was higher with topiramate 1,000 mg per day compared with 100 mg per day. Seizure reductions of 50%, 75%, or 100% were achieved in 46%, 25%, and 13% of the 1,000 mg per day treated group, as compared with 13%, 8%, and 0% of the 100 mg per day treated group, respectively.

*Comments*

RCTs have demonstrated the efficacy of topiramate as adjunctive therapy in adults and children with partial and generalized epilepsies and as a sole drug in partial epilepsies. The main drawbacks of these RCTs are an erroneous estimation of tolerated dosages, leading to a pessimistic judgment of drug tolerability. A dosage of 200 mg per day is considered to be the minimally effective dosage. No appreciable increase in responder rate was found at dosages above 400 mg per day. It is possible, however, that individual patients may benefit from higher dosage, but with a potential risk for toxicity.

Vigabatrin

*Summary*

Vigabatrin has been licensed as adjunctive treatment in many countries since 1989, but not in the United States.

138    *Clinical Trials in Neurologic Practice*

Clinical trials began with two short-term single-blind studies in adult patients, rapidly followed by six RCTs.[105–110] The objective of these studies was to document effects of vigabatrin as add-on therapy over a period of 7–12 weeks. Patients ranging in age from 10 to 63 years had uncontrolled partial or generalized seizures. Design was as follows: (1) an initial 5-week observation phase with constant doses of pre-existing therapy; (2) a first treatment period, with vigabatrin or placebo randomly added in a blinded fashion; (3) a 1-week transition; (4) a second treatment period with placebo or vigabatrin; and (5) a final 5-week single-blind period on placebo to evaluate any potential carryover or withdrawal effects in patients receiving placebo during the second double-blind period. Approximately one-half of patients experienced a greater than 50% decrease in seizure frequency with the active treatment; although five studies demonstrated a significant reduction in seizure frequency, one of them did not. This is likely due to the fact that the persons in this latter study were institutionalized patients with very refractory epilepsies. Tolerability of vigabatrin in these short-term studies was good except for some drowsiness.

An enrichment design strategy was used in two additional trials. One of these, performed in adults with refractory partial seizures, was divided into three phases: (1) a baseline period; (2) an open phase, in which vigabatrin was progressively added to previous therapy with individualization of optimal dose; and (3) a double-blind phase, in which only responders in open phase were randomly allocated to continue active treatment or switched to placebo.[111] Patients on vigabatrin maintained a 54.7% reduction of seizure frequency, whereas those on placebo showed an 18.6% increase in seizure frequency compared with baseline, which is a highly significant difference between the two groups. The most common side effects were drowsiness, depression, mood instability, and headaches.

A slightly different protocol was used in a Finnish study; patients were randomly allocated in the double-blind phase to vigabatrin 3 g per day or 1.5 g per day.[112] The dosage of 3 g per day appeared to be more effective than 1.5 g per day. However, even with the low dosage, the seizure frequency was significantly reduced as compared to baseline.

The question of an optimal effective vigabatrin dosage was addressed in an add-on, placebo-controlled crossover study of vigabatrin in 24 refractory adult patients with mixed seizure types.[113] The vigabatrin dosage was 1 g twice daily for 6 weeks, followed by 1.5 g twice daily for 6 weeks. An overall reduction in the number of seizures failed to reach statistical significance. As for partial seizures, a significant reduction was noted with 2 g vigabatrin, but not with 3 g. A deterioration in control of partial seizures as compared with the equivalent placebo phase was observed when patients were changed from 2 to 3 g per day, as if a dosage upper limit existed, above which vigabatrin could be useless or even noxious. This trial is not cited in the discussion of a dose-response study published 6 years later in the same journal.[114] Percentages of responders were 24%, 51%, and 54% for vigabatrin doses of 1, 3, and 6 g per day, respectively. Vigabatrin was generally well tolerated; dropouts, due to adverse events, were higher in the 6 g per day group.

Drowsiness was the most frequent side effect of vigabatrin in controlled trials. Probably for this reason, a placebo-controlled, crossover trial was undertaken with the aim of documenting the effect of vigabatrin on mental functioning.[115] Vigabatrin dosage was 2 g per day for 6 weeks, and 3 g per day for an additional

*Clinical Trials in Epilepsy* 139

6 weeks. No significant differences were found between vigabatrin and placebo at baseline and at weeks 2, 6, and 12 of both treatment periods for any measure of a battery of neuropsychologic tests. A greater degree of sedation was noted after 2 and 6 weeks on vigabatrin than during the placebo phase, but not at 12 weeks nor later, during an open follow-up period. This suggests development of tolerance to sedation, and this side effect should be minimized with a slow-dose escalation.

Double-blind trials are problematic in children. However, such a trial was performed with an unusual design.[116] Twenty-eight children, treated on an open basis with vigabatrin as co-medication for refractory epilepsy of various types and having had incomplete improvement after at least 3 months of treatment, were included for randomization. The protocol comprised two phases, each of 2 months' duration. In the first phase (double-blind), patients were allocated to vigabatrin or placebo. In the second phase (single-blind), all patients received placebo after vigabatrin was blindly stopped at 3 weeks. Escape criterion was more than 50% increase of seizure frequency or increased severity of seizures. Patients remaining in the study were more numerous on vigabatrin (93%) than on placebo (46%) ($p < .001$), and seizure frequency was lower on vigabatrin than on placebo ($p < .05$).

Two additional multicenter, placebo-controlled, parallel-group studies addressed the efficacy and safety of vigabatrin as adjunctive therapy among children aged 3–16 years with drug-resistant complex partial seizures. In the first study, patients were titrated over 10 weeks from 0.5 or 1 g per day to doses ranging from 1.5 to 4 g per day and maintained on that dose for 7 weeks.[117] Of 88 children randomized and included in the intent-to-treat analysis, 55.8% were responders in the vigabatrin group and 26.7% in the placebo group ($p = .01$). The most common adverse events were somnolence, increased seizure frequency, headache, and dizziness. In the second study, children were randomized to receive placebo or vigabatrin 20, 60, or 100 mg per day.[118] They were titrated over 6 weeks and maintained on the randomized dose for a total of 8 weeks. There was a strong linear response across the three doses that was only marginally significant due to the low power of the trial. Reduction in seizure frequency in the 100 mg/kg per day group was significantly superior to that in the placebo group ($p = .01$). Adverse reactions were similar to those of the previous study.

*Comments*

Vigabatrin has been studied mainly in adults with refractory partial seizures. Its efficacy in generalized epilepsies is dubious; vigabatrin can worsen myoclonic seizures.[119] Its efficiency in symptomatic infantile spasms was discovered outside RCTs. Vigabatrin tolerability in the short-term add-on trials was fair, and in comparative studies, better, than that of conventional drugs.[120] Side effects have been mainly transient and dose-related. Drowsiness is the most frequent complaint. No significant cognitive impairment in vigabatrin-treated patients has been reported.[121] An unusually high incidence of depression first noted in one trial was later confirmed.[122] Long-term vigabatrin studies demonstrated a somewhat annoying weight gain but no idiosyncratic adverse reactions. Withdrawal effects were documented in the first controlled trials. Visual field defects are, at present, the most concerning safety issue associated with vigabatrin use.[123]

140    *Clinical Trials in Neurologic Practice*

## Zonisamide

*Summary*

Zonisamide is presently marketed only in Japan and Korea. Some trials have been published only in abstract form, or in Japanese, and their results summarized in *Antiepileptic Drugs*, Fourth Edition.[124]

An add-on trial performed in the United States included adult patients with refractory partial seizures randomized to zonisamide (n = 78) or placebo (n = 74).[125] After an observation period of 12 weeks, the percentage of responders was 28.6% in the zonisamide-treated group, as compared to 13.2% in the placebo-treated group ($p$ = .03). The most commonly observed adverse reactions were lethargy and somnolence that occurred early during treatment. Some patients on zonisamide developed irritability or "bizarre thoughts." Another trial with a similar design included adult patients with four complex partial seizures per month randomized to zonisamide (n = 71) or placebo (n = 68).[126] An initial dose of zonisamide of 1.5 mg/kg per day was increased to 3 mg/kg per day in the second week and 6 mg/kg per day for the third and fourth weeks. Percentages of responders were 29.9% in the zonisamide-treated group and 9.4% in the placebo-treated group. Complete remission was observed only in 6.2% of patients in the zonisamide group. Adverse events, mostly fatigue, somnolence, dizziness, and ataxia, occurred in 59.2% of zonisamide-treated patients compared to 27.9% on placebo.

Adults with untreated or refractory partial seizures received zonisamide (n = 55) or carbamazepine (n = 64).[124] No significant differences in efficacy were found. The incidence of adverse effects was 51.7% in the zonisamide-treated group and 56.9% in the carbamazepine-treated group. Anorexia was only observed with zonisamide; ataxia was more frequent in the carbamazepine-treated group.

In an 8-week duration study in pediatric patients (15 years of age or younger) with untreated or uncontrolled convulsive or nonconvulsive seizures, or a combination of both, Oguni et al.[124] compared zonisamide (n = 18) with valproate (n = 16). The decreased frequency of generalized tonic-clonic seizures was 81.2% in the zonisamide-treated group and 66.7% in the valproate-treated group.

*Comments*

Zonisamide appears to have a broad spectrum of activity, but this is not completely documented. Favorable results have been published in childhood myoclonic epilepsies and in symptomatic generalized epilepsies, such as Lennox-Gastaut syndrome. Data analysis of the 1,008 patients exposed to zonisamide before its launch showed the occurrence of adverse effects in almost half of treated patients, and approximately 20% of patients had to discontinue the drug.[124] Neurotoxicity (dose-related) and gastrointestinal symptoms were less frequent with monotherapy open trials. Kidney stones were not reported in Japan. The ultimate positioning of zonisamide in the treatment of epilepsy awaits a better definition of its efficacy and tolerability profiles. AEDs have tra-

*Clinical Trials in Epilepsy* 141

ditionally been developed against different seizure types, whereas responsiveness to medication and prognosis depend on the type of epilepsy syndrome. Pivotal RCTs performed mainly in patients with partial seizures poorly define the spectrum of activity of a new compound and may overlook its major interest (e.g., lamotrigine and generalized epilepsies). An erroneous evaluation of target dosage could have deleterious consequences, such as an underestimation of efficiency (gabapentin) or overestimation of adverse events (topiramate). Too rapid a dose titration could also give a pessimistic impression of poor tolerability (transient side effects) or safety (e.g., lamotrigine and skin rash).

Caution and alertness are needed due to the fact that patient exposure during premarketing studies is limited. These studies are insufficient in their assurance that all life-threatening, rare, adverse reactions have been calculated. Experience with these rare but potentially fatal adverse effects requires that at least 30,000–100,000 patients be actively treated.[127] Blood (felbamate) or ocular (vigabatrin) toxicity has been missed by RCTs.

## REFERENCES

1. Mattson RH, Cramer JA, Collins JF, et al. Comparison of carbamazepine, phenobarbital, phenytoin, and primidone in partial and secondarily generalized tonic-clonic seizures. N Engl J Med 1985;313:145–151.
2. Dichter MA, Brodie MJ. New antiepileptic drugs. N Engl J Med 1996;334:1583–1590.
3. Commission on Antiepileptic Drugs of the International League Against Epilepsy. Guidelines for clinical evaluation of antiepileptic drugs. Epilepsia 1989;30:400–408.
4. French JA. The Art of Antiepileptic Trial Design. In JA French, IE Leppik, MA Dichter (eds), Antiepileptic Drug Development. Philadelphia: Lippincott–Raven, 1998;113–123.
5. Gram L, Schmidt D. Innovative designs of controlled clinical trials in epilepsy. Epilepsia 1993;34(Suppl 7):S1–S6.
6. Leber PD. Hazards of inference: the active control investigation. Epilepsia 1989;30(Suppl 1):S57–S63.
7. Wilensky AJ, Ojemann LM, Temkin NR, et al. Chlorazepate and phenobarbital as antiepileptic drugs: a double-blind study. Neurology 1981;31:1271–1276.
8. Bird CAK, Griffin BP, Miklazewska JM, Galbraith AW. Tegretol (carbamazepine): a controlled trial of a new anticonvulsant. Br J Psychiatry 1966;112:737–742.
9. Pryse-Phillips WEM, Jeavons PM. Effect of carbamazepine (Tegretol) on the electroencephalogram and ward behavior of patients with epilepsy. Epilepsia 1970;1:263–279.
10. Rodin EA, Rim CS, Rennick PM. Effect of carbamazepine on patients with psychomotor epilepsy: result of a double-blind study. Epilepsia 1974;15:547–561.
11. Kutt H, Solomon G, Wasterlain C, et al. Carbamazepine in difficult to control epileptic outpatients. Acta Neurol Scand 1975;(Suppl 60):27–32.
12. Marjerrisson G, Jedlicki SM, Keogh RET, et al. Carbamazepine: behavioral, anticonvulsant and EEG effects in chronically-hospitalized epileptics. Dis Nerv Syst 1968;29:133–136.
13. Rajotte P, Jilek W, Jilek L, et al. Propriétés antiépileptiques et psychotropes de la carbamazépine (Tégrétol). Union Med Can 1967;96:1200–1206.
14. Simonsen N, Olsen IZ, Kuhl V, Lund M, Wendelboe J. A comparative controlled study between carbamazepine and diphenylhydantoin in psychomotor epilepsy. Epilepsia 1976;17:169–176.
15. Troupin AS, Ojeman LM, Halpern L, et al. Carbamazepine—a double-blind comparison with phenytoin. Neurology 1977;27:511–519.
16. Cereghino JJ, Brock JT, Van Meter JC, et al. Carbamazepine for epilepsy: a controlled prospective evaluation. Neurology 1974;24:401–410.
17. Kosteljanetz M, Christiansen J, Dam AM, et al. Carbamazepine vs. phenytoin: a controlled trial in focal motor and generalized epilepsy. Arch Neurol 1979;36:22–24.
18. Ramsay RE, Wilder BJ, Berger JR, Bruni J. A double-blind study comparing carbamazepine with phenytoin as initial therapy in adults. Neurology 1983;33:904–910.

142    *Clinical Trials in Neurologic Practice*

19. Mikkelsen B, Berggreen P, Joensen P, et al. Clonazepam (Rivotril) and carbamazepine (Tegretol) in psychomotor epilepsy: a randomized multicenter trial. Epilepsia 1981;22:415–420.
20. Gram L, Wulff K, Rasmussen KE, et al. Valproate sodium: a controlled clinical trial including monitoring of drug levels. Epilepsia 1977;18:141–148.
21. Gram L, Flachs H, Würtz-Jorgensen A, et al. Sodium valproate, serum level and clinical effect in epilepsy: a controlled study. Epilepsia 1979;20:303–312.
22. Sato S, White BG, Penry JK, et al. Valproic acid versus ethosuximide in the treatment of absence seizures. Neurology 1982;32:157–163.
23. Mattson RH, Cramer JA, Collins JF. A comparison of valproate with carbamazepine for the treatment of complex partial seizures and secondarily generalized tonic-clonic seizures. N Engl J Med 1992;327:765–771.
24. So EL, Lai CW, Pellock J, et al. Safety and efficacy of valproate and carbamazepine in the treatment of complex partial seizures. J Epilepsy 1992;5:149–152.
25. Chadwick D. Valproate in the treatment of partial epilepsies. Epilepsia 1994;35(Suppl 5):S96–S98.
26. Seino M. A comment on the efficacy of valproate in the treatment of partial seizures. Epilepsia 1994;35(Suppl 5):S101–S104.
27. Leppik IE, Dreifuss FE, Pledger GW, et al. Felbamate for partial seizures: results of a controlled clinical trial. Neurology 1991;41:1785–1789.
28. Theodore WH, Raubertas RF, Porter RJ, et al. Felbamate: a clinical trial for complex partial seizures. Epilepsia 1991;32:392–397.
29. Bourgeois B, Leppik IE, Sackellares JC, et al. Felbamate: a double-blind controlled trial in patients undergoing presurgical evaluation of partial seizures. Neurology 1993;43:693–696.
30. Sachdeo R, Kramer LD, Rosenberg A, Sachdeo S. Felbamate monotherapy: controlled trial in patients with partial onset seizures. Ann Neurol 1992;32:386–392.
31. Faught E, Sachdeo RC, Remler MP, et al. Felbamate monotherapy for partial-onset seizures: an active-control trial. Neurology 1993;43:688–692.
32. The Felbamate Study Group in Lennox-Gastaut Syndrome. Efficacy of felbamate in childhood epileptic encephalopathy (Lennox-Gastaut syndrome). N Engl J Med 1993;328:29–33.
33. Leppik IE. Felbamate. Epilepsia 1995;36(Suppl 2):S66–S72.
34. Crawford P, Ghadiali E, Lane R, et al. Gabapentin as an antiepileptic drug in man. J Neurol Neurosurg Psychiatry 1987;50:682–686.
35. Sivenius J, Kälviäinen R, Ylinen A, Riekkinen P. Double-blind study of gabapentin in the treatment of partial seizures. Epilepsia 1991;32:539–542.
36. UK Gabapentin Study Group. Gabapentin in partial epilepsy. Lancet 1990;335:1114–1117.
37. US Gabapentin Study Group No 5. Gabapentin as add-on therapy in refractory partial epilepsy: a double-blind, placebo-controlled, parallel-group study. Neurology 1993;43:2292–2298.
38. Anhut H, Ashman P, Feuerstein TJ, et al. and The International Gabapentin Study Group. Gabapentin (Neurontin) as add-on therapy in patients with partial seizures: a double-blind, placebo-controlled study. Epilepsia 1994;35:795–801.
39. Chadwick D, Leiderman DB, Sauermann W, et al. Gabapentin in generalized seizures. Epilepsy Res 1996;25:191–197.
40. Leiderman D, Garofalo E, LaMoreaux L. Gabapentin patients with absence seizures: two double-blind, placebo-controlled studies. Epilepsia 1993;34(Suppl 6):45.
41. Appleton R, Fichtner K, Murray G, et al. Gabapentin (Neurontin) as add-on therapy in children with refractory partial seizures: a 12-week, double-blind, placebo-controlled study. Epilepsia 1998;39(Suppl 6):163.
42. Bergey GK, Morris HH, Rosenfeld W, et al. Gabapentin monotherapy: I. An 8-day, double-blind, dose-controlled, multicenter study in hospitalized patients with refractory complex partial or secondarily generalized seizures. Neurology 1997;49:739–745.
43. Beydoun A, Fischer J, Labar DR, et al. Gabapentin monotherapy: II. A 26-week, double-blind, multicenter study of conversion from polytherapy in outpatients with refractory complex partial seizures or secondarily generalized seizures. Neurology 1997;49:746–752.
44. Chadwick DW, Anhut H, Greiner MJ, et al. A double-blind trial of gabapentin monotherapy for newly diagnosed partial seizures. Neurology 1998;51:1282–1288.
45. Leach JP, Girvan J, Paul A, Brodie MJ. Gabapentin and cognition: a double-blind, dose ranging, placebo-controlled study in refractory epilepsy. J Neurol Neurosurg Psychiatry 1997;62:372–376.
46. Beydoun A, Fakhoury T, Nasreddine W, Abou-Khalil B. Conversion to high dose gabapentin monotherapy in patients with medically refractory partial epilepsy. Epilepsia 1998;39:188–193.
47. Wilson EA, Sills GJ, Forrest G, Brodie MJ. High dose gabapentin in refractory partial epilepsy: clinical observations in 50 patients. Epilepsy Res 1998;29:161–166.

## Clinical Trials in Epilepsy    143

48. McLean MJ. Gabapentin. Epilepsia 1995;36(Suppl 2):S73–S86.
49. Jawad S, Richens A, Goodwin G, Yuen WC. Controled trial of lamotrigine (Lamictal) for refractory partial seizures. Epilepsia 1989;30:356–363.
50. Binnie CD, Debets RMC, Engelsman M, et al. Double-blind crossover trial of lamotrigine (Lamictal) as add-on therapy in intractable epilepsy. Epilepsy Res 1989;4:222–229.
51. Sander JWAS, Patsalos PN, Oxley JR, et al. A randomised double-blind placebo-controlled add-on trial of lamotrigine in patients with severe epilepsy. Epilepsy Res 1990;6:221–226.
52. Loiseau P, Yuen AWC, Duché B, et al. A randomised double-blind placebo-controlled crossover add-on trial of lamotrigine in patients with treatment-resistant partial seizures. Epilepsy Res 1990;7:136–145.
53. Schapel GJ, Beran RG, Vajda FJE, et al. Double-blind, placebo-controlled, crossover study of lamotrigine in treatment resistant partial seizures. J Neurol Neurosurg Psychiatry 1993;56:448–453.
54. Smith D, Baker G, Davies G, et al. Outcomes of add-on treatment with lamotrigine in partial epilepsy. Epilepsia 1993;34:312–322.
55. Schmidt D, Ried S, Rapp P. Add-on treatment with lamotrigine for intractable partial epilepsy: a placebo-controlled cross-over trial. Epilepsia 1993;34(Suppl 2):66.
56. Messenheimer J, Ramsay RE, Willmore LJ, et al. Lamotrigine therapy for partial seizures: a multicenter, placebo-controlled, double-blind, cross-over trial. Epilepsia 1994;35:113–121.
57. Boas J, Cooke EA, Yuen AWC. Controlled trial of lamotrigine (Lamictal) for treatment-resistant partial seizures. Epilepsia 1995;36(Suppl 3):S113.
58. Matsuo F, Bergen D, Faught E, et al. Placebo-controlled study of the efficacy and safety of lamotrigine in patients with partial seizures. Neurology 1993;43:2284–2291.
59. Matsuo F, Gay P, Madsen J, et al. Lamotrigine high-dose tolerability and safety in patients with epilepsy: a double-blind, placebo-controlled, eleven-week study. Epilepsia 1996;37:857–862.
60. Steiner TJ, Silveira C, Yuen WC. Comparison of lamotrigine (Lamictal) and phenytoin monotherapy in newly diagnosed epilepsy. Epilepsia 1994;35(Suppl 7):61.
61. Brodie MJ, Richens A, Yuen AWC. Double-blind comparison of lamotrigine and carbamazepine in newly diagnosed epilepsy. Lancet 1995;245:476–479.
62. Chang G, Vazquez B, Gilliam F, et al. Lamictal (lamotrigine) monotherapy is an effective treatment for partial seizures. Neurology 1997;48:A335.
63. Beran RG, Berkovic SF, Dunagan FM, et al. Double-blind, placebo-controlled, crossover study of lamotrigine in treatment-resistant generalised epilepsy. Epilepsia 1998;39:1329–1333.
64. Graf WD, Pellock JM, Duchowny M, et al. Lamictal is effective for add-on treatment of partial seizures in children and adolescents. Epilepsia 1997;38(Suppl 8):193.
65. Motte J, Trevathan E, Arvidsson JFV, et al. Lamotrigine for generalized seizures associated with the Lennox-Gastaut Syndrome. N Engl J Med 1997;337:1807–1812.
66. Stolarek I, Blacklaw J, Forrest G, Brodie MJ. Vigabatrin and lamotrigine in refractory epilepsy. J Neurol Neurosurg Psychiatry 1994;57:921–924.
67. Reinikainen KJ, Keraanen T, Halonen T, et al. Comparison of oxcarbazepine and carbamazepine: a double-blind study. Epilepsy Res 1987;1:284–289.
68. Houtkooper MA, Lammertsma A, Meyer JWA, et al. Oxcarbazepine (GP 47 680): A possible alternative to carbamazepine? Epilepsia 1987;28:693–698.
69. Scandinavian Oxcarbazepine Study Group. A double-blind study comparing oxcarbazepine and carbamazepine in patients with newly diagnosed, previously untreated epilepsy. Epilepsy Res 1989;3:70–76.
70. Bill PA, Vigonius U, Pohlmann H, et al. A double-blind controlled clinical trial of oxcarbazepine versus phenytoin in adults with previously untreated epilepsy. Epilepsy Res 1997;27:195–204.
71. Guerreiro MM, Vigonius U, Pohlmann H, et al. A double-blind controlled clinical trial of oxcarbazepine versus phenytoin in children and adolescents with epilepsy. Epilepsy Res 1997;27:205–213.
72. Christe W, Krämer G, Vigonius U, et al. A double-blind controlled clinical trial: oxcarbazepine versus sodium valproate in adults with newly diagnosed epilepsy. Epilepsy Res 1997;26:451–460.
73. Schachter SC, Vasquez B, Fisher RS, et al. Monotherapy trial of oxcarbazepine for partial seizures in hospitalized presurgical patients. Epilepsia 1996;37(Suppl 5):202.
74. Beydoun AA, Sachdeo R, Rosenfeld W, et al. Safety and efficacy of oxcarbazepine monotherapy in patients with medically refractory partial epilepsy. Epilepsia 1998;39(Suppl 6):48.
75. Vigonius U, Moore A, Krämer G, et al. Oxcarbazepine: results of a clinical trial designed to assess the feasibility of a twice-daily administration. Epilepsia 1995;36(Suppl 3):S119.
76. Richens A, Chadwick DW, Duncan JS, et al. Adjunctive treatment of partial seizures with tiagabine: a placebo-controlled trial. Epilepsy Res 1995;21:37–42.
77. Crawford PM, Engelsman M, Brown SW et al. Tiagabine: phase II study of efficacy and safety in adjunctive treatment of partial seizures. Epilepsia 1993;34(Suppl 2):182.

## 144 Clinical Trials in Neurologic Practice

78. Uthman BM, Rowan AJ, Ahmann PA, et al. Tiagabine for complex partial seizures. Arch Neurol 1998;55:56–62.
79. Kälviäinen R, Brodie M, Duncan J, Chadwick D, Edwards D, Lyby K, for the Northern European Tiagabine Study Group. A double-blind, placebo-controlled trial of tiagabine given three-times daily as add-on therapy for refractory partial seizures. Epilepsy Res 1998;30:31–40.
80. Sachdeo RC, Leroy RF, Krauss GL, et al. Tiagabine therapy for complex partial seizures: a dose-frequency study. Arch Neurol 1997;54:595–601.
81. Ben-Menachem E. International experience with tiagabine. Epilepsia 1995;36(Suppl 6):S14–S21.
82. Lassen LC, Sommerville K, Mengel HB, et al. Summary of five controlled trials with tiagabine as adjunctive treatment of patients with partial seizures. Epilepsia 1995;36(Suppl 3):S148.
83. Leppik IE. Tiagabine: the safety landscape. Epilepsia 1995;36(Suppl 6):S10–S13.
84. Kälviäinen R, Äokiä M, Riekinen PJ. Cognitive adverse effects of antiepileptic drugs. Incidence, mechanism and therapeutic implications. CNS Drugs 1996;5:358–368.
85. Sveinbjornsdottir S, Sander JWAS, Patsalos PN, et al. Neuropsychological effects of tiagabine, a potential new antiepileptic drug. Seizure 1994;3:29–35.
86. Dodrill CB, Arnett JL, Sommerville KW, Shu V. Cognitive and quality of life effects of differing dosages of tiagabine in epilepsy. Neurology 1997;48:1025–1031.
87. Krauss G, Carlson HA, Deaton R, Sommerville KW. Beneficial results of tiagabine therapy in patients with psychiatric history. Epilepsia 1997;38(Suppl 8):105.
88. Hogan RE, Lenz GT, Deaton R, Sommerville KW. Weight changes with adjunctive therapy of phenytoin, carbamazepine, or tiagabine in a multicenter trial of partial seizures. Epilepsia 1998;39(Suppl. 6):125.
89. Biton V, Vasquez B, Sachdeo RC, et al. Adjunctive tiagabine compared with phenytoin and carbamazepine in the multicenter, double-blind trial of complex partial seizures. Epilepsia 1998;39(Suppl 6):125.
90. Schachter SC. Tiagabine monotherapy in the treatment of partial epilepsy. Epilepsia 1995;36(Suppl 6):S2–S6.
91. Uldall P, Bulteau C, Pedersen SA, et al. Single-blind study of safety, tolerability and preliminary efficacy of tiagabine as adjunctive treatment in children with epilepsy. Epilepsia 1995;36(Suppl 3):S147.
92. Dulac O, Bulteau C, Pedersen S, Uldall P. The challenges of epilepsy in children. Epilepsia 1997;38(Suppl 2):S1–S4.
93. Sommerville KW, Hearell M, Deaton R, Leppik IE. Adverse events with long-term tiagabine therapy. Epilepsia 1997;38(Suppl 8):106.
94. Collins SD, Brun S, Kirstein YG, Sommerville KW. Absence of visual field defects in patients taking tiagabine. Epilepsia 1998;39(Suppl 6):146–147.
95. Sharief M, Viteri C, Ben-Menachem E, et al. Double-blind, placebo-controlled study of topiramate in patients with refractory partial epilepsy. Epilepsy Res 1996;25:217–224.
96. Tassinari CA, Michelucci R, Chauvel P, et al. Double-blind, placebo-controlled trial of topiramate (600 mg daily) for the treatment of refractory partial epilepsy. Epilepsia 1996;37:763–768.
97. Ben-Menachem E, Henriksen O, Dam M, et al. Double-blind, placebo-controlled trial of topiramate as add-on therapy in patients with refractory partial seizures. Epilepsia 1996;37:539–543.
98. Faught E, Wilder BJ, Ramsey RE, et al. Topiramate placebo-controlled dose-ranging trial in refractory partial epilepsy using 200, 400 and 600 mg daily dosages. Neurology 1996;46:1684–1690.
99. Privitera M, Fincham R, Penry JK, et al. Topiramate placebo-controlled dose-ranging trial in refractory partial epilepsy using 600, 800 and 1000 mg daily dosages. Neurology 1996;46:1678–1683.
100. Reife RA, Pledger GW. Topiramate as adjunctive therapy in refractory partial epilepsy: pooled analysis of data from five double-blind, placebo-controlled trials. Epilepsia 1997;38(Suppl 1):S31–S33.
101. Elterman R, Glauser TA, Ritter FJ, et al. Topiramate as adjunctive therapy in pediatric patients with partial-onset seizures. Epilepsia 1997;38(Suppl 8):98.
102. Biton V, Montouris GD, Riviello JD, Reife R. Efficacy and safety of topiramate in generalized seizures of non-focal onset. Epilepsia 1997;38(Suppl 8):206–207.
103. Glauser TA, Sachdeo RC, Ritter FJ, et al. Topiramate as adjunctive therapy in Lennox-Gastaut syndrome. Epilepsia 1997;38(Suppl 8):207.
104. Sachdeo RC, Reife RA, Lim P, Pledger G. Topiramate monotherapy for partial onset seizures. Epilepsia 1997;38:294–300.
105. Rimmer EM, Richens A. Double-blind study of gamma-vinyl-GABA in patients with refractory epilepsy. Lancet 1984;1:189–190.
106. Gram L, Klosterkov P, Dam M. Gamma-vinyl-GABA: a double-blind placebo-controlled trial in partial epilepsy. Ann Neurol 1985;17:262–266.

## Clinical Trials in Epilepsy  145

107. Loiseau P, Hardenberg JP, Pestre M, et al. Double-blind placebo-controlled study of vigabatrin (gamma-vinyl-GABA) in drug-resistant epilepsy. Epilepsia 1986;27:115–120.
108. Tartara A, Manni R, Galimberti CA, et al. Vigabatrin in the treatment of epilepsy: a double-blind placebo-controlled study. Epilepsia 1986;27:717–723.
109. Remy C, Favel P, Tell G, et al. Étude en double-aveugle contre placebo en permutations croisées du vigabatrin dans l'épilepsie de l'adulte résistant à la thérapeutique. Boll Lega It Epil 1986;54/55:241–243.
110. Tassinari CA, Michelluci R, Ambrosetto G, Salvi F. Double-blind study of vigabatrin in the treatment of drug-resistant epilepsy. Arch Neurol 1987;44:907–910.
111. Ring HA, Heller AJ, Farr IN, Reynolds EH. Vigabatrin: rational treatment for chronic epilepsy. J Neurol Neurosurg Psychiatry 1990;53:1051–1055.
112. Sivenius MR, Ylinen A, Murros K, et al. Double-blind dose reduction study of vigabatrin in complex partial epilepsy. Epilepsia 1987;28:688–692.
113. McKee PJW, Blacklaw J, Friel E, et al. Adjuvant vigabatrin in refractory epilepsy: a ceiling to effective dosage in individual patients? Epilepsia 1993;34:937–943.
114. Dean C, Mosier M, Penry K. Dose-response study of vigabatrin as add-on therapy in patients with uncontrolled complex partial seizures. Epilepsia 1999;40:74–82.
115. Gilham RA, Blacklaw J, McKee PJW, Brodie MJ. Effect of vigabatrin on sedation and cognitive function in patients with refractory epilepsy. J Neurol Neurosurg Psychiatry 1993;56:1271–1275.
116. Chiron C, Dulac O, Gram L. Vigabatrin withdrawal randomized study in children. Epilepsy Res 1996;25:209–215.
117. Valentine C, Mettert N, Mosier M, Michon AM. A parallel group study comparing oral adjunctive vigabatrin with placebo in children with uncontrolled complex partial seizures. Epilepsia 1998;39(Suppl 6):166.
118. Van Orman CB, Ruckh S, Mosier M. Efficacy and safety of vigabatrin in children with uncontrolled complex partial seizures: a dose-response study. Epilepsia 1998;39(Suppl 6):166.
119. Perucca E, Gram L, Avanzini G, Dulac O. Antiepileptic drugs as a cause of worsening of seizures. Epilepsia 1998;39:5–17.
120. Kälviäinen R, Mervaala E, Sivenius J, Riekkinen PJ. Vigabatrin. Clinical Use. In RH Levy, RH Mattson, BS Meldrum (eds), Antiepileptic Drugs (4th ed). New York: Raven Press, 1995;925–930.
121. Monaco F. Cognitive effects of vigabatrin. Neurology 1996;47(Suppl 1):S6–S11.
122. Reynolds EH, Ring HA, Farr IN, et al. Open, double-blind and long-term study of vigabatrin in chronic epilepsy. Epilepsia 1991;32:530–538.
123. Eke T, Talbot JF, Lawden MC. Severe persistent visual field constriction associated with vigabatrin. BMJ 1997;314:180–181.
124. Seino M, Naruto S, Ito T, Miyazaki H. Zonisamide. In RH Levy, RH Mattson, BS Meldrum (eds), Antiepileptic Drugs (4th ed). New York: Raven Press, 1995;1011–1023.
125. Wilder BJ, Ramsay RE, Browne T, Sackellares JC. A multicenter double-blind, placebo-controlled study on zonisamide on medically refractory patients with complex partial seizures. Epilepsia 1985;26:545.
126. Schmidt D, Jacob R, Loiseau P, et al. Zonisamide for add-on treatment of refractory partial epilepsy: a European double-blind trial. Epilepsy Res 1993;15:67–73.
127. Pellock JM, Brodie MJ. Felbamate: 1997 update. Epilepsia 1997;38:1261–1264.

# 8
# Dementia
Florence Pasquier and Jean-Marc Orgogozo

Dementia is becoming a major concern worldwide, because its prevalence and incidence rise exponentially with increasing age. The prevalence rates are doubled with every 5.1 years of age, from approximately 5% in those aged 65 and older (4–12%) to 40% in those older than 90 years,[1] and up to 58% in those 95 and older.[2] The annual incidence rate of dementia is 2.2% per year for those older than 65 years.[3] According to 1996 United Nations projections, the number of individuals aged 65 and older in the more developed countries will increase from 169 million (14.2% of the population) to 287 million (24.7% of the population) in 2020.[3] Besides the human and social costs, the economic burden of dementia is enormous in industrialized countries,[3] both from direct costs (i.e., those that result in actual monetary expenditures, such as hospital care, physician visits, medications, home health care workers, and institutional care) and indirect costs (i.e., those that do not result in actual monetary expenditures, such as time spouses spend helping and caring). A major issue in treatment research is that delaying the onset or progression of dementia by 5–7 years would reduce the prevalence of the disease by half in persons of this age group (i.e., those near the end of their lives).[4]

Dementia may be of several origins, including the following: degenerative, vascular, infectious, inflammatory, metabolic, and neoplastic, and treatment depends on the cause. However, Alzheimer's disease (AD) together with cortical Lewy bodies (as their clinical distinction is often difficult) accounts for three-fifths to three-quarters of those with dementia; the second most frequent type is vascular dementia (VaD). We focus on AD, which is the main target of clinical trials, for obvious public health and marketing reasons, and on VaD, which could be preventable. A major problem is that, except for rare genetic conditions, there is not any definite marker for diagnosing AD and for differentiating VaD during life. The diagnosis is, therefore, made on clinical or cerebral imaging criteria whose reliability for AD is, at best, 85–90%. The accuracy of diagnosis of VaD is sometimes as low as 50%.[5] The criteria for frontotemporal dementias (FTD) and dementia with Lewy bodies (DLB) is recent; these conditions are still poorly recognized. Moreover, 40–50% of

147

148    *Clinical Trials in Neurologic Practice*

demented patients have a combination of neuropathologic lesions (mainly degenerative and vascular).[6,7] The concomitant presence of other neurologic conditions may significantly influence the severity of the cognitive deficit.[6,8] In addition, AD and VaD have common risk factors and could be associated more often than expected by chance.[9] Another problem is that dementia is a progressive disease, but progression is not absolutely linear[10] because it has a great interindividual heterogeneity.[11] Furthermore, many concomitant somatic disorders (e.g., infections—cardiovascular, digestive, or urinary), which are frequent at the age when dementia occurs, may interfere with the clinical expression of dementia, mainly in behavior but also in cognitive symptoms.

Thus, large trials are needed to minimize the consequences of diagnostic errors, heterogeneity of clinical presentation and disease progression, and to provide adequate statistical power while allowing for subject dropout.

## DEFINITION OF DEMENTIA

According to the International Classification of Diseases,[12] dementia is defined by evidence of a decline in memory and other cognitive abilities, characterized by deterioration in judgment and thinking, such as planning and organizing, and in the general processing of information, in the absence of clouding of consciousness. These symptoms should be present for at least 6 months. There is also a decline in emotional control or motivation, or a change in social behavior. The diagnosis is further supported by evidence of damage to other higher cortical functions, such as aphasia, apraxia, or agnosia. The most common screening test used is the Mini-Mental State Examination (MMSE),[13] with a cutoff score of 26.

Treatments have different goals, and clinical trials may focus on treating the disease to arrest or slow its progression, treating the cognitive or behavioral symptoms, or a combination of these approaches. The way to assess treatment efficacy may be direct, using "objective" scales as much as possible to quantify symptoms, or indirect, measuring the symptoms' impact on patients' activities of daily living, caregiver burden, or economic consequences of patient management.

Dementia therapy has largely focused on amelioration of cognitive impairment, but, additionally, regulatory guidelines demand an assessment of global or functional status of patients, or both.

## DIAGNOSTIC CRITERIA

### Alzheimer's Disease

The most widely used criteria for AD trials are the National Institute of Neurologic and Communicative Disorders and Stroke–Alzheimer's Disease and Related Disorders Association criteria.[14] These criteria are broad and are compatible with a number of other degenerative diseases, such as DLB, which are often underdiagnosed. Postmortem[15,16] and clinical[17] studies have suggested that DLB accounts for 10–20% of dementia cases in hospital settings. Many patients have pathologic features of both AD and DLB (Lewy body variant of AD), and 36% of patients clinically diagnosed as AD had Lewy bodies at autopsy.[16] The criteria of DLB[18] do not exclude the possible concomitant presence of AD. Therefore, the diagnosis of AD with the National Institute of Neurologic and Communicative Disorders and Stroke–Alzheimer's Disease and Related Disorders Association criteria is far from ideal.

## Vascular Dementia

A review of various sets of criteria of VaD concluded that only the criteria of the State of California Alzheimer Disease Diagnostic and Treatment Centers[19] and of the National Institute of Neurological and Communicative Disorders and Stroke—Association Internationale pour le Recherche et l'Enseignement en Neurosciences[20] provide sufficient operational criteria for dementia in patients with cerebrovascular disease and for the establishment of a relationship between dementia and vascular disease.[21] The National Institute of Neurological and Communicative Disorders and Stroke—Association Internationale pour le Recherche et l'Enseignement en Neurosciences[20] criteria include recommendations for the use of computed tomography and magnetic resonance imaging. VaD is heterogeneous, and the reliability of the criteria is modest: 18–54% of VaD patients have Alzheimer lesions at autopsy. It is plausible that the availability of specific diagnostic tests for the various degenerative diseases, from which VaD has to be differentiated, will improve the reliability of the diagnosis of VaD.[21]

## CLINICAL TRIALS

### History

Early trials with vasodilators in dementia have been reviewed by Yesavage et al.,[22] and by Orgogozo and Spiegel.[23] The original rationale was that dementia resulted from impaired cerebral blood flow caused by narrowing of arteries. In AD, the impaired cerebral blood flow is now thought to be a consequence rather than the cause of the disease, although microvascular changes occur in AD, and indicators of atherosclerosis were associated with AD in a cross-sectional analysis from the Rotterdam study.[24,25] However, if blood flow could be increased, it would be unlikely to improve the primary neuronal degeneration.[23] In VaD, vasodilators would not be expected to reverse atherosclerotic changes or to improve perfusion through occluded vessels or through infarcted tissue. Early trials experienced many methodologic problems, and precise information was often lacking. Before research, diagnostic criteria, and assessment scales were made available, study populations and judgment criteria were highly heterogeneous. Based on these studies, constructive criticisms and topical recommendations were made.[26]

150    *Clinical Trials in Neurologic Practice*

## Assessment of Therapeutic Efficacy in Alzheimer's Disease

The main goals of AD treatments are as follows:

1. Symptomatic improvement, which may manifest in enhanced cognition, more autonomy, improvement in behavioral dysfunction autonomy, or a combination of these
2. Slowing or arrest of symptom progression
3. Primary prevention by intervention in key pathogenic mechanisms at a pre-symptomatic stage

The United States and particularly the European regulatory guidelines concentrate on assessment of symptomatic improvement in three domains: (1) cognition, as measured by objective tests (cognitive end-point); (2) activities of daily living (functional end-point); and (3) overall clinical response, as reflected by global assessment (global end-point). Other end-points of interest may include behavioral symptoms.

The European Medical Evaluating Agency recommends identifying the therapeutic target, choosing a primary criterion, and defining individual responders. The protocol should specify the minimal degree of improvement required on the primary criterion, evaluating the lack of worsening on secondary criteria (including side effects). The responder analysis allows an overall estimate of use by transforming individual responses in group benefits through odds ratios.

## Efficacy Variables and Outcome Measures

Rating scales determine disease severity and serve as primary outcome measures to assess the therapeutic efficacy of investigational compounds. Outcome measures in AD have been reviewed.[27] The main rating scales used in AD follow.

Staging Measures

Global Deterioration Scale[28]
Clinical Dementia Rating Scale (CDR)[29]
Functional Assessment Staging[30]

Cognitive Measures

A test is defined by the quantification of a set of tasks that patients must perform by following instructions under the control of the examiner. Some conditions in the design of dementia tests are that they need to be simple, short, and sensitive enough to assess changes across a wide range of severity to avoid floor or ceiling effect. They require inter-rater reliability and face validity (i.e., direct applicability of the result of the test to the function being measured). Commonly proposed criteria are as follows: (1) to be culture-free, or at least appropriate for different languages and cultures; (2) to correlate well with universally accepted estimates of a function; (3) to relate closely to the cognitive problems for which the trial treatment is being undertaken; and (4) to have several (four or more) parallel forms available to avoid a training effect. The choice of instruments should remain open, provided that these conditions are respected. The following are the most widely used cognitive tests:

MMSE[13]
Mattis Dementia Rating Scale[31]
Consortium to Establish a Registry for Alzheimer's Disease[32]
Alzheimer's Disease Assessment Scale (ADAS).[33]

The ADAS includes 21 items, which are divided into two sections: an 11-item cognitive subscale (ADAS-Cog) evaluating memory, language, and praxis functions, and a 10-item noncognitive subscale (ADAS-Noncog) that rates mood, autonomic function, agitation, delusions, hallucinations, tremor, concentration, and distractibility. Scores on the ADAS-Cog range from 0 (no impairment) to 70 (errors in all subtests); on the ADAS-Noncog, they range from 0 to 50. The ADAS-Cog has become the standard instrument for demonstrating cognitive improvement in short-term efficacy AD drug trials since it was used for the approval of tacrine and donepezil (see the section Symptomatic Studies). In tacrine studies, an improvement of 4 points (which corresponds to 6-month average spontaneous decline) was found in approximately 40% of treated patients, and an improvement of 8 points (1-year decline) was found in 10–12%.[34,35] A mean difference between the active treatment and placebo group of at least 2.5 points is considered desirable for symptomatic trials.[36] The double-blind design of a clinical trial allows a direct comparison with the placebo group; however, few data are available on the effects of various demographic or clinical variables[37] and on the natural decline of performance[11] on the ADAS-Cog. An improvement of even 8 points means little in a severely demented patient, whereas the same improvement in a mild case may result in a return to a more independent life. Thus, positive findings with the ADAS must be validated by a concurrent improvement in a measure of activities of daily living, or at least in a global assessment of change. The ADAS is not sensitive to change in very early or mild cases of dementia (ceiling effect).

## Clinical Global Outcome Measure

The rationale of this assessment, recommended by the U.S. Food and Drug Administration (FDA)[38] is that a clinically meaningful antidementia drug effect should be detectable by a clinician interviewing the patient in isolation from other sources of information, such as psychometric performance and information provided by the caregiver.

### Clinician's Interview-Based Impression of Change

The Clinician's Interview-Based Impression of Change (CIBIC) rating must be made by the physician, without input from the family or caregiver, and without knowledge of the patient's performance on rating scales or neuropsy-

152    *Clinical Trials in Neurologic Practice*

chologic tests. The domains on which the CIBIC should be based are as follows: (1) observation of appearance and behavior; (2) speech, with form being more important than content; (3) mood, based on observation and not on report; (4) thought content, based mainly on report; (5) insight, based on capacity of self-perception; and (6) cognitive state (e.g., orientation, consciousness, alertness).

### Clinician's Interview-Based Impression of Change-Plus

The Clinician's Interview-Based Impression of Change-Plus (CIBIC-Plus) includes input from the caregiver. It is a more useful version, but strong biases may come from the attitude of the informant toward the patient.[39]

In both cases, the integrative estimation is based on an interview by the observer, whose global impression is rated on a seven-point scale going from "markedly worse" to "markedly improved." These global estimates have a high inter-rater variability and a lack of sensitivity (or responsiveness) to drug effect, so that they should be used only with large numbers of patients or for prolonged periods of follow-up,[40] or both.

**Activities of Daily Living**    Activities of daily living are grouped under basic self-care activities (e.g., moving, dressing, and personal hygiene) and instrumental activities (e.g., housework, cooking, using household devices, telephoning, shopping, using transportation, and driving). The following are scales used to measure the disease's effect on daily living:

> Progressive Deterioration Scale[41]
> Interview for Deterioration in Daily Living Activities in Dementia[42]
> Cleveland Scale for Activities of Daily Living[43]
> Bayer-Activities of Daily Living Scale[44]
> Disability Assessment for Dementia[45]

**Behavioral Rating Scales**    The behavioral and psychological signs and symptoms of dementia are the most important contributors to psychological distress in families and are important predictors of institutionalization, more rapid decline, and earlier death.[46] They include mood, delusions, affectivity, and interpersonal relations. They may produce more disability at the personal level, and more handicap at the social level, than cognitive symptoms. Some drugs that are efficacious for cognition can worsen the global outcome if behavioral symptoms (e.g., agitation or aggressiveness) increase. Conversely, some drugs that improve behavior may impair cognition (e.g., sedatives or neuroleptics). They are gaining increasing attention in clinical trials and research. Different sources of information (family caregiver, professional caregiver, observation by clinicians, and patient self-report) may result in different conclusions regarding the frequency and severity of behavioral disturbance. Family caregivers are intimately familiar with the behavior of patients and well positioned to report behavioral data. Observations, however, may be biased by caregiver mood, the lack of sophistication of the caregiver as an observer, or the previous relationship of the patient and caregiver.[47] The

*Dementia* 153

following two scales are examples of caregiver-based assessment instruments for behavioral disturbances:

Behavioral Pathology in Alzheimer's Disease[48]
Neuropsychiatric Inventory with Caregiver Distress Scale (NPI-D)[49,50]

Professional caregivers can provide information for rating scales, particularly for patients who are hospitalized or institutionalized. Members of the nursing staff are the usual reporters and have the advantage of being more experienced in behavioral observation. Examples of behavioral scales using professional caregiver reports include the following:

Nurses' Observation Scale for Inpatient Evaluation[51]
Ward Daily Behavioral Scale[52]
NPI-Nursing Home Version[47]
Multidimensional Observation Scale for Elderly Subjects[53]

Direct observation of patients by clinicians is relevant for acute changes in behavior, but not for clinical trials. Patient report is typically useful only in the early phases of a dementing illness, because later insight is often compromised, and the patients can reliably report only on their immediate circumstances.

**Caregiver Burden**    *Caregiver burden* refers to the physical and psychological or emotional, social, and financial problems that can be experienced by family members caring for an impaired older adult. The impact of caring has been found to persist even after the patient has been institutionalized. Instruments to measure this dimension are as follows:

Screen for Caregiver Burden[54]
Revised Memory and Behavior Problem Checklist[55]

**Quality of Life**    Quality of Life (QOL) measures are an established outcome in many therapeutic areas, but they have been recently developed for patients with dementia, for whom they raise specific methodologic difficulties. Use of disease-specific instruments is recommended to take into account the staging of the disease and to include the views and values of each patient and his or her caregivers.[56] Some instruments available are as follows[57]:

Quality of Life-AD[58]
Blau QOL[59]
Caregivers' time use[60] and cost data

It is assumed that a change in score on a test reflects a similar change in performance. However, all these continuous measures suffer from lack of linearity across their entire spectrum and are susceptible to ceiling and floor effects depending on the severity of dementia. Subjects who drop out of a clinical trial early cannot provide the correct change score needed for the statistical analysis.

**Rate of Progression to End-Point**    Clinically relevant pivotal changes in patient status can be used as end points in a longitudinal analysis, provided that

154 *Clinical Trials in Neurologic Practice*

they are irreversible. Such milestones were used as a measure of progression in one study.[61,62] Survival analysis allows the consideration of censored subjects. Survival methods may also include prognostic variables in the analysis (e.g., Cox proportional hazards model) that adjust for potential baseline differences between groups. The end points should be clinically meaningful, well-recognized, and stable and should occur consistently with the progression of the disease, frequently enough during the period of follow-up. Examples are as follows:

Prespecified drop in a cognitive measure
Transition from a CDR of 2–3
Loss of independence/institutionalization
Mortality

Because of the high inter- and intrapatient variability, measures of changes have to be very responsive. The choice of tools should remain open: Cognitive assessments are culture biased, functional outcomes are environment biased, global assessment is subjective, and others, such as handicap or quality of life, are still research items.

As the main objective of treatments for dementia, whatever the mechanism of action, is to slow the progression of the cognitive and functional decline, the assessment of the course of the disease is essential.


## Factors to Be Considered

Prognostic factors such as early age at onset,[63] male gender, low education, and ApoE 4 genotype, all potential factors of shorter survival, and other vascular risk factors must all be considered in clinical trial. ApoE4 may modify the response to pharmacologic treatment.[64,65] There may be an interaction between gender and ApoE genotype.[66] In addition, estrogen replacement therapy, which was associated with a reduced risk of AD,[67–69] may have a positive influence on cognition, and especially on memory.[70,71] The age at menopause should also be considered.[71,72]

The clinical presentation may also be related to the prognosis and course of the disease, although the data are controversial. Severe language impairment,[73] extrapyramidal signs, and psychotic symptoms,[74] myoclonus,[75] and seizures[76] have been shown to be associated with faster cognitive decline. Extrapyramidal symptoms and psychosis, especially visual hallucinations, could mark the presence of Lewy body disease or vascular pathology. The faster progression and the good response to tacrine of DLB[77] make an accurate diagnosis of such cases desirable. Early involvement of frontal lobes (severe impairment in executive functions and frontal hypometabolism on functional imaging studies) is associated with a more rapid clinical course,[78] whereas temporal lobe dysfunction could predict a lower rate of cognitive decline.[79] Apraxia does not seem to influence the rate of progression, but it is associated with early death.[80] Patients with AD have increased susceptibility to infections, particularly pneumonia and urinary tract infections, that may interfere with the course of the disease.[81]

*Dementia* 155

It is desirable to avoid any treatment likely to impair alertness, intellectual function, or behavior, such as benzodiazepines and older neuroleptics. If they cannot be avoided, the acceptable level of use of these treatments should be set *a priori* and remain constant throughout the trial.

## Rationale and Different Classes of Compounds

The brain of patients with AD is characterized by a dramatic loss of neurons and synapses, neurofibrillary tangles, and senile amyloid plaques and a severe reduction of numerous neurotransmitters, particularly acetylcholine (ACh). Amyloid aggregation and deposition involve oxygen radicals, oxidative stress, and lipid peroxidation, among others. Several studies have also shown inflammatory reactions in AD. These changes usually begin in the entorhinal cortex and the nucleus basalis and progress in an orderly topographic fashion.[82]

### Cholinergic Treatment

A selective loss of cholinergic cells has been shown to be highly correlated with intellectual impairment in AD[83,84]; therefore, the basal forebrain cholinergic system is a key therapeutic target. The cholinergic hypothesis states that a decrease of ACh in the brain of AD patients plays an important role in the deterioration of cognitive functioning.[85] Strategies to enhance the transmission of ACh have included ACh precursors, ACh releasers, M1-, M3-, or M4-ACh receptor agonists, nicotinic agonists, and particularly the use of acetylcholinesterase inhibitors (AChEIs).[86] AChEIs (tacrine, donepezil, and rivastigmine) were the first drugs approved for the treatment of AD. These are discussed in more detail in the sections Tacrine, Donepezil, and Rivastigmine. Acetylcholinesterase inhibitors may also reduce the secretion of amyloid precursor protein (APP), so that their long-term administration could reduce the process of β-amyloid deposition.

The use of ACh precursors such as choline or phosphatidylcholine (lecithin) failed to produce positive results.[87] ACh releasers, including pyridine derivatives, were tried with limited success in animals and humans; most of the direct-acting ACh agonists on postsynaptic cholinergic (muscarinic) receptors, which are relatively unaffected in AD, are short acting or do not cross the blood-brain barrier.[88] Muscarinic agonists could regulate amyloid metabolism.[89] As the M1-muscarinic receptor is predominant in the brain, selective M1-muscarinic agonists such as xanomeline, milameline, and SB 202026 have been the most actively studied, but they failed to show efficacy in phase III trials.

Interventions to prevent the destruction of neurons and the disruption of brain function by β-amyloid include the administration of antioxidants and of free-radical scavengers. Their administration reduces further neuronal damage from β-amyloid deposits, activates various growth factors to repair damaged cells and restore their functions, stimulates the normal processing of the precursor protein that aids in neuronal repair, and, more importantly, prevents the formation of additional β-amyloid.[90]

156    *Clinical Trials in Neurologic Practice*

### Antioxidants and Free-Radical Scavengers

Based on the hypotheses that free radicals are involved in neuronal damage after ischemia and that they are implicated in the inflammatory process, drugs acting as antioxidants or as free-radical scavengers have been tried in AD. The MAO-B inhibitor/antioxidant selegiline (L-deprenyl) has shown a retardation of worsening in AD patients as assessed by loss of independence and nursing home placement progression in AD, as did alpha-tocopherol, one isoform of vitamin E.[61] Other MAO-B inhibitors are being studied, but lazabemide, one of the most advanced, was recently dropped from development. An extract of Gingko biloba, with antioxidant and free radical–scavenging properties, is also being tested in dementia.[91]

### Neuroprotective and Neurotrophic Agents

Propentofylline, a phosphodiesterase inhibitor and an adenosine uptake inhibitor, interferes with the neuroinflammatory process and acts as a neuroprotective glial cell modulator. It was assessed in clinical trials in AD and VaD with promising results: Four early phase III multinational, double-blind studies involving 901 patients with AD and 359 patients with VaD showed efficacy that was maintained through an 8-week withdrawal segment, suggesting an impact on disease progression.[92] Later studies applied a combination of a withdrawal and delayed onset of treatment design in a second segment, with an overall active treatment period of 72 weeks, and showed beneficial effects on cognitive and global functions.[93] Propentofylline stimulates nerve growth factor synthesis, which has an important role in the maintenance of cholinergic and other neurons in the central nervous system. Idebenone also stimulates nerve growth factor synthesis, scavenges free radicals, and protects cell membranes against lipid peroxidation. It can also protect against glutamate and β-amyloid–induced neurotoxicity and has been investigated in a number of clinical trials.[94] The development of this molecule is ongoing, whereas propentofylline was dropped.

### Attenuating Potentiation of Glutamate Toxicity

The search for neuroprotective agents to prevent neuronal loss includes the development of drugs that inhibit excitatory amino acid neurotransmission. Potent antagonists at the *N*-methyl-D-aspartate glutamate receptor are associated with psychotomimetic side effects. The use of low-affinity, noncompetitive *N*-methyl-D-aspartate receptor antagonists, such as memantine, is promising.[95]

### Anti-Inflammatory Agents

The use of anti-inflammatory drugs is based on evidence of activated inflammatory processes in AD brains, which may contribute to neurodegeneration, and on

*Dementia*   157

clinical and epidemiologic observations suggesting that nonsteroidal anti-inflammatory drugs (NSAIDs) could be protective against AD[96] and associated with preserved cognitive functions.[97] A study even suggested a time-of-exposure dependent protective effect of NSAIDs on the occurrence of AD,[98] which suggests a causal relationship. Several clinical trials support the idea that anti-inflammatory therapy may be beneficial in AD through several mechanisms.[99] Cyclooxygenase-2 inhibitors, a well-tolerated class of NSAIDs, are currently being assessed for their effect in slowing the progression of the disease.

## Estrogens

The mechanism of action of estrogens remains to be clarified; antidepressive effect, improvement of cerebral blood flow, direct stimulation of neurons, development of glial cells, and modulation of apolipoprotein E expression have been suggested.[100] Estrogens also have anti-inflammatory properties and could prevent the action of free radicals.[101] Estrogens could modify the natural course of dementia[102] and improve performance in demented women.[66,103] Estrogens promote the growth and survival of cholinergic neurons and could decrease cerebral amyloid deposition, both of which may delay the onset of or prevent AD.[102] Finally, they may also enhance the response to cholinesterase inhibitors.[104]

In a preliminary open trial, Fillit et al.[104] demonstrated that some older women with AD experienced clear cognitive benefit (attention, orientation, and mood) from oral estradiol treatment. In a subsequent placebo-controlled study using low-dose transdermal estradiol, no cognitive benefits were found.[106] A controlled, randomized long-term clinical trial to test the hypothesized role of hormone replacement therapy in the onset and progression of dementia in women began in 1996.[101]

## Study Goals

Most therapeutic trials have dealt with mild to moderate stages of the disease (MMSE between 10 and 26) (Figure 8.1).

## Symptomatic Studies

The goal of symptomatic studies is to demonstrate improvement in the symptoms of the disease, mainly cognitive impairment. Usually, these trials require at least 100 subjects per treatment arm depending on the assumptions involved in power analysis, most often designed with a 90% power. These trials also require assessments in other domains (i.e., functional and global assessments must be performed as well). Such studies were used to test AChEIs (see below). Controlled clinical trials aimed at demonstrating short-term symptomatic improvement should last at least 6 months. However, studies of 1 year or more would be desirable to evaluate the maintenance of efficacy. Open-label follow-up of at least 12 months is recommended for the demonstration of long-

158  *Clinical Trials in Neurologic Practice*

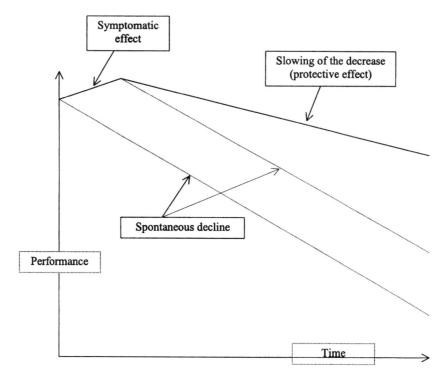

*Figure 8.1*  Study goals.

term safety and to estimate the maximal duration of the symptomatic effects. The following sections discuss symptomatic studies with acetylcholinesterase inhibitors.

*Tetrahydroaminoacridine (Tacrine)*

The first report on improvement of cognitive function in AD patients with tacrine was published in 1986.[107] The drug was the first to be approved by the FDA in 1993 and has since been used therapeutically in the United States, and since 1994 in France. More than 2,000 patients have been studied in five double-blind, placebo-controlled trials. Overall, 30–40% demonstrated improvement, compared to 10% of those taking placebo. The highest dose was the most effective. Ten to 20% of patients developed cholinergic side effects that generally diminished within a few days; 30% of patients taking tacrine developed reversible and asymptomatic elevation in liver enzymes, and 5–10% needed to discontinue the drug.

Studies have shown that the use of tacrine will reduce overall costs by reducing and delaying admission to nursing homes or other long-term care facilities.[108,109]

*Donepezil*

Donepezil is a reversible selective central AChEI; at clinical doses, it has only minor side effects, and its long half-life allows once-a-day dosing. A comprehensive worldwide, clinical double-blind, placebo-controlled trials program involving approximately 2,000 patients demonstrated significant improvement in both cognition and global function (ADAS-Cog and CIBIC-Plus).[110] Long-term investigations have shown that treatment benefits are maintained for more than 4.5 years and that the size of treatment effect in comparison with untreated patients seems to become larger over time. A cost-effectiveness analysis, performed to assess the economic impact of donepezil in the treatment of mild or moderate AD, showed that for mild AD, if the drug effect exceeds 2 years, the drug would pay for itself in terms of cost offsets.[111]

*Rivastigmine*

Rivastigmine inhibits cholinesterase pseudoirreversibly. Its development program included approximately 40 clinical studies with an enrollment of more than 5,000 patients in the active treatment group. It demonstrated an effect on the ADAS-Cog, CIBIC-Plus, MMSE, Global Deterioration Scale, and ADL.[112] It has been used clinically in Europe since 1997 and in North America since 2000. Long-term efficacy is apparent for at least 1 year, thus far.

Conclusions

Other AChEIs are under development. Based on more than 30 phase II clinical trials in more than 6,000 subjects from comparable patient populations during a 6-month treatment period, one can demonstrate significant cognitive effects measured with the ADAS-Cog scale for three different reversible (tacrine, donepezil, and galanthamine), and three irreversible, or pseudoirreversible (eptastigmine, rivastigmine, and metrifonate) AChEIs.[113] The magnitude of these clinical effects, expressed as the difference between drug- and placebo-treated patients at 6 months, or as the difference between 6 months and baseline assessment in drug-treated patients, is rather similar for the six drugs in a range of 3–5 ADAS-Cog points after 6 months. Differences among the various drugs studied concern chemical structure, enzymatic mechanism of action, pharmacokinetic and pharmacodynamic properties, selectivity for acetylcholinesterase (versus butyrylcholinesterase), and cholinergic receptor affinities. These characteristics may explain the observed differences in severity of side effects, number of patient dropouts, and general cholinergic toxicity in clinical trials. The mode of administration (dosage and titration) has to be adapted accordingly. Certain patients are high responders, whereas other patients respond very little (or not at all) to the drug. In addition to positive cognitive effects, AChEIs show significant behavioral effects. Long-term studies show that clinical efficacy can be extended to 12 months or more, followed by a progressive decrease in clinical efficacy. The immediate challenge is to investigate whether

160    *Clinical Trials in Neurologic Practice*

AChEIs can be useful at early stages of the disease or in subjects with mild cognitive impairment who are at risk for developing AD.[113]

## Studies That Test a Slowing of Decline

Drug trials that result in a slowing of cognitive decline could be expected to demonstrate an increase in the size of treatment effect over time that is proportional to the duration of the study. Longer studies require fewer patients but are at higher risk for dropouts. A global impression of change is less reliable in these studies, because baseline examination becomes increasingly difficult to recall over time. Based on the estimate of a deterioration rate of 7 points per year on the ADAS-Cog in placebo-treated patients, a 1-year trial designed to detect a 50% reduction in the rate of decline would require only 75–125 subjects per treatment arm.[36] A greater number of subjects is needed if detection of a smaller treatment difference is expected. Such studies need at least 1 year of follow-up, and a 2–3 year follow-up is preferred, which makes the use of a placebo-controlled arm problematic.

## Study Design

Several designs have been used in AD trials.[36]

## Crossover Design

In a simple two-period crossover design, every patient is treated twice, once with the active agent and once with placebo, in random order.[107,114,115] The main advantage of this design is that patients are their own controls, reducing the variance contributed by between-subject heterogeneity. However, it has several drawbacks. One is that period and order effects may occur, according to the treatment (placebo or active drug) with which the patients started the trial, and patients entering the second treatment period may not have returned to the initial clinical state. They may necessitate washout periods to prevent carryover effects. Another drawback is that patient dropouts are more common due to the long period of treatment, because patients must have received both treatments to analyze an effect. Crossover designs should therefore be avoided, except perhaps in short-term phase II symptomatic trials.

## Enrichment Design

During the first stage of enrichment designs, a dose-titration with the active drug is performed in all patients to identify optimal dose for responders. Non-responders are dropped out. During the second stage, responders of the first stage are randomized to active drug or placebo.[116,117] Because all patients receive the active drug, it is difficult to determine true adverse effects of the compound; carryover effects may occur in patients crossed over to placebo. Moreover, it is difficult to generalize the trial results from a preselected population. The advantage is to determine the most effective dose during the dose-titration phase.

## Parallel Group Designs

Parallel group designs are now the most widely used designs, as they have proven to be more efficient.[95,117–121] The participants are divided at random into as many groups as there are treatment arms. The problem of between-subject variability remains the requirement of a large population to gain statistical power. The comparability of treatment groups must be verified, especially regarding prognostic factors. With these provisos, parallel group placebo-controlled trials are, by far, the most reliable way to demonstrate efficacy.

## Randomized Withdrawal Design

In the randomized withdrawal design, subjects on active drug at the end of the first part of the study are switched to placebo, whereas those on placebo remain on placebo. In the case of purely symptomatic effects, the slope of the group that receives the active drug rapidly joins that of the placebo group during the second part of the study. On the contrary, the slopes remain more or less parallel during the second phase if the drug slowed the progression of the disease.

# Guidelines

Phase III large, multicenter, double-blind, randomized, and placebo-controlled trials are needed for drug approval in many countries. The hypothesis tested in a study should be stated explicitly, and the population size is calculated to test this hypothesis. Study end points are chosen for being clinically meaningful and objective. In AD trials, demonstration of efficacy is needed on multiple end points, including at least a cognitive test instrument and a clinician's global impression, or a functional scale. This is because a statistically significant change of a few points on the ADAS-Cog score may not be clinically relevant by itself. Efficacy for behavior or economic impact is an additional end point that may be desirable.

For the purpose of clinical trials, the severity of the dementia syndrome must be measured at baseline (before starting treatment) and at follow-up to assess treatment effect. This can be made by quantitative or qualitative evaluation or through global estimates, structured questionnaires, rating scales, or neuro-psychologic tests. Important requirements for assessment scales include correlation with widely accepted criteria, sensitivity to change responsiveness, availability of several parallel forms, avoidance of ceiling or floor effects, and applicability in different languages and cultures. It is recommended that each domain be assessed by a different investigator who should be independent of and blind to all other rating outcomes.

162    *Clinical Trials in Neurologic Practice*

Run-In Period

The screening and run-in period preceding randomization of treatment is used for washout of previously administered medicinal products that are incompatible with the trial and for the qualitative and quantitative baseline assessment of patients. Patients with major short-term fluctuations of their condition should be excluded. Placebo may be given during this period to assess compliance with medication.

Guidelines for the clinical evaluation of antidementia drugs published by the FDA[122] assert a preference for placebo as an internal control and for parallel rather than crossover studies. Similarly, the European Agency for the Evaluation of Medicinal Products Human Medicines Evaluation Unit published guidelines[123] that became operational in January 1998. Companies can submit new drug applications centrally, the approval then being granted for all European Union member states, or through an individual country, in which case the company seeks approval from each other member state. European guidelines differ from FDA guidelines mainly in recommending longer trial periods and using three primary outcome measures (adding activities of daily living as an important dimension of assessment).[123,124] The Canadian guidelines are the most comprehensive[125]: They address disease stage and dementias other than AD. The Japanese guidelines are notable for explicitly including vascular dementia and for being influenced by the International Working Group on Harmonization of Dementia Drug Guidelines.[126]

## Clinical Trials on Behavioral Symptoms

There have been surprisingly few controlled trials of conventional psychotropic agents in patients with AD. Antipsychotic drugs, antidepressants, and anxiolytics have been administered to these patients because of the similarity of delusions, mood changes, and anxiety symptoms in AD to those of the idiopathic psychiatric illnesses for which these agents were developed. These symptoms, however, may have different or only partially overlapping pathophysiologies, and treatment responses cannot be confidently extrapolated from one condition to another.[46] Few studies were designed to detect solely an improvement in behavior in AD patients, although many case reports and case series have indicated improvement with several psychotropic compounds.[127] A number of randomized clinical trials with benzodiazepines for the treatment of behavioral symptoms of dementia have been published, most of them comparing the effect of long-lasting benzodiazepine with antipsychotic agents. They all had methodologic limitations.[128] A double-blind study compared the efficacy and side effects of trazodone and haloperidol for treating agitated behaviors associated with dementia.[129] A meta-analysis of controlled trials of conventional neuroleptic treatment of dementia did not show a large benefit of neuroleptics compared with placebo and demonstrated severe adverse effects.[130] Assessment of selective serotonin reuptake inhibitors and new antipsychotic agents (atypical neuroleptics, e.g., clozapine, risperdal, and olanzapine) are ongoing or awaited.

There is preliminary evidence that behavioral and psychological signs and symptoms of AD may be reduced by AChEIs. Raskin et al.[131] showed that cooperation, delusion, and pacing, assessed on the ADAS-Noncog, improved with tacrine.[131] An open-label study designed to assess the effects of tacrine on behavioral changes in AD patients with the neuropsychiatric inventory (NPI) showed a decrease of anxiety, apathy, hallucinations, aberrant motor behaviors, and disinhibition.[132] In a double-blind, 6-month placebo-controlled clinical trial of xanomeline, a muscarinic receptor agonist, Bodick et al.[133] observed in the treated group a significant reduction in vocal outbursts, suspiciousness, delusions, agitation, hallucinations, wandering, fearfulness, compulsiveness, tearfulness, mood swings, and threatening behavior.[133]

## Other Interventions

### Rehabilitation

Rehabilitation strategies, aimed at optimizing patient functioning at every stage of the disease course by exploiting preserved abilities and performance-enhancing factors, have been tried in case reports.[134] Assessment of these interventions is very difficult, however, given all of the factors involved.

### Psychosocial and Behavioral Interventions

In a meta-analysis of 11 studies in which blind intervention was carried out on caregivers, intervention proved more beneficial than the placebo comparison in nine studies. Two suggested that early treatment might delay nursing home placement; both educational and emotional support were effective, especially emotional support, and the combination may be more effective than either alone.[135] A randomized controlled trial on behavioral management in nursing and residential homes showed that residents can benefit from improved quality of care achieved by training from a hospital outreach team.[136]

## Variants of Alzheimer's Disease and Other Dementias

### Dementia with Lewy Bodies

DLB typically has prominent attentional deficits with relative preservation of episodic memory, especially in the early stages. Executive dysfunction and visuospatial impairments may be disproportionately severe.[18] Hallucinations and delusions occur particularly early and are often disruptive; conventional neuroleptics are not tolerated. Spontaneous fluctuations may complicate assessment of the efficacy of a compound. Responses to new antipsychotic drugs and to L-dopa therapy were published as case reports or pilot studies.[137,138] Preliminary observations suggested that patients with DLB may benefit particularly from cholinergic treatment.[76,139] Some have speculated that DLB, which may represent approximately 25% of all clinically diagnosed AD, explains the minority of responders to treatment of AD with tacrine.[140] Actually, an improvement with tacrine does not appear more frequently in DLB than in pure-AD but may be

164    *Clinical Trials in Neurologic Practice*

qualitatively different.[141] AChEIs are currently being assessed in placebo-controlled trials for this indication.

Vascular Dementia

Idebenone,[142] propentofylline,[143] memantine,[94] and Gingko biloba extracts[90] have been tested in VaD. However, VaD is heterogeneous in pathogenesis and clinical manifestation, and the progression of the disease is not linear. The main focus of the third International Conference on Harmonization of Dementia Drug Guidelines, held in Osaka, Japan in November 1998, was the spectrum of vascular causes of cognitive impairment and VaD with special reference to practical VaD drug guidelines.[144]

Frontotemporal Dementia

FTD, one of the clinical syndromes of frontotemporal degeneration,[145] is characterized by profound alteration in personality and social conduct with inertia and loss of volition or social disinhibition and distractibility, or a combination of these. Emotions are blunted and insight is lost. Cognitive deficits occur in the domains of abstraction, planning, problem solving, and attention, whereas primary tools of perception and spatial functions are well preserved. Patients are not clinically amnesic and remain oriented in place. Memory performance testing is, however, typically inefficient, its impairment arising secondary to patients' frontal regulatory disturbances rather than because of a primary amnesia. At first, FTD manifests itself in behavioral changes with relatively stable global cognition; however, language, verbal fluency, and memory tests are reliable tools to follow the progression of the disease. When the MMSE is lower than 18, mutism and apathy generally prevent neuropsychological testing within the next 6 months.[146] There is no evidence of cholinergic abnormality, unlike the situation in AD; rather, serotonin receptors are lost.[147] Only a few open-label trials with small sample sizes have been performed in FTD.[148,149]

## OTHER PERSPECTIVES

### Primary and Secondary Prevention

True preventive or very early treatment in patients with risk factors, including vascular risk factors, could be effective in the near future. Estrogens are currently under assessment: 8,300 women aged 65–79 during a 2-year period will be randomized and followed annually for 6–9 years.[100] An antihypertensive drug (nitrendipine) has already shown a preventive action on the incidence of dementia (degenerative as well as vascular) in a double-blind, placebo-controlled trial in subjects at least 60 years of age with isolated systolic hypertension,[150] but the absolute risk reduction was very small. Other putative disease-modifying agents, such as neuroprotectors, should be tested in the near future. A first pragmatic attitude could be to test such agents in patients with mild cognitive impairment (MCI), which is a strong predictor of dementia.[151] As 10–15% of subjects with MCI evolve to AD each year,[152] they may be considered as being in a preclinical stage of dementia. It is estimated that a clinical trial to prevent dementia in subjects with MCI will require at least 3 years of follow-up and several hundred subjects. Once an agent is proven safe and effective in subjects with MCI, it might be tested in a larger and longer prevention trial in normal individuals. Subjective memory complaints may predict dementia within 3 years, particularly when there are objective signs of memory deterioration.[153] However, memory complaints may lack validity as a predictor of AD in subjects with normal cognition.[154] Another strategy is to test putative neuroprotectors first in advanced forms of AD, which may respond more easily despite a lower clinical relevance at this stage.[61]

## Other Issues

Comparison of two symptomatic drugs in a direct comparison for efficacy and tolerance could be done, as well as combinations of drugs. Development of drugs that prevent the abnormal phosphorylation of τ-protein and, hence, neurofibrillary tangle formation, would have great therapeutic potential. Recent data on the genetics and molecular biology of AD should provide the premises for more rational and physiopathologically oriented treatments of the disease.[155]

Clinical symptoms appear to correlate with the spread of the disease from the hippocampus into the association areas of the neocortex.[156] Disruption of hippocampal circuitry has been suggested as an explanation of the impairments of memory that are characteristic of AD. Therapeutic efforts to treat the early cognitive decline in AD could be directed toward restoration of these circuits, which, for the most part, use glutamate as their main neurotransmitter.[157]

Trials could also address the question of heterogeneity and could be performed in subgroups of patients. An International Working Group on Harmonization of Dementia Drug Guidelines was formed to standardize the assessment of dementia in clinical trials; its position papers are published regularly in *Alzheimer's Disease and Associated Disorders.*

All AD guidelines state that the cognitive tests must cover more than memory alone, as impairments in domains other than memory are mandatory for the diagnosis. However, because memory dysfunction is generally the first cognitive impairment in AD and may be present even in the preclinical stages, future trials may need more sensitive tools.[158]

Hippocampal atrophy was shown to be present in presymptomatic individuals at risk of autosomal-dominant familial AD.[159] Medial temporal lobe atrophy is also a predictor of dementia in subjects with mild cognitive impairment.[160] This measurement might therefore be useful as an efficacy variable in the future. The progression of global brain atrophy may also be useful for the assessment of disease progression and the evaluation of treatments.[161,162]

## ETHICAL ISSUES

Considering the widely acknowledged benefit of AChEIs, the question of further long-term, double-blind studies against placebo is debatable,[163] particularly in

166   *Clinical Trials in Neurologic Practice*

countries where these treatments are paid for by social care services. Is it ethical to propose a placebo when a well-tolerated, affordable treatment is available? Most trials available suggest that the earlier the treatment, the better the stabilization of the clinical course.

Another important issue is the ability to provide active drug after a double-blind study to participants who did not worsen during the trial and *a fortiori* if they improved during the trial. To cope with this, it is increasingly common for trial patients to be enrolled in an open-label, long-term follow-up study once the double-blind, placebo-controlled period has ended, which answers the ethical issue in an acceptable regulatory way and allows collection of safety data on long-term use of the drug.

The question of informed consent is becoming increasingly tricky. The diagnosis of Alzheimer's disease by definition includes the criteria for dementia, which is characterized by loss of insight and impaired judgment. Therefore, it is implicitly understood that patients with dementia may not be competent to make decisions regarding themselves and others and indeed may not even recognize their impairment. The policies are not the same in all countries. Some major issues remain unresolved, including how to assess competence to consent and how to assess the relative risks and benefits of a protocol for a patient with dementia.[124] However, participation in clinical trials is associated with a lower risk of nursing home admission, whereas mortality, risk of hospitalization, and onset of severe functional deficits are not different.[164]

Inconclusive and negative study results should be published.[165] In many sensitive areas, such as conflict of interest and mechanisms of informed consent, there is cultural disparity. The position paper from the International Working Group on Harmonization of Dementia Drug Guidelines raised questions for discussion in any cultural context.[166] Few studies have been conducted in severely demented patients.[94]

To overcome the drawback of heterogeneous study population, a strict selection of patients is often made, which may bias the results and deprive future patients from efficacious drugs.

## CONCLUSIONS

Dementia is a heterogeneous syndrome with no explicit criteria other than clinical criteria. Therefore, it is necessary for any clinical trial to be cautious regarding the diagnostic criteria used and the experience of the investigators in diagnosing dementia. Patterns of clinical presentation, rates of progression, and prognostic factors should be considered in the design and analysis of clinical trials. Although AD is the most common form of dementia, other types may be amenable to trials, because clinical criteria are becoming more operational and practitioners more familiar with dementia and involved in the management of demented patients. Pharmacoeconomics is a relatively new science that is likely to become more important. The present guidelines are suggestive, but not normative. Innovative designs are explicitly encouraged in the European Medical Evaluating Agency guidelines.

# REFERENCES

1. Jorm AF, Korten AE, Henderson AS. The prevalence of dementia: a quantitative integration of the literature. Acta Psych Scand 1987;76:464–479.
2. Ebly EM, Parhad IM, Hogan DB, et al. Prevalence and types of dementia in the very old: results from the Canadian Study of Health and Aging. Neurology 1994;44:1593–1600.
3. Katzman R, Fox PJ. The World-Wide Impact of Dementia. Projections of Prevalence and Costs. In R Mayeux, Y Christen (eds), Epidemiology of Alzheimer's Disease: From Gene to Prevention. New York: Springer-Verlag, Berlin Heidelberg, 1999;1–17.
4. American Federation for Aging Research and the Alliance for Aging Research. Putting aging on hold: delaying the diseases of old age. An official report of the White House Conference on Aging. Washington: American Federation for Aging Research, 1995.
5. Galasko D, Hansen LA, Katzman RP, et al. Clinical-neuropathological correlations in Alzheimer's disease and related dementias. Arch Neurol 1994;51:888–895.
6. Nagy Z, Esiri MM, Jobst KA, et al. The effects of additional pathology on the cognitive deficit in Alzheimer disease. J Neuropathol Exp Neurol 1997;56:165–170.
7. Berg L, McKeel D, Miller JP, et al. Clinicopathological studies in cognitively healthy aging and Alzheimer's disease. Relation of histologic markers to dementia severity age, sex, and apolipoprotein E genotype. Arch Neurol 1998;55:326–335.
8. Snowdon DA, Greiner LH, Mortimer JA, et al. Brain infarction and the clinical expression of Alzheimer disease. The Nun Study. JAMA 1997;277:813–817.
9. Pasquier F, Leys D. Why are stroke patients prone to develop dementia? J Neurol 1997;244:135–42.
10. Helmes E, Merskey H, Fox H, et al. Patterns of deterioration in senile dementia of the Alzheimer type. Arch Neurol 1995;52:306–310.
11. Piccini C, Bracco L, Amaducci L. The Natural Progression of Alzheimer's Disease. In S Gauthier (ed), Pharmacotherapy of Alzheimer's Disease. London: Martin Dunitz, 1998;7–32.
12. World Health Organization. The ICD-10 Classification of Mental and Behavioural Disorders. Diagnostic criteria for research. World Health Organization, Geneva, 1993.
13. Folstein MF, Folstein SE, McHugh PR. "Mini-mental state". A practical method for grading the cognitive state of patients for the clinician. J Psych Res 1975;12:189–198.
14. McKhann G, Drachman D, Folstein M, et al. Clinical diagnosis of Alzheimer's disease: report of the NINCDS-ADRDA Work Group under the auspices of Department of Health and Human Services Task Force on Alzheimer's disease. Neurology 1984;34:939–944.
15. Burns A, Luthert P, Levy R, et al. Accuracy of clinical diagnosis of Alzheimer's disease. Br Med J 1990;301:1026.
16. Hansen L, Salmon D, Galasko D, et al. The Lewy body variant of Alzheimer's disease: a clinical and pathological entity. Neurology 1990;40:1–8.
17. Shergill S, Mullan E, D'Ath P, et al. What is the clinical prevalence of Lewy body dementia? Int J Geriatr Psychiatr 1994;9:907–912.
18. McKeith IG, Galasko D, Kosaka K, et al. Consensus guidelines for the clinical and pathologic diagnosis of dementia with Lewy bodies (DLB). Neurology 1996;47:1113–1124.
19. Chui HC, Victoroff JI, Margolin D, et al. Criteria for the diagnosis of ischemic vascular dementia proposed by the State of California Alzheimer's Disease Diagnostic and Treatment Centers. Neurology 1992;42:473–480.
20. Roman GC, Tatemichi TK, Erkinjuntti T, et al. Vascular dementia: diagnostic criteria for research studies. Report of the NINDS-AIREN International Workshop. Neurology 1993;43:250–260.
21. Scheltens P, Hijdra AH. Diagnostic criteria for vascular dementia. Haemostasis 1998;28:151–157.
22. Yesavage JA, Tinklenburg JR, Hollister LE, et al. Vasodilatators in senile dementias—a review of the literature. Arch Gen Psychiatr 1979;36:220–223.
23. Orgogozo JM, Spiegel R. Critical review of clinical trials in senile dementia—II. Postgrad Med J 1987;63:337–343.
24. Hofman A, Ott A, Breteler MMB, et al. Atherosclerosis, apolipoprotein E and the prevalence of dementia and Alzheimer's disease in the Rotterdam Study. Lancet 1997;349:151–154.
25. Buée L, Hof PR, Delacourte A. Brain microvascular changes in Alzheimer's disease and other dementias. Ann N Y Acad Sci 1997;826:7–24.
26. Dartigues JF. Methodology of Clinical Trials in Dementia. Part II: Future Trials—Recommendations. In R Capildeo, JM Orgogozo (eds), Methods in Clinical Trials in Neurology. Vascular and Degenerative Brain Disease. London: The Macmillan Stockton Press, 1988;295–301.

## 168  *Clinical Trials in Neurologic Practice*

27. McKeith IG, Cummings JL, Lovestone S, et al. Outcome measures in Alzheimer's disease. London: Martin Dunitz, 1999.
28. Reisberg B, Ferris SH, de Leon MJ, et al. The global deterioration scale for assessment of primary degenerative dementia. Am J Psychiatry 1982;139:1136–1139.
29. Hughes CP, Berg L, Danziger WL, et al. A new clinical scale for the staging of dementia. Br J Psychiatry 1982;140:566–572.
30. Reisberg B. Functional assessment staging (FAST). Psychopharmacol Bull 1988;24:653–659.
31. Mattis S. Dementia Rating Scale Professional Manual. Odessa: Psychological Assessment Resources, 1988.
32. Morris JC, Heyman A, Mohs RC, et al. The Consortium to Establish a Registry for Alzheimer's Disease (CERAD). Part I. Clinical and neuropsychological assessment of Alzheimer's disease. Neurology 1989;39:1159–1165.
33. Rosen WWG, Mohs RC, Davis KL. A new rating scale for Alzheimer's disease. Am J Psychiatry 1984;141:1356–1364.
34. Davies KL, Than LJ, Gamzu ER, et al. A double-blind, placebo-controlled multicenter study of tacrine for Alzheimer's disease. The Tacrine Collaborative Study Group. N Engl J Med 1992;327:1253–1259.
35. Farlow M, Gracon SI, Hershey LA, et al. A controlled trial of tacrine in Alzheimer's disease. The Tacrine Study Group. JAMA 1992;268:2523–2529.
36. Grundman M, Thal LJ. Trial Designs. In S Gauthier (ed), Pharmacotherapy of Alzheimer's Disease. London: Martin Dunitz, 1998;43–56.
37. Doraiswamy PM, Bieber F, Kaiser L, et al. The Alzheimer's Disease Assessment Scale: pattern and predictors of the baseline cognitive performance in multicentre Alzheimer's disease trials. Neurology 1997;48:1511–1517.
38. Food and Drug Administration. Letter to the Industry by P. Leber, Director of Regulator Affairs, 1991;22:1–8.
39. Schneider LS, Olin JT. Clinical global impressions in Alzheimer's clinical trials. Int Psychogeriatr 1996;8:277–290.
40. Knopman DS, Knapp MJ, Gracon SI, et al. The Clinician Interview-Based Impression (CIBI): a clinician's global change rating scale in Alzheimer's disease. Neurology 1994;44:2315–2321.
41. DeJong R, Osterlund OW, Roy GW. Measurement of quality-of-life changes in patients with Alzheimer's disease. Clin Ther 1989;11:545–554.
42. Teunisse S, Derix MM, van Crevel H. Assessing the severity of dementia. Patient and caregiver. Arch Neurol 1991;48:274–277.
43. Patterson MB, Mack JL, Neundorfer MM, Martin RJ, et al. Assessment of functional ability in Alzheimer disease: a review and a preliminary report on the Cleveland Scale for Activities of Daily Living. Alzheimer Dis Assoc Disord 1992;6:145–163.
44. Hindmarch I, Lehfeld H, de Jongh P, et al. The Bayer Activities of Daily Living Scale (B-ADL). Dement Geriatr Cogn Disord 1998;9 (Suppl 2):20–26.
45. Gelinas I, Gauthier L, McIntyre M, et al. Development of a functional measure for persons with Alzheimer's disease: the disability assessment for dementia. Am J Occup Ther 1999;53:471–481.
46. Steel C, Rovner B, Chase GA, et al. Psychiatric symptoms and nursing home placement of patients with Alzheimer's disease. Am J Psychiatry 1990;145:1049–1051.
47. Cummings JL, Masterman DL. Assessment of treatment-associated changes in behavior and cholinergic therapy of neuropsychiatric symptoms in Alzheimer's disease. J Clin Psychiatry 1998;59(Suppl 13):23–30.
48. Reisberg B, Borenstein J, Salob SP, et al. Behavioral symptoms in Alzheimer's disease: phenomenology and treatment. J Clin Psychiatry 1987;48:9–15.
49. Cummings JL, Mega M, Gray K, et al. The Neuropsychiatric Inventory: comprehensive assessment of psychopathology in dementia. Neurology 1994;44:2308–2314.
50. Kaufer DI, Cummings JL, Christine D, et al. Assessing the impact of neuropsychiatric symptoms in Alzheimer's disease: the Neuropsychiatric Inventory Caregiver Distress Scale. J Am Geriatr Soc 1998;46:210–215.
51. Honigfeld G, Klett CJ. The Nurses' Observation Scale for Inpatient Evaluation. J Clin Psychol 1965;21:65–71.
52. Blunden J, Hodgkiss A, Klemperer F, et al. The Ward Daily Behaviour Scale. Br J Psychiatry 1994;165:87–93.
53. Helmes E, Csapo K, Short JA. Standardization and validation of the Multidimensional Observation Scale for Elderly Subjects (MOSES). J Gerontol 1987;42:395–405.
54. Vitaliano PP, Russo J, Young HM, et al. The screen for caregiver burden. Gerontologist 1991;31:76–83.

*Dementia* 169

55. Teri L, Truax P, Logsdon RG, et al. Assessment of behavioral problems in dementia: the Revised Memory and Behavior Problems Checklist. Psychol Aging 1992;7:622–631.
56. Rabins PV, Kasper JD. Measuring quality of life in dementia: conceptual and practical issues. Alzheimer Dis Assoc Disord 1997;11(Suppl 6):100–104.
57. Whitehouse PJ, Orgogozo JM, Becker RE, et al. Quality of life assessment in dementia drug development. Position paper from the International Working Group on Harmonization of Dementia Drug Guidelines. Alzheimer Dis Assoc Disord 1997;11(Suppl 3)56–60.
58. Logsdon RG. Quality of life in Alzheimer's disease: implications for research. Gerontologist 1996;36(Special issue 1):278.
59. Blau TH. Quality of life, social indicators, and criteria of change. Prof Psychol 1977;11:464–473.
60. Clipp EC, Moore MJ. Caregivers time use: an outcome measure in clinical trial research on Alzheimer's disease. Clin Pharmacol Ther 1995;58:228–236.
61. Sano M, Ernesto C, Klauber MR, et al. Rationale and design of a multicenter study of selegiline and alpha-tocopheral in the treatment of Alzheimer disease using novel clinical outcomes. Alzheimer's Disease Cooperative Study. Alzheimer Dis Assoc Disord 1996;10:132–140.
62. Sano M, Ernesto C, Thomas RG, et al. A controlled trial of selegiline, alpha-tocopherol, or both as treatment for Alzheimer's disease. The Alzheimer's Disease Cooperative Study. N Engl J Med 1997;336:1216–1222.
63. Koss E, Edland S, Fillenbaum G, et al. Clinical and neuropsychological differences between patients with earlier and later onset of Alzheimer's disease: a CERAD analysis, Part XII. Neurology 1996;46:136–141.
64. Poirier J, Delisli MC, Quirion R, et al. Apolipoprotein E4 allele as a predictor of cholinergic deficits and treatment outcome in Alzheimer's disease. Proc Natl Acad Sci U S A 1995;92:12260–12264.
65. Richard F, Helbecque N, Neuman E, et al. APOE4 genotyping and response to drug treatment in Alzheimer's disease. Lancet 1997;349:539.
66. Duara R, Barker WW, Lopez-Alberola R, et al. Alzheimer's disease: interaction of apolioprotein E, genotype, family history of dementia, gender, education, ethnicity, and age of onset. Neurology 1996;46:1575–1579.
67. Henderson VW, Paganini-Hill A, Emanuel CK, et al. Estrogen replacement therapy in older women. Comparisons between Alzheimer's disease cases and non-demented control subjects. Arch Neurol 1994;51:896–900.
68. Kawas C, Resnick S, Morrison A, et al. A prospective study of estrogen replacement therapy and the risk of developing Alzheimer's disease: the Baltimore Longitudinal Study of Aging. Neurology 1997;48:1517–1521.
69. Waring SC, Rocca WA, Petersen RC, et al. Post-menopausal estrogen replacement therapy and risk of AD. A population-based study. Neurology 1999;52:965–970.
70. Sherwin B. Estrogen effects on cognition in menopausal women. Neurology 1997;48(Suppl 7):S21–S26.
71. Costa A, Nappi RE, Sinforiani E, et al. Cognitive function at menopause: neuorendocrine implications for the study of the aging brain. Funct Neurol 1997;12:175–180.
72. Sobow TM, Kutter EP, Kloszewska I. Hormonal decline indicator in women (age at menopause) modifies age of onset in sporadic Alzheimer's disease. Alzheimer's Reports 1999;2:27–29.
73. Bracco L, Gallato R, Grigoletto F, et al. Factors affecting course and survival in Alzheimer's disease. A 9-year longitudinal study. Arch Neurol 1994;51:1213–1219.
74. Chui HC, Lyness SA, Sobel E, et al. Extrapyramidal signs and psychiatric symptoms predict faster cognitive decline in Alzheimer's disease. Arch Neurol 1994;51:676–681.
75. Kaye JA, May C, Atack JR, et al. Cerebrospinal fluid neurochemistry in the myoclonic subtype of Alzheimer's disease. Ann Neurol 1988;24:647–650.
76. Volicer L, Smith S, Volicer BJ. Effect of seizures on progression of dementia of the Alzheimer type. Dementia 1995;6:258–263.
77. Liberini P, Valerio A, Memo M, et al. Lewy-body dementia and responsiveness to cholinesterase inhibitors: a paradigm for heterogeneity of Alzheimer's disease? Trends Pharmacol Sci 1996; 17:155–160.
78. Mann UM, Mohr E, Gearing M, et al. Heterogeneity in Alzheimer's disease: progression rate segregated by distinct neuropsychological and cerebral metabolic profiles. J Neurol Neurosurg Psychiatry 1992;55:956–959.
79. Butters MA, Lopez OL, Becker JT. Focal temporal lobe dysfunction in probable Alzheimer's disease predicts a slow rate of cognitive decline. Neurology 1996;46:687–692.
80. Burns A, Jacoby R, Levy R. Progression of cognitive impairment in Alzheimer's disease. J Am Geriatr Soc 1991;39:39–45.
81. Volicer L, Hurley AC. Physical status and complications in patients with Alzheimer disease: implications for outcome studies. Alzheimer Dis Assoc Disord 1997;11(Suppl 6):60–65.

# 170    Clinical Trials in Neurologic Practice

82. Delacourte A, David J-P, Buée L, et al. The biochemical pathway of neurofibrillary degeneration during aging and Alzheimer Disease. Neurology 1999;52:1158–1165.
83. Whitehouse PJ, Price DL, Struble RG, et al. Alzheimer's disease and senile dementia: loss of neurons in the basal forebrain. Science 1982;215:1237–1239.
84. Lehéricy S, Hirsch E, Cervera-Pierot P, et al. Heterogeneity and selectivity of the degeneration of cholinergic neurons in the basal forebrain of patients with Alzheimer's disease. J Comp Neurol 1993;330:15–31.
85. Francis PT, Palmer AM, Snape M, et al. The cholinergic hypothesis of Alzheimer's disease: a review of progress. J Neurol Neurosurg Psychiatry 1999;66:137–147.
86. Lemiere J, Gool DV, Dom R. Treatment of Alzheimer's disease: an evaluation of the cholinergic approach. Acta Neurol Belg 1999;99:96–106.
87. Becker R, Giacobini E, Elbe R, et al. Potential pharmacotherapy of Alzheimer disease. A comparison of various forms of physostigmine administration. Acta Neurol Scand Suppl 1988;116:19–32.
88. Forette F, Boller F. Drug Development in Alzheimer's Disease: A Review of Its History and a Preview of Its Future. In S Gauthier (ed), Pharmacotherapy of Alzheimer's Disease. London: Martin Dunitz, 1998;1–15.
89. Growdon JH. Muscarinic agonists in Alzheimer's disease. Life Sci 1997;60:993–998.
90. Nikolov R, Richardson. Antiamyloid strategies for the treatment of Alzheimer's disease. Drugs Today 1998;34:673–689.
91. Le Bars PL, Katz MM, Berman N, et al. A placebo-controlled, double-blind, randomized trial of an extract of Gingko biloba for dementia. North American EGb Study Group. JAMA 1997;278:1327–1332.
92. Marcusson J, Rother M, Kittner B, et al. A 12-month, randomized, placebo-controlled trial of propentofylline (HWA 285) in patients with dementia according to DSM III-R. The European Propentofylline Study Group. Dement Geriatr Cogn Disord 1997;8:320–328.
93. Kittner B. Effect of Propentofylline on disease progression in Alzheimer disease and vascular dementia—results of studies using the combined randomized start/withdrawal design. Neurobiol Aging 1998;18(Suppl 2):S302–S303.
94. Gutzmann H, Hadler D. Sustained efficacy and safety of idebenone in the treatment of Alzheimer's disease: update on a 2-year double-blind multicentre study. J Neural Transm Suppl 1998;54:301–310.
95. Winblad B, Poritis N. Memantine in severe dementia, results of the 9M-Best Study (benefit and efficacy in severely demented patients during treatment with memantine). Int J Geriat Psychiatry 1999;14:135–146.
96. Rogers J, Kirby LC, Hempelman SR, et al. Clinical trial of indomethacin in Alzheimer's disease. Neurology 1993;43:1609–1611.
97. Peacock JM, Folsom AR, Knopman DS, et al. for the Atherosclerosis Risk in Communities (ARIC) Study Investigators. Association of nonsteroidal anti-inflammatory drugs and aspirin with cognitive performance in middle-aged adults. Neuroepidemiology 1999;18:134–143.
98. Stewart WF, Kawas C, Corrada M, et al. Risk of Alzheimer's disease and duration of NSAID use. Neurology 1997;48:626–632.
99. Aisen PA. Inflammation and Alzheimer's disease: mechanisms and therapeutic strategies. Gerontology 1997;43:143–149.
100. Honjo H, Tanaka K, Kashiwagi T, et al. Senile dementia-Alzheimer's type and Estrogen. Horm Metab Res 1995;27:204–207.
101. McBee WL, Dailey ME, Dugan E, et al. Hormone replacement therapy and other potential treatments for dementia. Endocrinol Metab Clin North Am 1997;26:329–345.
102. Tang MX, Jacobs D, Stern Y, et al. Effect of oestrogen during menopause on risk and age at onset of Alzheimer's disease. Lancet 1996;348:429–432.
103. Henderson VW, Watt L, Buckwalter JG. Cognitive skills associated with estrogen replacement in women with Alzheimer's disease. Psychoneuroendocrinology 1996;21:421–430.
104. Birge ST. Is there a role for oestrogen replacement therapy in the prevention and treatment of dementia? J Am Geriatr Soc 1996;44:865–870.
105. Fillit H, Weinreb H, Cholst I, et al. Observations in a preliminary open trial of estradiol therapy for senile dementia-Alzheimer's type. Psychoneuroendocrinology 1986;11:337–345.
106. Fillit H. Estrogens in the pathogenesis and treatment of Alzheimer's disease in post-menopausal women. Ann N Y Acad Sci 1994;743:233–239.
107. Summers WK, Majovski IV, Marsch GM, et al. Oral tetrahydroaminoacridine in long-term treatment of senile dementia, Alzheimer-type. N Engl J Med 1986;315:1241–1245.
108. Knopman D, Schneider L, Davis K, et al. Long-term tacrine (Cognex) treatment: effects on nursing home placement and mortality, Tacrine Study Group. Neurology 1996;47:166–177.
109. Henke CJ, Birchmore MJ. The economic impact of tacrine in the treatment of Alzheimer's disease. Clin Ther 1997;19:330–344.
110. Burns A, Rossor M, Hecker J, et al. The effects of Donepezil in Alzheimer's disease—results from an multinational trial 1. Dement Geriatr Cogn Disord 1999;10:237–244.

*Dementia* 171

111. Neumann PJ, Hermann RC, Kuntz KM, et al. Cost-effectiveness of donepezil in the treatment of mild or moderate Alzheimer's disease. Neurology 1999;52:1138–1145.
112. Rosler M, Anand R, Cicin-Sain A, et al. Efficacy and safety of rivastigmine in patients with Alzheimer's disease: international randomised controlled trial. BMJ 1999;318:633–638.
113. Giacobini E. Invited review: Cholinesterase inhibitors for Alzheimer's disease therapy: from tacrine to future applications. Neurochem Int 1998;32:413–419.
114. Stern Y, Sano M, Mayeux R. Long-term administration of oral physostigmine in Alzheimer's disease. Neurology 1988;38:1837–1841.
115. Gauthier S, Bouchard R, Lamontagne A, et al. Tetrahydroaminoacridine-lecithin combination treatment in patients with intermediate-stage Alzheimer's disease. Results of a Canadian double-blind, crossover, multicenter study. N Engl J Med 1990;322:1272–1276.
116. Davis KL, Thal LJ, Gamzu ER, et al. The Tacrine Collaborative Study Group. A double-blind, placebo-controlled multicenter study of tacrine for Alzheimer's disease. N Engl J Med 1992;327:1253–1259.
117. Thal LJ, Schwartz G, Sano M, et al. Physostigmine Study Group. A multicenter double-blind study of controlled-release physostigmine for the treatment of symptoms secondary to Alzheimer's disease. Neurology 1996;47:1389–1395.
118. Farlow M, Gracon SI, Hershey LA, et al. A controlled trial of tacrine in Alzheimer's disease. The Tacrine Study Group. JAMA 1992;268:2523–2529.
119. Burke WJ, Roccaforte WH, Wengel SP, et al. L-Deprenyl in the treatment of mild dementia of the Alzheimer type: results of a 15-month trial. J Am Geriatr Soc 1993;41:1219–1225.
120. Bodick NC, Offen WW, Levey AI, et al. Effects of xanomeline, a selective muscarinic receptor agonist on cognitive function and behavioral symptoms in Alzheimer's disease. Arch Neurol 1997;54:465–473.
121. Rogers SL, Friedhoff LT. The efficacy and safety of donepezil in patients with Alzheimer's disease: results of a US multicentre randomized, double-blind, placebo-controlled trial. The Donepezil Study Group. Dementia 1996;7:293–303.
122. Becker RE, Colliver JA, Markwell SJ, et al. Double-blind, placebo-controlled study of metrifonate, an acetylcholinesterase inhibitor, for Alzheimer's disease. Alzheimer Dis Assoc Disord 1996;10:124–131.
123. Leber P. Guidelines for Clinical Evaluation of Antidementia Drugs. Washington: U.S. Food and Drug Administration, 1990.
124. CPMP Working Party on Efficacy of Medicinal Products. Note for Guidance. The European Agency for the Evaluation of Medicinal Products Human medicines Evaluation Unit, London: 1997.
125. Whitehouse PJ. Regulatory Issues in Anti-Dementia Drug Development. In S Gauthier (ed), Pharmacotherapy of Alzheimer's Disease. London: Martin Dunitz, 1998;57–74.
126. Mohr E, Feldman H, Gauthier S. Canadian guidelines for the development of antidementia therapies, a conceptual summary. Can J Neurol Sci 1995;22:62–71.
127. Report of the International Working group on Harmonization of Dementia Drug Guidelines. Alzheimer Dis Assoc Disord 1997;11(Suppl 3):1–64.
128. Kumar V, Durai NB, Jobe T. Pharmacologic management of Alzheimer's disease. Clin Geriatr Med 1998;14:129–146.
129. Practice guideline for the treatment of patients with Alzheimer's disease and other dementias of late life. Am J Psychiatry 1997;154:20–25.
130. Sultzer DL, Gray KF, Gunay I, et al. A double-blind comparison of trazodone and haloperidol for treatment of agitation in patients with dementia. Am J Geriatr Psychiatry 1997;5:60–69.
131. Schneider LS, Pollock VE, Lyness SA. A metaanalysis of controlled trials of neuroleptic treatment of dementia. J Am Geriatr Soc 1990;38:553–563.
132. Raskin MA, Sadowsky CH, Sigmund WR, et al. Effect of tacrine on language, praxis, and noncognitive behavioral problems in Alzheimer's disease. Arch Neurol 1997;54:836–840.
133. Kaufer DI, Cummings, JL, Christine D. Effect of tacrine on behavioral symptoms in Alzheimer's disease: an open-label study. J Geriatr Psychiatry Neurol 1996;9:1–6.
134. Bodick NC, Offen WW, Levey AI, et al. Effects of xanomeline, a selective muscarinic receptor agonist, on cognitive function and behavioral symptoms in Alzheimer disease. Arch Neurol 1997;54:465–473.
135. Van der Linden M, Juillerat AC. Management of cognitive deficits in patients with Alzheimer's disease. Rev Neurol (Paris) 1998;154(Suppl 2):S137–S143.
136. Rabins PV. The caregiver's role in Alzheimer's disease. Dement Geriatr Cogn Disord 1998; 9(Suppl 3):25–28.
137. Proctor R, Burns A, Powell HS, et al. Behavioural management in nursing and residential homes: a randomised controlled trial. Lancet 1999;354:26–29.

## 172  Clinical Trials in Neurologic Practice

138. Williams SW, Byrne EJ, Stokes P. Treatment of diffuse Lewy body disease: a pilot study. Int J Geriat Psychiatry 1993;8:731–739.
139. Walker Z, Grace J, Overshot R, et al. Olanzapine in dementia with Lewy bodies: a clinical study. Int J Geriatr Psychiatry 1999;14:459–466.
140. Perry EK, Haroutunian V, Davis KL, et al. Neocortical cholinergic activities differentiate Lewy body dementia from classical Alzheimer's disease. Neuroreport 1994;5:547–549.
141. Hansen LA. The Lewy body variant of Alzheimer disease. J Neural Transm 1997;(Suppl 51):83–93.
142. Lebert F, Souliez L, Pasquier F, et al. Tacrine efficacy in Lewy body dementia. Int J Geriat Psychiatr 1998;13:516–519.
143. Parnetti L, Senin U, Mecocci P. Cognitive enhancement therapy for Alzheimer's disease. The way forward. Drugs 1997;53:752–768.
144. Rother M, Erkinjuntti T, Roessner M, et al. Propentofylline in the treatment of Alzheimer's disease and vascular dementia: a review of phase III trials. Dement Geriatr Cogn Disord 1998;9(Suppl 1):36–43.
145. Alzheimer Disease and Related Disorders, Supplement ("Osaka VaD"). Summary of the 1st International Conference on Development of Drug Treatment for Vascular Dementia. 1999, In press.
146. Neary D, Snowden JS, Gustafson L, et al. Frontotemporal lobar degeneration. A consensus on clinical diagnostic criteria. Neurology 1998;51:1546–1554.
147. Pasquier F, Lebert F, Lavenu I, et al. The clinical picture of frontotemporal dementia: diagnosis and follow-up. Dement Geriatr Cogn Disord 1999;10(Suppl 1):10–14.
148. Procter AW, Qurne M, Francis PT. Neurochemical features of frontotemporal dementia. Dement Geriatr Cogn Disord 1999;10(Suppl 1):80–84.
149. Coull JT, Sahakian BJ, Hodges JR. The a2 antagonist idazoxan remediates certain attentional and executive dysfunction in patients with dementia of frontal type. Psychopharmacology 1996;123:239–249.
150. Swartz JR, Miller BL, Lesser IM, et al. Frontotemporal dementia: treatment response to serotonin selective reuptake inhibitors. J Clin Psychiatry 1997;58:212–216.
151. Forette F, M, Staessen JA, et al. on behalf of the Syst-Eur Investigators. Prevention of dementia in randomised double-blind placebo-controlled Systolic Hypertension in Europe (Syst-Eur) trial. Lancet 1998;352:1347–1351.
152. Flicker C, Ferris SH, Reisberg B. Mild cognitive impairment in the elderly: predictors of dementia. Neurology 1991;41:1006–1009.
153. Petersen RC, Smith GE, Waring SC, et al. Aging, memory, and mild cognitive impairment. Int Psychogeriatr 1997;9(Suppl 1):65–69.
154. Schmand B, Jonker C, Hooijer C, et al. Subjective memory complaints may announce dementia. Neurology 1996;46:121–125.
155. Schofield PW, Marder K, Dooneief G, et al. Association of subjective memory complaints with subsequent cognitive decline in community-dwelling elderly individuals with baseline cognitive impairment. Am J Psychiatry 1997;154:609–615.
156. Aisen P, Davis K. The search for disease-modifying treatment for Alzheimer's disease. Neurology 1997;48:35–41.
157. Bancher C, Braak H, Fischer P, et al. Neuropathological staging of Alzheimer lesions and intellectual status in Alzheimer's and Parkinson's disease patients. Neurosci Lett 1993;162:179–182.
158. Davies P. Challenging the cholinergic hypothesis in Alzheimer's disease. JAMA 1999;281:1433–1434.
159. Simard M, van Reekum R. Memory assessment in studies of cognition-enhancing drugs for Alzheimer's disease. Drugs Aging 1999;14:197–230.
160. Fox NC, Warrington EK, Freeborough PA, et al. Presymptomatic hippocampal atrophy in Alzheimer's disease. A longitudinal MRI study. Brain 1996;119:2001–2007.
161. Visser PJ, Scheltens P, Verhey FR, et al. Medial temporal lobe atrophy and memory dysfunction as predictor of dementia in subjects with mild cognitive impairment. J Neurol 1999;246:477–485.
162. Fox NC, Freeborough PA, Rossor MN. Visualisation and quantification of rates of atrophy in Alzheimer's disease. Lancet 1996;348:94–97.
163. Fox NC, Freeborough PA. Brain atrophy progression measured from registered serial MRI: validation and application to Alzheimer's disease. JMRI 1997;7:1069–1075.
164. Farlow MR. New treatments in Alzheimer disease and the continued need for placebo-controlled trials. Arch Neurol 1998;55:1396–1398.
165. Albert SM, Sano M, Marder K, et al. Participation in clinical trials and long-term outcomes in Alzheimer's disease. Neurology 1997;49:38–43.
166. Post SG, Beerman B, Brodaty H, et al. Ethical issues in dementia drug development. Position paper from the International Working Group on Harmonization of Dementia Drug Guidelines. Alzheimer Dis Assoc Disord 1997;11(Suppl 3):26–28.

# 9
# Clinical Trials in Parkinson's Disease
Ergun Y. Uc, Andrea J. DeLeo, and Robert L. Rodnitzky

Applied clinical therapeutics in hypokinetic movement disorders dates to the treatment of parkinsonian tremor with belladonna alkaloids by Charcot in 1877.[1] Today, new therapies are subject to the scrutiny of rigorous testing in the form of clinical trials. Clinical trials in hypokinetic movement disorders are the primary method by which investigators prospectively measure disease outcome in response to pharmacologic or surgical interventions. The origin of clinical trials can be traced to the eighteenth century,[2] but the methodology to conduct this form of clinical research continued to evolve and within the later half of the twentieth century came to include the following basic principles: a clearly defined study hypothesis; accurate definition and measurement of primary and secondary outcome variables; and avoidance of systematic error and bias through randomization, blinding, and the use of a control group.[3,4] In this chapter, we review the conduct of clinical trials investigating hypokinetic movement disorders, with particular focus on therapeutic interventions for Parkinson's disease (PD).

PD represents the prototypic hypokinetic movement disorder. It is the most commonly seen hypokinetic movement disorder in clinical practice, affecting 100–105 individuals per 100,000, or approximately 1% of the U.S. population 60 years of age and older.[5] Clinical trials involving PD present several unique challenges. One of the difficulties encountered in conducting clinical trials in PD is the accuracy of clinical diagnosis of study participants, as no validated diagnostic test for the condition exists,[6] rather, the diagnosis is made on clinical grounds alone. Other neurodegenerative parkinsonian syndromes, such as progressive supranuclear palsy, multisystem atrophy,[7] and corticobasal ganglionic degeneration, can be misdiagnosed as idiopathic PD. In an autopsy study of 100 patients diagnosed with PD during life, diagnostic clinicopathologic correlation was demonstrated in only 82% of cases.[8] Another challenge in clinical trials involving PD is the accurate assessment of improvement or deterioration. Because there is no readily available reliable biologic marker of disease severity, clinical trials have largely depended on clinical assessment as measures of improvement or progression. In this regard, difficulty can be encountered when evaluating therapeutic efficacy or disease progression in PD because of the lack of correlation between the various rating scales used to

174    *Clinical Trials in Neurologic Practice*

assess clinical domains of the disease and the lack of inter-rater reliability among clinical examiners who apply these scales.

Several PD rating scales had been applied before 1987, at which time the Unified Parkinson's Disease Rating Scale (UPDRS) was instituted as a standard means of PD assessment.[9] This instrument has emerged as the preferred vehicle for PD assessment in most clinical trials. The UPDRS includes the following domains:

Subscale I—mentation, behavior, and mood
Subscale II—activities of daily living when "on/off"
Subscale III—motor examination
Subscale IV—motor complications of therapy
Subscale V—modified Hoehn and Yahr Staging
Subscale VI—modified Schwab and England Activities of Daily Living Scale (ADL)

The UPDRS identifies both self-reported disability (subscale II) and objective estimates of motor disability (subscale III), although there may be a discrepancy between the two.[10] On balance, the UPDRS is a reliable, reproducible, and valid scale with demonstrated internal consistency.[11]

Clinical trials in PD also present a major challenge in that the efficacy of an investigational treatment must often be measured on an hour to hour basis, typically at home, over long periods of time. These data are normally collected from daily diaries kept by study participants, and are subject to the inconsistent understanding and cooperation of individual study subjects.

## CLINICAL TRIALS INVOLVING SPECIFIC THERAPEUTIC MODALITIES

### Levodopa

The advent of levodopa (LD) in the treatment of PD and the demonstration of its efficacy in the late 1960s were landmark events in the history of clinical trials for this condition.[12] But before long, it became apparent that complications associated with long-term LD therapy and means of counteracting them would require further intense investigation. LD-induced dyskinesias and end-of-dose wearing off, for example, were identified within several years of the introduction of the drug.[13] One of the most basic putative complications of LD is its possible toxic effect on dopaminergic neurons,[14,15] an issue that generates spirited controversy.

Mortality data in PD have been used to address the question of LD neurotoxicity. The results of some mortality studies argue against a neurotoxic effect of LD. The mortality rate for PD patients before LD treatment was nearly 200% higher than in the general population. However, in studies of cohorts treated with LD, it was only 33–85% higher and most of the deaths were seen in patients with severe disease at study entry.[16,17] In a population-based study of PD between 1967 and 1979, the total mortality among patients was significantly higher than in controls; however, the mortality rate noted in LD-treated patients was compa-

*Clinical Trials in Parkinson's Disease*    175

rable to that found in controls.[18] An acknowledged limitation of this study is the fact that selection bias for treatment could not be ruled out.

Further evidence against a toxic effect of chronic LD therapy appeared in a study demonstrating that motor fluctuations were not influenced by early LD treatment in 125 consecutive, newly diagnosed patients treated with LD and followed for 2–10 years.[19] Although not truly a clinical trial, an autopsy analysis in five patients who used LD for 9–26 years for indications other than idiopathic PD suggested that LD administered in ordinary doses was not toxic to substantia nigra neurons.[20] Although not definitely proven to have cytotoxic effects, LD therapy is associated with a variety of adverse clinical effects, and the bulk of clinical trials involving LD since then have, in some way, addressed issues such as dyskinesias, loss of efficacy in PD over time, and techniques of altering the drug's pharmacokinetic profile to positively impact these issues.

## Peripheral Dopa-Decarboxylase Inhibitors

To increase bioavailability and prevent systemic side effects of LD, the aromatic amino acid decarboxylase inhibitors carbidopa (CD) or benserazide (BZ) were added to LD formulations in North America and Europe, respectively. A double-blind study showed that a CD/LD combination was more effective in treating motor fluctuations compared to placebo and LD.[21] Similar plasma LD levels were produced with formulations containing 200-mg LD/50-mg BZ or 250-mg LD/25-mg of CD. In various blinded trials, both combinations were found to have similar efficacy in the relief of parkinsonian symptoms and did not differ with regard to influence on blood pressure, liver function, renal function, and hematologic parameters. However, the frequency and severity of gastrointestinal side effects were significantly higher with the CD formulation, which was attributed to the smaller ratio of CD to LD compared to the BZ to LD ratio.[22–24] Increasing the CD to LD ratio from 1:10 to 1:5 in a randomized, double-blind trial reduced adverse effects and improved the efficacy of LD in mild to moderate disease.[24,25]

One of the clinical maneuvers that evolved to combat complications associated with LD was the drug holiday. *Drug holiday* has come to mean complete withdrawal of all LD compounds for a period of at least 1 week in severely disabled patients in an attempt to "resensitize" dopamine receptors. It was widely practiced in the early days of treatment with LD, but has largely fallen out of favor, although used occasionally to treat intractable psychiatric side effects. In a review of 24 patients undergoing 31 holidays, significant benefit persisted as long as 1 year in only six individuals, despite early transient improvements in several individuals.[26] Given the significant morbidity associated with severe akinesia during a drug holiday, most clinicians have concluded that in most instances the practice carries an unfavorable risk to benefit ratio.

Competition with LD for absorption from the gut and for transport from plasma to brain by dietary large neutral amino acids may be partly responsible for the fluctuating clinical response seen in some patients receiving this agent. In a study attempting to demonstrate these effects, protein meals reduced peak plasma LD concentrations by 29% and delayed absorption by 35 minutes during oral administration of the drug. However, bypassing intestinal absorption by intravenous infusion of LD produced stable plasma levels.[27] In the same study,

176    *Clinical Trials in Neurologic Practice*

competition at the blood-brain barrier (BBB) level was demonstrated by documenting that high-protein meals or infused leucine reversed the therapeutic effect of infused LD without reducing plasma LD concentrations. The practical clinical benefit of increased "on" time, resulting from the reduction or redistribution of dietary protein intake in patients receiving LD, was subsequently demonstrated.[28]

### Controlled Release versus Immediate Release Levodopa Preparations

Controlled release (CR) formulations of LD were developed in an attempt to ameliorate motor fluctuations associated with this drug by producing more sustained plasma LD levels after oral dosing. Initial clinical trials provided mixed results on the overall efficacy of these formulations. A 14-week double-blind crossover comparison of CD/LD-immediate release (IR) and -CR formulations did not reveal a significant difference in efficacy and tolerability.[29] In some studies, a minority of patients were not satisfied with CR because of the unpredictable time at which the medication first took effect, despite the prolongation of daily "on" time.[30,31] A double-blind, 6-month crossover study found no significant difference in disability ratings, motor response fluctuations, or safety between CD/LD 25/100 and CR 50/200, although the CR formulation was superior in patients' ratings of percent "on" time and ADL during the open-label phase of the study.[32] In a later multicenter, double-blind, controlled trial of CR versus IR formulations in advanced PD patients, CR significantly reduced daily "off" time and improved function according to both physician and patient global ratings. In those receiving CR, daily dosing frequency was 33% less, whereas daily intake of LD was increased by 25%.[33] With this study, CD/LD-CR began to emerge as an effective means of enhancing "on" time in PD. Subsequent studies established its effect over a longer time course. Exposure to CD/LD-CR for at least 3 years was not associated with any increase in incidence of adverse effects.[34] In another early study assessing the long-term benefit of CR formulations, patients with motor fluctuations were followed for 36–39 months on open-label CD/LD-CR. At the end of this time, disability scores remained essentially unchanged and 62% of patients had increased daily "on" time compared with baseline.[35]

Another question explored regarding CR-LD formulations is whether the more stable plasma LD levels they produce prevent fluctuations associated with chronic LD administration. The CR FIRST trial randomized 618 de novo patients to required dosages of CD/LD-CR 50/200 or -IR 25/100 and followed them for 5 years.[36] The primary end point was the presence of wearing off or dyskinesias. After 5 years, the response, safety, and side-effect profiles of IR- and CR-LD were similar. The incidence of wearing off or dyskinesias was low in both groups (16–20%), but there was no significant difference between them. ADL scores were better in the CR group, although it has since been questioned whether this could be partly explained by the higher mean LD dose in the CR group, even after adjustment for CR's lower bioavailability. The fact that both treatment regimens were associated with a lower incidence of motor fluctuations and dyskinesias compared to other long-term trials provided a somewhat different perspective of the natural history of chronic LD therapy.[36] Although this study did not prove that early administration of a CR formulation prevents the development of motor fluctuations, it was widely regarded as an example of the reduction in incidence of these adverse events accomplished by careful administration of either LD formulation.

A sustained-release formulation of BZ/LD (Madopar hydrodynamically balanced system [HBS]) was also developed. In a study comparing BZ/LD HBS to CD/LD-CR, equivalent bioavailability of LD was demonstrated in both formulations, but the former drug was associated with a higher fluctuation index, presumably due to its somewhat higher $C_{max}$ and a slightly lower $C_{min}$.[37] A 5-year study comparing IR BZ/LD to HBS in de novo PD patients, similar to the CR FIRST study, was also conducted.[38] In this study, as in CR FIRST, similar efficacy and no difference in occurrence of motor fluctuations or dyskinesias was noted between the two formulations.

Another proposed method to alleviate fluctuations in PD is to administer LD in liquid form. A study of liquid LD/CD in ascorbic acid solution versus LC/CD tablets in PD patients with severe fluctuation showed that those receiving the liquid drug had reduced bradykinesia, decreased dyskinesia, and increased "on" time when compared to those receiving standard tablet therapy.[39]

LD remains the most effective treatment for PD. There are no convincing experimental or clinical data to indicate that neurodegeneration is accelerated by LD, although a large North American clinical trial (ELLDOPA) is under way to further examine this issue. It does seem that LD increases life expectancy among patients with PD. Motor fluctuations and dyskinesias appearing in LD-treated patients are not influenced by the time-release properties of the tablet and are most likely related to the severity of the underlying disease, as well as to treatment-related factors such as the duration and dose of LD therapy. However, most clinicians agree that introduction of LD should not be delayed if comparable comfort and improved quality of life cannot be provided by alternative agents.

## Selegiline

Selegiline (SLG) is a selective monoamine-oxidase-B (MAO-B) inhibitor that benefits PD by inhibiting the central catabolism of dopamine and enhancing the effect of administered LD. In double-blind, placebo-controlled trials, SLG was shown to decrease motor fluctuations and reduce LD requirement.[40,41] When administered as monotherapy in the initial stage of PD, however, SLG was only of minimal symptomatic benefit.[42] Selegiline, also known as *deprenyl*, has also been evaluated as a possible neuroprotective agent in PD based on its ability to reduce the formations of oxyradicals derived from dopamine metabolism and its potential to neutralize exogenous neurotoxins. Deprenyl and Tocopherol Antioxidative Therapy of Parkinsonism (DATATOP) was a landmark clinical trial in PD that evaluated these putative properties of SLG. In this study, conducted by the North American Parkinson Study Group, 800 de novo PD patients were randomly assigned to one of four treatments: tocopherol and placebo, deprenyl and placebo, deprenyl and tocopherol, or double placebo; and analyzed in a $2 \times 2$ factorial design. In the absence of a reliable biomarker for progression of PD, a novel end point was chosen—an increase in parkinsonian disability sufficient to require treatment with LD. An analysis of the correlation of this end point to UPDRS

178   *Clinical Trials in Neurologic Practice*

scores and other conventional rating scales revealed that the need for LD therapy correlated with functional (Schwab-England ADL, UPDRS ADL) scores rather than ratings reflecting clinical examination criteria.[43] In an interim analysis, only 97 subjects who received SLG had reached the end point during an average of 12 months follow-up, as compared to 176 subjects who did not receive SLG (57% risk reduction).[44] Based on this interim observation, revealing a marked apparent benefit of SLG, all study participants were then assigned to open-label SLG, and continued the tocopherol blind. Patients were then followed for an additional 14 ± 6 months, which revealed that there was no beneficial effect of tocopherol or any interaction between tocopherol and SLG.[45] Also noted was that UPDRS motor scores improved during the first 3 months of SLG treatment and worsened after it was withdrawn. This raised the question that the delayed need for LD associated with SLG might be the result of a symptomatic effect of the drug rather than neuroprotection, an issue that remains unsettled. The subjects maintained the blindness of their original deprenyl and tocopherol treatment assignments, and were followed for an additional 1.5–2.0 years on open-label SLG after the conclusion of the DATATOP study. Among patients who did not reach the end point during the study, there was no significant difference in regard to future LD requirement between the original treatment assignments.[46] Similarly, there was no difference in ultimate Hoehn-Yahr, Schwab-England, or UPDRS scale scores; wearing off; dyskinesias; and freezing among patients who had reached the end point of LD requirement in the DATATOP study.[47]

In contrast to the 4-week SLG washout period in the DATATOP trial, several later studies used an 8-week washout for analysis of the drug's effect after the end point was reached in hopes of eliminating any residual symptomatic effect.[48,49] These studies were more supportive of the notion that SLG has a neuroprotective effect. A 14-month double-blind, placebo-controlled study randomized 101 untreated PD patients to four treatment groups: SLG and CD/LD, placebo and CD/LD, SLG and bromocriptine (BRC), and placebo and BRC.[49] UPDRS scores obtained at 14 months, 2 months after withdrawal of SLG or its placebo, or 7 days after withdrawal of Sinemet or BRC showed significant clinical deterioration in the placebo group versus SLG, suggesting that SLG had indeed slowed the progression of disease. The Swedish Parkinson Study Group randomized 157 untreated patients to SLG or placebo in a double-blind study using the initial need for LD therapy as the end point. SLG significantly delayed the need for LD therapy. As analyzed by the UPDRS total and motor scores, the progression of symptoms from baseline to the end of the 8-week washout period was significantly slower in the SLG group, when the progression was adjusted by the time to reach the end point.[48]

Beyond the controversy surrounding the possible neuroprotective properties of SLG, a study in the UK raised the concern that SLG actually increases mortality in PD. In an open, long-term, prospective trial, 782 de novo PD patients, who were not receiving dopaminergic treatment, were randomized to treatment with LD/dopa decarboxylase inhibitor alone (arm 1), LD/decarboxylase inhibitor in combination with SLG (arm 2), or BRC alone (arm 3).[50] After an average 5–6 year follow-up, the hazard ratio for mortality in arm 2 compared with arm 1 was 1.57. The reason for the apparent increased mortality when SLG was added to LD was not apparent to the authors, but they concluded that extreme caution must be exercised in using this combination therapy. Other investigators questioned the findings of this study, noting such unexplained data as the markedly disparate dropout rates among the three treatment arms.[51] The possibility that excess mortality might be related to cardiovascular toxicity related to the use of SLG in combination with LD was raised because of observed orthostatic hypotension in some patients.[52,53] However, a subsequent analysis of the excess mortality seen in this study revealed that neither revised diagnoses, autonomic or cardiovascular events, nor drug interactions could explain this finding. Falls and possible dementia were the only factors that were more common in the group receiving SLG and LD.

In contrast to the United Kingdom (UK) study, a meta-analysis of five long-term, prospective, randomized trials of SLG in patients with untreated PD demonstrated no increase in mortality associated with SLG treatment, whether patients also received LD or did not.[54] In another study contradicting the UK study, mortality analysis of the DATATOP cohort after an average of 8.2 years of observation revealed that the death rate in PD was unaffected by SLG, tocopherol, or combined treatment assignments and was similar to that expected for an age- and gender-matched U.S. population without PD.[55] The UK investigators, on the other hand, questioned whether the absence of a link between SLG/LD and mortality in DATATOP was related to inexact ascertainment of the number of deaths or to an atypical selection process for study participants.[56]

Selegiline remains a controversial drug. It cannot be stated with certainty whether it is neuroprotective or whether it increases mortality in PD. For those not convinced of its link to increased mortality, the drug may be useful for delaying the need for LD therapy.

## Dopamine Agonists

Dopamine agonists exert their clinical effect through direct stimulation of dopamine receptors. Clinical trials have attempted to evaluate their efficacy, both as monotherapy and as adjunctive treatment, as well as to establish the relative use of the different agents in this class of drugs. There are five orally administered dopamine agonists currently in use: bromocriptine (Parlodel), pergolide (Permax), pramipexole (Mirapex), ropinirole (Requip), and cabergoline (Dostinex). Cabergoline is not marketed in North America for the treatment of Parkinson's disease. Although there are differences between these agents, there are even more similarities. There are, however, some basic questions of use and efficacy that can be raised about this entire class of agents. One of the most controversial issues is whether early use of these agents alone or as an adjunct to LD results in any long-term benefit, especially a reduced incidence of motor complications. Retrospective surveys[57] were the first studies to suggest that this might be true. Later, double-blind studies comparing dopamine agonist monotherapy with LD monotherapy in early PD also concluded that the risk of developing motor complications was significantly less in those receiving agonists.[58] However, this notion is not universally accepted. It is generally noted that monotherapy with dopamine agonists, although associated with less risk of dyskinesia, has a more limited duration of benefit because only approximately 30% of PD patients continue to be adequately treated by this approach for more than 3 years without requiring LD.[59] A 4-year double-blind study of BRC versus LD versus combination therapy concluded that early

180    *Clinical Trials in Neurologic Practice*

combination therapy with LD plus BRC did not prevent or delay the onset of motor fluctuations.[60] In this study, as in most others, LD was found to have superior efficacy in relieving motor symptoms of PD. Another benefit of dopamine agonist therapy that became apparent early is its ability to ameliorate end-of-dose deterioration in patients receiving LD. In an early open-label study, a mean dosage of 22 mg of BRC resulted in a 43% reduction in wearing off, accompanied by a 15% reduction in LD dosage.[61]

These general observations regarding the potential benefits and shortcomings of dopamine agonist monotherapy, as well as their role in treating motor fluctuations, apply to each of the available agents in this class. There are, however, slight differences between the agents in terms of efficacy, side-effect profile, and, possibly, their relative use as long-term monotherapy.

## Bromocriptine

The efficacy of BRC in PD and its potential to exert an LD-sparing effect have been demonstrated in double-blind, randomized crossover studies.[62,63] In a 3-year double-blind multicenter study of 129 de novo PD patients,[64] low-dose LD-carbidopa (less than 600/150 mg/day) was found to be a more effective treatment than low-dose monotherapy with BRC (less than 30 mg/day), although more prone to cause dyskinesias.[60] The potential benefit of BRC's LD-sparing effect was demonstrated in a 42-month study in which a 30% substitution of LD by BRC in early PD reduced the risk of motor fluctuations by one-third compared to LD monotherapy.[65] A slow-release BRC formulation has been evaluated and found to have similar efficacy in the treatment of PD with a slightly less severe side effect profile than standard BRC.[66]

## Pergolide

The efficacy of pergolide (PRG) as an adjunctive treatment to LD in patients with advanced PD has been demonstrated in several double-blind, placebo-controlled randomized trials.[67–69] PRG improved motor fluctuations and decreased "off" periods significantly in a 6-month study evaluating its efficacy as adjunctive therapy in patients receiving LD.[68] A 3-year follow-up of this cohort revealed that 56% remained on PRG therapy, and for those who discontinued treatment, confusion and hallucinations were the most frequent reasons.[70] A 6-month double-blind trial enrolling 376 subjects showed that PRG added to LD resulted in significant improvement in total UPDRS score, ADL and motor scores, and number of "off" hours, and allowed a 25% mean reduction in LD dose.[69]

The advent of PRG prompted studies comparing it to BRC. BRC and PRG had a similar spectrum of clinical effects in 24 patients receiving monotherapy in a randomized, double-blind, two-period crossover study.[71] In another study, patients who had lost benefit from PRG were changed to BRC in open-label fashion, but no additional benefit was noted.[72] However, when 63 patients who failed BRC therapy for various reasons were changed to PRG, 31 experienced a good response and tolerated the new agent.[73]

*Clinical Trials in Parkinson's Disease* 181

## Pramipexole (PRM)

PRM is an orally active dopamine agonist with selective activity at the dopamine D2 receptor family and preferential affinity for the D3 receptor subtype. Unlike BRC and PRG, it is not an ergot derivative. A multicenter, parallel group, double-blind, placebo-controlled, 10-week clinical trial randomized 264 patients to placebo and monotherapy with different PRM doses ranging from 1.5 to 6.0 mg per day. Ninety-eight percent of the placebo group and 67–81% of the PRM group were able to complete the study depending on dosage assignment. The adverse experiences and withdrawals were more frequent in the highest dose group. All PRM groups showed significant improvement in total UPDRS scores compared to placebo.[74] The efficacy and safety of PRM monotherapy were confirmed in a multicenter, randomized, double-blind trial of 335 patients. After a 7-week dose-escalation phase, the subjects were followed for 24 weeks with a mean daily maintenance dose of 3.8 mg. Significant improvements in the UPDRS ADL and motor examination scale scores emerged at week 3 of the dose-escalation period and persisted throughout the study. Although approximately 80% of patients finished the study in both groups, adverse events such as nausea, insomnia, constipation, somnolence, and visual hallucinations were more frequent in the PRM group.[75]

The use of PRM as adjunctive therapy has also been demonstrated. Reduction of "off" period severity and duration, improvement of motor function in both "on" and "off" stages, and decrease in daily LD requirement were observed in a double-blind, placebo-controlled parallel group study.[76] The relative efficacy of BRC and PRM for this purpose has been studied. In a 6-month study of 247 moderate to advanced patients with "wearing off," subjects were randomized to placebo to as much as 4.5 mg per day of PRM or to 30 mg per day of BRC. UPDRS ADL scores improved significantly for PRM (27.7%) and for BRC (14%) versus placebo (4.8%). UPDRS motor scores also showed significant improvements for PRM (34%) and BRC (23.8%) versus placebo (5.7%). Although both BRC and PRM were superior to placebo, the study was not powered to show statistical differences between the BRC and PRM active treatment groups.

## Ropinirole

Ropinirole (RPN) is another nonergoline dopamine agonist that binds specifically to the D2 receptor family. RPN monotherapy has been shown to be efficacious and safe in patients with early PD in several randomized, double-blind, placebo-controlled clinical trials. In a 6-month study, 241 patients, stratified by concomitant use of SLG, were randomized to placebo or different doses of RPN (1.5–8.0 mg t.i.d.). The UPDRS motor score improved by 24% in the RPN group and deteriorated by 3% in the placebo group.[77] The 6-month extension of this study enrolled 147 patients who successfully completed the initial study and showed that RPN was still effective at the end of 12 months. The combined results indicated that after 12 months, 19% of the RPN group required initiation of LD therapy, compared to 46% of the placebo group. Another study of 63 patients showed that, compared to placebo, the RPN group had significantly more improvement

182    *Clinical Trials in Neurologic Practice*

in the UPDRS motor score (43.4% versus 21.0%), a greater number of responders, and more improvement in the clinician's global evaluation.[78] As is the case for other agonists, LD has been shown to be more efficacious than RPN monotherapy. In a planned 6-month interim analysis of a 5-year study comparing RPN and LD, UPDRS motor scores improved significantly more with LD (44% versus 32%), although there was no significant difference in the frequency of "responders." Of importance, improvement in clinical global impression scores for those on RPN or LD were similar in mild patients (Hoehn-Yahr stages II and less), but LD resulted in greater improvement for advanced patients (stages II and III).[79] This observation suggests that monotherapy with an agonist, in this case, RPN, can be satisfactory for mild PD patients but may not be sufficient once significant motoric disability supervenes. Although no direct comparisons between RPN and PRM have been made, RPN has been compared to BRC. In a planned 6-month interim analysis of a 3-year double-blind, randomized, multicenter study, 335 patients were stratified by concomitant use of SLG and randomized to RPN or BRC. UPDRS motor examination scores and the proportion of responders were significantly better in the RPN group. However, in the subgroup analysis, this difference was not detected in those taking SLG concomitantly.[80]

RPN, similar to other agonists, is also effective in improving motor fluctuations. In a 3-month randomized, placebo-controlled trial, RPN administered as adjunctive therapy along with LD significantly reduced the duration of "off" periods in 46 patients with moderate motor disability and motor fluctuations.[81]

The benefit of RPN in delaying the onset of dyskinesias was demonstrated in a 5-year, prospective, randomized, double-blind study comparing its safety and efficacy with that of LD in 268 patients with early Parkinson's disease.[82] Forty-seven percent in the RPN group and 51% in the LD group completed the study. In the RPN group, 34% of the patients received no LD supplementation. The analysis of the time of onset of dyskinesia showed a significant difference in favor of RPN. At 5 years, the cumulative incidence of dyskinesia, regardless of LD supplementation, was 20% in the RPN group and 45% in the LD group. There was no significant difference between the two groups in the mean change of the UPDRS activities of daily living score among those who completed the study. However, the difference in improvement of the UPDRS mean motor-function scores was significant in favor of the LD group, which needs to be taken into consideration when interpreting the results.

Cabergoline

Cabergoline (CBG) is an ergoline dopamine agonist with a half-life exceeding 48 hours, allowing it to be administered once a day. Its efficacy as monotherapy in mild PD has been investigated and compared to that of LD. No significant difference in clinical improvement or adverse events between the CBG monotherapy and LD groups were noted at the end of the first year in 413 de novo patients studied in a randomized, double-blind study.[83] A greater number of CBG-treated patients than LD-treated patients required supplemental LD, yet at the end of 1 year, 62% could still be maintained on CBG alone. The continuation of this study for 3–5 years demonstrated more than a 50% lower relative risk for motor fluctuations and dyskinesia for those in the CBG group (22%), compared to subjects randomized to LD (34%).[58]

The long-term efficacy of adjunctive CBG therapy in patients with motor fluctuations and dyskinesias on chronic LD therapy was initially demonstrated in open-label trials of 6–12 months duration.[84–86] In one of these studies,[86] CBG was added to the LD regimen of 17 patients with persistent motor fluctuations, during which LD was slightly reduced. The UPDRS motor score and the proportion of "off" time spent during waking hours improved significantly in the eight patients who were able to complete 1 year of study. Seven of these patients were followed for as many as 39 months without any subsequent increase in the percentage of "off" hours.[87]

Other studies have also demonstrated the efficacy of CBG as adjunctive therapy in LD-treated patients with fluctuating responses.[88,89] In a 6-month placebo-controlled trial of patients experiencing short-duration LD responses,[89] the CBG group had significantly improved UPDRS motor scores and timed hand-tapping test scores, compared to those receiving placebo. Reflecting the extremely long half-life of CBG, this effect was consistently observed before the first LD and CBG dose of the day, throughout the LD interdose interval, and as long as 48 hours after the last CBG dose. In a subsequent open-label dose-escalation phase, further improvement was documented as the dosage was gradually raised to 10 mg daily without significantly increased dyskinesias as long as LD was concomitantly reduced.

The relative efficacy of CBG compared to other agonists has been infrequently evaluated. In a study comparing CBG and BCR, CBG (up to 6 mg/day) was given as a single morning dose and was found to be at least as effective as BCR (up to 40 mg/day). The improvement in motor UPDRS scores and the frequency of adverse events were similar in both groups. However, the percentage of awake hours "on" was higher in those treated with CBG.[90]

Sudden irresistible attacks of sleep (mostly without warning) deserve attention as a possible side effect of PRM and RPN. Eight PD patients taking PRM and one taking RPN fell asleep while driving, causing accidents. The attacks ceased when the drugs were stopped.[91] Subsequent reports have suggested that virtually all dopamine agonists have the potential to result in this adverse effect.[92]

Another dopamine agonist, apomorphine, can be an effective, and relatively immediate, rescue agent for parkinsonian off-states, when administered intranasally, as documented in a double-blind, placebo-controlled crossover trial.[93]


Summary

Most studies suggest that dopamine agonists used as monotherapy result in fluctuations and dyskinesias, less frequently than LD, possibly by more closely mimicking the physiologic tonic release of dopamine from normal nigral neurons as a result of their longer duration of action. Their use as monotherapy in early PD may help to retard the onset of motor fluctuations of dyskinesias, although there is no certain clinical evidence of a neuroprotective effect. Despite these positive features, in the majority of patients, dopamine agonist monotherapy provides less clinical benefit than LD, requires a longer time to titrate to an

184    *Clinical Trials in Neurologic Practice*

effective dose than LD, and usually must be supplemented with LD within a variable period of time.

Dopamine agonists are very useful as adjunctive therapy to LD in patients with advanced PD, often improving end-of-dose deterioration, allowing a reduction in LD dosage, and, as a consequence, reducing dyskinesias. A general criticism of clinical trials evaluating the effect of dopaminergic agonists in advanced PD is patient selection. Typically, patients with dementia, orthostasis, random on/off oscillations, or diphasic dyskinesia are excluded from these studies, leaving the clinician without objectively determined suggestions as to the proper role of these agents in the management of the most complicated PD patients.

## Catechol-O-Methyltransferase Inhibition

The enzyme catechol-O-methyltransferase (COMT) is localized in glial cells of the brain, in addition to extracerebral tissues, with the highest representation in the gut and liver. It is responsible for the peripheral degradation of LD to 3-O-methyldopa (3-OMD), through the transfer of a methyl group from *S*-adenosyl-L-methionine to the 3-hydroxyl group of LD.[94] LD that escapes this conversion can cross the BBB and be metabolized to dopamine. The primary role of peripheral COMT inhibition lies in its ability to enhance LD entry into the brain by increasing its bioavailability and lowering plasma concentrations of 3-OMD.[95] Drugs that inhibit this peripheral enzymatic degradation process extend the duration of action of LD, resulting in less severe motor fluctuations and "wearing off" associated with LD monotherapy.[96] However, it has been postulated, but not proven, that high plasma 3-OMD levels resulting from the action of COMT may play a role in the development of motor fluctuations and dyskinesias in PD.

Two reversible COMT inhibitors, tolcapone (Tasmar) and entacapone (Comtan), have been the focus of recent investigation. They represent an exclusively adjunctive therapy used to slow the elimination of LD, thus extending its plasma half-life and duration of effect. Both agents possess peripheral COMT-inhibitory effects; however, TC exhibits an additional central effect through its ability to cross the BBB,[97] the clinical benefit of which has yet to be elucidated. The addition of COMT inhibitors to LD therapy does not increase peak plasma LD concentrations, but pharmacokinetic studies have demonstrated that both agents[98,99] increase the plasma LD area under the curve (AUC). Increasing the plasma LD AUC may allow for a reduction of total daily LD dosage by as much as 30%, and offers smoother LD availability to the central nervous system.

### Tolcapone

Clinical trials examined the pharmacokinetic and pharmacodynamic efficacy of tolcapone (TC) in humans. A double-blind, randomized, placebo-controlled, two-way crossover study design[100] demonstrated excellent tolerability of single TC dosages between 10 and 800 mg in combination with a fixed LD/BZ dosage (100/25) in healthy volunteers. In addition, this trial demonstrated that the maximum effect on LD occurred at a TC dosage of 200 mg. Although the LD AUC and elimination half-life increased twofold on TC, the drug had no effect on LD $C_{max}$. TC was rapidly absorbed, with an average $T_{max}$ of 1.5 hours and a half-life of 2.3 hours. No appreciable hepatic toxicity was noted in any of the treatment arms.

A later trial[101] assessed the clinical pharmacology of t.i.d. TC doses of 100, 200, 400, or 800 mg among 48 elderly subjects. At dosages of 400 and 800 mg t.i.d., an increased $C_{max}$ and AUC for TC were noted. These studies, suggesting a stable, predictable, and well-tolerated TC response profile at 100 mg and 200 mg t.i.d. dosing in healthy human subjects, and a salutary effect on the LD AUC, paved the way for subsequent trials in PD patients.

A multicenter, randomized, double-blind, parallel group, placebo-controlled, dose-finding study evaluated the safety and efficacy of TC doses at 50, 200, and 400 mg t.i.d. for 6 weeks in PD patients experiencing end-of-dose LD-dependent motor fluctuations.[102] At 6 weeks, there was an extension of duration of LD benefit ("on" time) by 25% at all dosage levels compared to placebo, and an average 40% decrease in "off" time. An increase in the LD AUC was noted among all subjects within the three TC treatment arms. TC 200 mg and 400 mg t.i.d. treatment arms demonstrated the most significant improvement in UPDRS motor scores and allowed for the greatest reduction in daily LD. No dose-limiting effects were experienced by participants; however, TC was noted to increase the prevalence, frequency, and intensity of LD-induced dyskinesia during the first week of therapy, necessitating a subsequent reduction in daily LD dosage.

TC's adjunctive efficacy and safety has also been demonstrated in PD patients receiving LD but not experiencing motor fluctuations. In a multicenter, randomized, double-blind, parallel-group, placebo-controlled trial conducted over 12 months, participants with a stable response to LD were randomized to treatment of placebo, TC 100 mg t.i.d., or TC 200 mg t.i.d.[103] This study demonstrated a clear improvement in UPDRS ADL and motor disability scores in both TC treatment groups when compared to placebo controls. Both TC treatment groups had a decrease in mean daily LD dose, whereas the placebo group required an increase in dosage. Over the 12 months, both TC treatment groups demonstrated reduction in the physical scale of the sickness impact profile score, but not in the total or psychosocial scales.

Of the adverse effects experienced in this study, only diarrhea (13%) resulted in more terminations in treated patients than controls. Although TC was generally well tolerated at both treatment dosages, a significant elevation in the liver enzymes, alanine aminotransferase, and aspartate aminotransferase developed in eight patients, requiring their withdrawal from the study. Liver functions returned to normal levels within 2–4 weeks after withdrawal of TC. Roche laboratories has issued an alert regarding four reported cases of fatal fulminant hepatic failure in patients receiving TC. Based on this experience, it has been suggested that patients who are candidates for TC therapy have normal liver function tests documented before treatment, and agree to undergo biweekly liver enzyme blood sampling thereafter. In view of this potentially serious adverse event, the published treatment guidelines suggest that patients not demonstrating clear symptomatic clinical benefit within 3 weeks of treatment initiation have TC withdrawn.

The results of this multicenter study raise the question as to whether the same degree of benefit seen in patients receiving this LD-enhancing agent could have been achieved as easily by simply administering more LD. The authors address

186    *Clinical Trials in Neurologic Practice*

this issue by pointing out that the placebo group did, in fact, receive more LD and did not fare as well in most efficacy measures as those receiving TC. Although pharmacokinetic studies were not performed in this trial, TC's ability to increase the AUC without an increase in the LD $C_{max}$ may be the basis of the improvement noted, in part by avoiding the putative adverse effects of more variable plasma LD levels that might result from LD alone.

To determine whether this new agent is truly superior to existing therapies in improving motor fluctuations, an 8-week open-label, randomized, multicenter trial was conducted to examine the relative efficacy of TC 200 mg t.i.d. and the dopamine agonist, BRC, in LD-treated PD patients experiencing "end-of-dose" deterioration.[104] The dosage of LD was adjusted in the TC group to minimize LD-induced adverse events. In the BRC treatment group, dosages of LD were adjusted to manage adverse motor events, and BRC was adjusted in response to nonmotor dopaminergic complications. Both TC and BRC treatment groups experienced a reduction in total daily LD dosage of 33% and 11%, respectively, although the difference in reduction of total daily LD dosage was not statistically significant. Similarly, no statistically significant difference between groups was noted in total "on" or "off" time. The greatest difference between the TC and BRC treatment groups was the side-effect profile, the former experiencing more muscle cramps and dystonia, and the latter demonstrating a higher incidence of hallucinations, orthostatic hypotension, and nausea.

## Entacapone

Entacapone (EC), in contrast to TC, is an exclusively peripheral COMT inhibitor. An early dose-response study of EC examined its effect on the pharmacokinetics of LD and the resulting clinical response in 20 advanced PD patients known to exhibit motor fluctuations.[105] This randomized, double-blind, placebo-controlled, single-graded dose, crossover design consisted of five 1-day treatment periods. During the 5 test days, patients received single doses of EC (50, 100, 200, or 400 mg) or placebo in combination with standard LD/decarboxylase inhibitor. The LD $C_{max}$ was virtually unchanged at all dosages of EC, but LD $T_{max}$ was delayed, and LD half-life was prolonged after a 200-mg dosage. The LD AUC demonstrated a 23% increase after 200 mg of EC compared to placebo, with similar results achieved at higher dosages. The highest increase in mean on-time (21%) and the greatest prolongation of dyskinesias (32%) were noted after administration of 200-mg EC, compared to placebo. However, the magnitude of dyskinesias was unaffected at all EC dosages, corresponding to an unchanged LD $C_{max}$. Similar results, suggesting improvement in "on" time were obtained when subjects were maintained on 200 mg of EC for 24 weeks in a randomized, placebo-controlled, double-blind, parallel group, multicenter trial, examining PD patients with end-of-dose wearing-off.[106]

The pharmacokinetic and pharmacodynamic effects of EC in patients receiving sustained-release LD were evaluated in a 5-week open-label, randomized, single-graded dose crossover design trial. Dosages of 100, 200, 400, and 800 mg were administered to 12 healthy volunteers receiving a fixed dose of controlled-release CD/LD (50/200 CR).[107] In this study, LD AUC was maximally increased by only 33% after a 400-mg dose of EC; other investigators[105] had demonstrated a much greater increase of 65% after a 400-mg dose in patients receiving the standard formulation of LD. The dissimilarity between these results may be due to the difference in absorption times of EC and controlled-release LD formulations, the former being absorbed much more rapidly than controlled-release LD, resulting in the almost complete elimination of EC at the time of maximal plasma LD concentration. These results suggest that an optimal dosage of 200-mg EC administered with controlled-release LD formulations is efficacious in increasing the LD AUC, although this effect on LD is slightly less than that with standard LD, owing to the mismatch in absorption profiles. The $T_{max}$ of EC is 0.4–0.9 hours and elimination half-life is 0.3–0.4 hours, both considerably shorter than that associated with TC, suggesting that serial dosing of EC may be required after a single dose of Sinemet CR, considering the prolonged plasma LD levels resulting from this formulation.

## SURGICAL TREATMENT OF PARKINSON'S DISEASE

The history of functional neurosurgery for PD has recently been reviewed.[108] It began in 1921, with bilateral cervical rhizotomy, followed in the 1930s by motor corticectomy and lesioning the corticospinal tract at different levels. Transventricular surgery of the basal ganglia was performed by Myers in 1939 but was associated with significant surgical morbidity. Spiegel and Wycis performed the first stereotactic functional surgery in 1947, initially targeting the globus pallidus and ansa lenticularis. The lateral thalamus then became the preferred target in the 1950s with a few surgeons preferring the subthalamic nucleus (STN). The number of stereotactic operations declined dramatically toward the end of the 1960s when LD became available, but intractable complications of LD kept interest in surgery alive. The interest in functional neurosurgery for PD accelerated in the 1990s as a result of better understanding of basal ganglia physiology and significant advances in neuroradiology and electrophysiology.

The major surgical approaches in PD include ablative surgery (pallidotomy, thalamotomy); deep brain stimulation (DBS) of the thalamus, globus pallidus interna, and STN; and grafting of human or porcine fetal mesencephalic cells into the striatum. Attempting a traditional double-blind, placebo-controlled clinical trial to evaluate surgical procedures such as these presents major procedural hurdles. Blinding the patient and including a placebo treatment often require that a sham procedure be performed, a step that may prompt ethical concerns. Blinding the investigator is also difficult, but can be accomplished by using blinded raters other than the treating surgeon. Various techniques have been used to accomplish this latter goal.

### Thalamus

Thalamotomy

This procedure had been the traditional surgical treatment for tremor, but is now being overtaken in use by DBS of the thalamus. In an open study of 36

188    *Clinical Trials in Neurologic Practice*

PD patients undergoing ventral intermediate (VIM) thalamotomy for tremor control in the post-LD era, 86% had complete abolition of tremor and another 5% had significant improvement. Significant complications including dyspraxia, dysarthria, dysphagia, or abulia were noted in 14% of patients, but were not disabling in most.[109] Other open-label studies of this therapy for PD tremor reported benefit as well.[110,111] One group of investigators used blinded rating of videotapes to determine the relative severity of tremor on each side of the body.[112] They observed that after thalamotomy the laterality of the most predominant tremor changed and remained so for the long term, indicating reduction in tremor amplitude or inhibition of tremor progression on the operated side, or both.

Radiosurgical VIM thalamotomy using the gamma knife has also been performed with mixed results. In one study, only 50% of PD patients had an excellent response or complete relief of tremor.[113] In contrast, in another study of 27 patients with PD, 88% of patients became tremor-free or nearly tremor-free without any serious complications after gamma knife VIM thalamotomy.[114] In this study, blind raters and nonoperated PD controls were used.

### Thalamic Deep Brain Stimulation

An 8-year open-label experience with DBS of the thalamus in 117 patients, including 80 with PD and 20 with essential tremor, demonstrated that the procedure is well tolerated even by patients undergoing bilateral surgery (74 of 117 patients) and by elderly patients.[115] Tremor, but not bradykinesia or rigidity, was selectively suppressed in PD for as long as 8 years with more than 30% reduction in LD requirement in 40 patients. In essential tremor patients, results were satisfactory but deteriorated with time in 18.5% of cases. In another study, unilateral DBS of the VIM nucleus was found to be safe and efficacious in 29 patients with essential tremor and 24 patients with PD. After 1 year, there was still significant reduction in both essential and PD tremor based on raters who were blind to the "stimulator ON" and "stimulator OFF" state.[116] It has been suggested that the greatest reduction in disability is associated with improved postural tremor for both ET (essential tremor) and PD.[117]

A retrospective comparison of thalamotomy and thalamic DBS was conducted.[118] In a total of 19 thalamic DBS implants (16 for PD, 3 for essential tremor) and 26 thalamotomies (23 for PD and 3 for ET) performed over 6 years and followed for at least 3 months, complete tremor abolition occurred in 42% of both groups, near abolition in 79% and 69%, respectively, and recurrence in 5% and 15%. To achieve these results, 15% of thalamotomies, but no DBS implantation, had to be repeated. Ataxia, dysarthria, and gait disturbance were more common after thalamotomy (42%) than DBS (26%), and with DBS these complications could often be resolved by adjusting stimulation parameters.[118] Another potential benefit of thalamic DBS in PD was illustrated in a study demonstrating that peak-dose LD dyskinesias were greatly improved in each of 10 cases, and biphasic dyskinesias improved in two of three cases during 22–34 months of follow-up after the procedure.[119]

## Globus Pallidus Interna

Pallidotomy

In PD, excessive inhibitory activity of the globus pallidus interna (GPI), in large part due to excessive drive from the STN, is thought to "brake" the motor thalamus and the cortical motor system to produce the bradykinesia and the rigidity that are characteristic of this disorder. Modern intraoperative techniques have allowed much more accurate localization of lesions within the GPI. Based on a distinct frequency and pattern of single cell activity, GPI can be identified and mapped with a high degree of precision through microelectrode recording and stimulation. Micro- and macrostimulation can be used to locate the adjacent optic tract and internal capsule to avoid undesired lesioning of these structures.[120]

In 1992, Laitinen[121] reported his experience in 38 patients who underwent stereotactic lesioning of the posteroventral region of the GPI with a mean follow-up period of 28 months (range, 2–71 months). Besides great improvement of LD-induced dyskinesias, 92% of patients experienced significant relief of rigidity and bradykinesia, and 81% noted improved tremor. Persistent partial homonymous hemianopsia was reported in six patients as a result of damage to the optic tract. In a later study,[122] 18 patients with marked response fluctuations and dyskinesia underwent unilateral posteroventral pallidotomy (PVP) and were evaluated for 1 year. This study demonstrated a finding that has been repeatedly demonstrated since, namely that "off" scores improve more than "on" scores after PVP. The "off" scores improved 65% in this study as measured by UPDRS in the contralateral limb, and improved by 24.2% in the ipsilateral limb. No morbidity or mortality was reported. Follow-up of 11 of these patients for as many as 4 years revealed persistent contralateral improvement, and continued mild ipsilateral benefits in motor symptoms and dyskinesia during which they maintained a relatively stable LD dosage.[123] In a trial using blinded videotape evaluators,[124] 14 patients who underwent microelectrode-guided PVP had a 30% improvement in UPDRS "off" motor scores and a similar benefit in akinesia and postural stability, with almost total elimination of contralateral dyskinesias. In an investigation using similar evaluation techniques, comparable success was reported in 34 patients at 3-month's follow-up.[125] Several additional PVP series have demonstrated contralateral benefit,[126,127] but at least one has shown that ipsilateral benefit is not only less substantial, but may also wane within the first year.[126]

The effect of age on the outcome of PVP has been investigated by several groups with conflicting results. In the Emory pilot study,[127] older patients fared worse than younger subjects. A similar trend was noted by other investigators,[123] although it did not reach statistical significance. On the other hand, an evaluation of 20 consecutive advanced PD patients found no difference in the safety and efficacy of PVP between patients older or younger than 65 years.[128] A study investigating other risk factors compared preoperative MRI and outcomes and found that mild to moderate degrees of cortical atrophy, ventriculomegaly, and ischemic encephalopathy did not predispose patients to less favorable outcomes after unilateral PVP, although the presence of status cribriformis and lacunes were associated with a higher risk of transient side effects.[129]

190    *Clinical Trials in Neurologic Practice*

A major, and as of yet unresolved, procedural question involving PVP has centered around the clinical usefulness of microelectrode recording during the procedure. An investigation using postoperative MRI analysis showed that intra-operative microelectrode recording helped to achieve accurate placement of the lesion. However, no consistent correlation was found between lesion size and location and clinical outcome as measured by UPDRS and global outcome scores.[130] Similar successful results with PVP have been reported when computed tomography rather than magnetic resonance imaging (MRI) was used,[131] and microelectrode recording was omitted.[131,132]

The motoric benefits of PVP must be weighed against modest cognitive and behavioral risks associated with the procedure. Forty-two patients (24 right and 18 left hemisphere) were evaluated in the "on" state before PVP and afterward for as long as 24 months.[133] Modest improvement in sustained attention, but a decline in working memory, was observed by 6 months after surgery. Left-hemisphere lesions were associated with the loss of verbal learning and fluency in 60% of patients by 3–4 months without recovery. Right-hemisphere lesions led to loss of visuospatial construction abilities that were resolved in almost all patients by 1 year. Behavioral changes reflecting frontal dysfunction were reported in 30 patients. The relative impact of bilateral versus unilateral PVP on psychometric tests was addressed in a retrospective review of a consecutive series of eight simultaneous bilateral (BPVP) and 12 unilateral procedures. Except for one case of generalized impairment after BPVP, cognitive sequelae were restricted to selective reductions in categorical verbal fluency after both unilateral procedures and BPVP, and a reduction in phonemic verbal fluency after BPVP.[134]

The proximity of GPI to the optic tract has raised concerns about visual field defects resulting from PVP. In an early series,[121] Laitinen noted a 14% incidence of visual field cuts, but in two subsequent larger series[135,136] this complication appeared in less than 3% of patients, most likely related to improved lesion localization techniques.

Other facets of PVP have received some attention in the literature, but have been tested widely. PVP in LD-unresponsive parkinsonism has been found to be of limited or no benefit.[137] The use of gamma knife functional radiosurgical lesioning for older patients and those with major systemic diseases or coagulopathies has been suggested and attempted with inconsistent results.[114,138,139]

## Globus Pallidus Interna Stimulation

As a reversible alternative to PVP, DBS of the GPI has been shown by several groups to have motoric benefits that are comparable to PVP.[140–142] In one study, semantic verbal fluency and visuoconstructional test scores declined 3 months after GPI DBS in five of nine patients. However, no significant decline in the overall level of cognitive functioning was documented.[143] The efficacy of pallidal DBS relative to that of PVP has been studied in a prospective randomized trial.[144] Patients assigned to DBS achieved comparable benefit on UPDRS rating scales and ADL scores compared to those receiving PVP, although dyskinesias were more improved in the latter group. In some patients, the two procedures can be combined. A recent double-blind study suggested that patients having undergone a previous unilateral PVP could benefit from subsequent contralateral pallidal DBS.[145]

## Subthalamic Nucleus

DBS of the STN in advanced PD with motor fluctuations is another surgical treatment option. In an open study, 20 of 24 patients with bilaterally implanted STN electrodes were followed for 12 months. The UPDRS ADL and motor scores off medication improved by 60%. In contrast to reports on PVP, when "on," the UPDRS motor scores also improved significantly. The mean dosage of dopaminergic drugs was reduced by one-half. Cognitive performance scores remained unchanged, but one patient developed aphasia related to an intraoperative cerebral hemorrhage.[146] A double-blind evaluation of efficacy 6–12 months after chronic STN DBS in seven patients revealed similar improvement in both "on" and "off" scores, improvement in dyskinesias, and reduction in LD dosage.[147]

A small number of studies have been reported comparing GPI and STN DBS. A retrospective comparison of chronic STN (n = 8) versus GPI DBS (n = 5) in consecutive young onset patients with motor fluctuations and dyskinesia favored STN rather than GPI stimulation. In off-drug phases, the UPDRS motor score was improved by 71% with STN DBS versus 39% with GPI stimulation. In the on-drug phases, there was a marked improvement in dyskinesias in the GPI group, whereas significantly less dyskinesia benefit was noted in the STN group. However, with STN stimulation, the LD-equivalent dose could be reduced by 56%, leading to an indirect reduction of dyskinesia similar to that achieved in the GPI group.[148] Similar results were noted at the 3-month follow-up in an open study with eight patients undergoing GPI DBS (four unilateral and four bilateral) and six patients treated with STN DBS (five bilateral and one unilateral) at the 3-month follow-up.[149] A randomized trial may ultimately be required to determine which procedure is most effective for patients with different clinical features.

## Tissue Graft Therapies

The first tissue transplantation therapy to attract interest in the LD era was the adrenal graft. Preliminary case studies and small series in the 1980s reported symptomatic benefit from transplantation of adrenal medullary tissue to the putamen[150] or caudate nucleus.[151] However, based on subsequent experience showing limited benefit and significant mortality,[152] the procedure was largely abandoned.

Human fetal nigral grafts have been performed in a limited number of PD patients, and the results have been subjected to careful examination. In early studies, two patients with advanced PD showed significant and sustained improvement of motor function after unilateral intraputaminal implantation of fetal ventral mesencephalic tissue (age 6–7 weeks postconception) during a 3-year follow-up. In both patients, positron emission tomography (PET) scans demonstrated that [18F]dopa uptake increased within the operated putamen despite a progressive decrease in tracer uptake in unoperated striatal structures, suggesting functional integrity within a surviving neural graft.[153] Similarly, two patients with MPTP-induced parkinsonism demonstrated sustained improvement in motor function and increased striatal uptake of fluorodopa as long as 2 years after bilateral fetal mesencephalic grafting.[154] Since these early open trials, relatively consistent success has been observed in subsequent trials,[155,156] although one with a mean follow-up

192    *Clinical Trials in Neurologic Practice*

of 21 months revealed a slight deterioration in benefit with time.[157] A great variety of issues relating to identification of the optimal surgical technique for nigral grafts remain to be resolved. These include donor age, tissue storage (fresh, cryopreserved, or storage in medium), graft preparation (solid or cell suspension), implantation site (postcommissural putamen or caudate or both), laterality (bilateral versus unilateral), and the need for immunosuppressive drugs.[158] One question that has been reasonably well resolved is that transplanted nigral cells survive. Direct evidence that fetal nigral tissue can survive and innervate the striatum has come from autopsy studies of two patients who had showed sustained improvement in motor function and increased fluorodopa uptake in PET scans, but died 18 months later from unrelated causes. Using tyrosine hydroxylase immunohistochemical methods, each of the large fetal grafts in these patients was shown to contain dense clusters of dopaminergic neurons that were integrated into the host striatum.[159–161]

Difficulty in obtaining human fetal tissue has generated interest in finding a nonhuman source of donor cells. Cross-species grafts have been explored. Postmortem histologic analysis in a PD patient 7 months after unilateral implantation of fetal porcine neural cells into the caudate-putamen region demonstrated graft survival and the presence of porcine dopaminergic neurons as well as other neural and glial cells.[162]

## Summary

Surgery is reserved for the treatment of disabling medically refractory fluctuations and dyskinesias in patients who do not have dementia or additional serious medical comorbidities. VIM thalamotomy or DBS is indicated exclusively for tremor and does not usually greatly improve other parkinsonian features. Pallidotomy often produces relief of LD-induced dyskinesias along with significant reduction in contralateral akinesia, rigidity, and tremor. Pallidal DBS, a reversible and adjustable alternative to pallidotomy, can be performed bilaterally to increase efficacy, with less risk of cognitive and bulbar dysfunction compared to ablative procedures. Bilateral STN DBS is reported to improve all motoric aspects of parkinsonism and reduce daily LD requirement. Although transplantation of autologous adrenal medulla to the striatum has been largely abandoned, transplantation of fetal mesencephalon has generated promising clinical results, as well as histologic and PET evidence of graft survival. Similar cell survival has been demonstrated in xenografts. Incorporating neurotrophic factors and gene therapy into these surgical approaches is being studied. Despite all these encouraging developments, it must be kept in mind that many reports of surgical treatment are the products of uncontrolled, nonrandomized studies, often with short follow-up periods. Although methodologies for blinded evaluation of videotapes and blinding the investigator to the stimulator "on" state have been developed, most studies of surgical treatment are open studies without control sham operations and with clear vulnerability to selection and evaluation bias.

An exception is a double-blind (sham surgery), controlled trial of embryonic dopaminergic tissue transplants in advanced Parkinson's disease that has been carried out. The results of this trial have not yet been published as of June 2000.[163] For most surgical procedures, however, randomized and controlled trials will be needed to establish their safety, efficacy, and proper indications.

## REFERENCES

1. Marshall FJ, Kieburtz K, McDermott M, et al. Clinical research in neurology. From observation to experimentation. Neurol Clin 1996;14:451–466.
2. Bull JP. The historical development of therapeutic trials. J Chron Dis 1959;10:218–248.
3. Ellwein LB, Drummond MF. Economic analysis alongside clinical trials. Bias in the assessment of economic outcomes. Int J Technol Assess Health Care 1996;12:691–697.
4. DeMets DL. Distinctions between fraud, bias, errors, misunderstanding, and incompetence. Controlled Clin Trials 1997;18:637–650.
5. Kurland LT. Epidemiology: Incidence, Geographic Distribution and Genetic Considerations. In WS Fields (ed), Pathogenesis and Treatment of Parkinsonism. Springfield, IL: 1985:5–43.
6. Wilson JM, Levey AI, Rajput A, et al. Differential changes in neurochemical markers of striatal dopamine nerve terminals in idiopathic Parkinson's disease. Neurology 1996;47:718–726.
7. Wenning GK, Tison F, Ben Shlomo Y, et al. Multiple system atrophy: a review of 203 pathologically proven cases. Mov Disord 1997;12:133–147.
8. Hughes AJ, Daniel SE, Kilford L, Lees AJ. Accuracy of clinical diagnosis of idiopathic Parkinson's disease: a clinico-pathological study of 100 cases. J Neurol Neurosurg Psychiatry 1992;55:181–184.
9. Fahn S, Elton RL, members of UPDRS Development Committee. Unified Parkinson's Disease Rating Scale. In S Fahn, CD Marsden, DB Calne, M Goldstein (eds), Recent Developments in Parkinson's Disease, Vol 2. Florham, NJ: MacMillan Health Care Information: 1987:153–164.
10. Gancher S. Scales for the Assessment of Movement Disorders. In RM Herndon (ed), Handbook of Neurologic Rating Scales. New York: Demos Verander, 1997:81–106.
11. Richards M, Marder K, Cote L, Mayeux R. Interrater reliability of the Unified Parkinson's Disease Rating Scale motor examination. Mov Disord 1994;9:89–91.
12. Cotzias GC, Papavasiliou PS, Gellene R. Modification of parkinsonism—chronic treatment with L-dopa. N Engl J Med 1969;280:337–345.
13. Mones RJ, Elizan TS, Siegel GJ. An analysis of L-dopa-induced dyskinesias in 152 cases of Parkinson's disease. Neurology 1970;20:405–406.
14. Cotzias GC. L-Dopa for Parkinsonism. N Engl J Med 1968;278:630.
15. Yahr MD, Duvoisin RC, Hoehn MM, et al. L-Dopa (L-3,4-dihydroxyphenylalanine)—its clinical effects in parkinsonism. Transactions of the American Neurological Association 1968;93:56–63.
16. Joseph C, Chassan JB, Koch ML. Levodopa in Parkinson disease: a long-term appraisal of mortality. Ann Neurol 1978;3:116–118.
17. Marttila RJ, Rinne UK, Siirtola T, Sonninen V. Mortality of patients with Parkinson's disease treated with levodopa. J Neurol 1977;216:147–153.
18. Rajput AH, Offord KP, Beard CM, Kurland LT. Epidemiology of parkinsonism: incidence, classification, and mortality. Ann Neurol 1984;16:278–282.
19. Caraceni T, Scigliano G, Musicco M. The occurrence of motor fluctuations in parkinsonian patients treated long term with levodopa: role of early treatment and disease progression. Neurology 1991;41:380–384.
20. Rajput AH, Fenton ME, Birdi S, Macaulay R. Is levodopa toxic to human substantia nigra? Mov Disord 1997;12:634–638.
21. Sweet RD, McDowell FH, Wasterlain CG, Stern PH. Treatment of "on-off effect" with a dopa decarboxylase inhibitor. Arch Neurol 1975;32:560–563.
22. Greenacre JK, Coxon A, Petrie A, Reid JL. Comparison of levodopa with carbidopa or benserazide in parkinsonism. Lancet 1976;2:381–384.
23. Pakkenberg H, Birket-Smith E, Dupont E, et al. Parkinson's disease treated with Sinemet or Madopar. A controlled multicenter trial. Acta Neurol Scand Suppl 1976;53:376–385.
24. Rinne UK, Molsa P. Levodopa with benserazide or carbidopa in Parkinson disease. Neurology 1979;29:1584–1589.
25. Tourtellotte WW, Syndulko K, Potvin AR, et al. Increased ratio of carbidopa to levodopa in treatment of Parkinson's disease. Arch Neurol 1980;37:723–726.
26. Kofman OS. Are levodopa "drug holidays" justified? Can J Neurol Sci 1984;11:206–209.
27. Nutt JG, Woodward WR, Hammerstad JP, et al. The "on-off" phenomenon in Parkinson's disease. Relation to levodopa absorption and transport. N Engl J Med 1984;310:483–488.
28. Carter JH, Nutt JG, Woodward WR, et al. Amount and distribution of dietary protein affects clinical response to levodopa in Parkinson's disease. Neurology 1989;39:552–556.

## 194    Clinical Trials in Neurologic Practice

29. Feldman RG, Mosbach PA, Kelly MR, Thomas CA, Saint Hilaire MH. Double-blind comparison of standard Sinemet and Sinemet CR in patients with mild-to-moderate Parkinson's disease. Neurology 1989;39:96–101;discussion 105.
30. Rondot P, Ziegler M, Aymard N, Teinturier A. Effect of controlled-release carbidopa/levodopa on motor performance in advanced Parkinson's disease. Neurology 1989;39:74–77;discussion 95.
31. Deleu D, Jacques M, Michotte Y, Ebinger G. Controlled-release carbidopa/levodopa (CR) in parkinsonian patients with response fluctuations on standard levodopa treatment: clinical and pharmacokinetic observations. Neurology 1989;39:88–92;discussion 95.
32. Hutton JT, Morris JL, Roman GC, et al. Treatment of chronic Parkinson's disease with controlled-release carbidopa/levodopa. Arch Neurol 1988;45:861–864.
33. Hutton JT, Morris JL, Bush DF, et al. Multicenter controlled study of Sinemet CR vs Sinemet (25/100) in advanced Parkinson's disease. Neurology 1989;39:67–72;discussion 72–73.
34. Hutton JT, Morris JL. Long-acting carbidopa-levodopa in the management of moderate and advanced Parkinson's disease. Neurology 1992;42:51–56;discussion 57–60.
35. Rodnitzky RL, Dickins QS, Dobson J. Long-term clinical efficacy of Sinemet CR in patients with Parkinson's disease. Neurology 1989;39:92–95;discussion 95.
36. Block G, Liss C, Reines S, et al. Comparison of immediate-release and controlled release carbidopa/levodopa in Parkinson's disease. A multicenter 5-year study. The CR First Study Group. Eur Neurol 1997;37:23–27.
37. Grahnen A, Eckernas SA, Collin C, et al. Comparative multiple-dose pharmacokinetics of controlled-release levodopa products. Eur Neurol 1992;32:343–348.
38. Dupont E, Andersen A, Boas J, et al. Sustained-release Madopar HBS compared with standard Madopar in the long-term treatment of de novo parkinsonian patients. Acta Neurol Scand Suppl 1996;93:14–20.
39. Kurth MC, Tetrud JW, Irwin I, et al. Oral levodopa/carbidopa solution versus tablets in Parkinson's patients with severe fluctuations: a pilot study. Neurology 1993;43:1036–1039.
40. Lees AJ, Shaw KM, Kohout LJ, et al. Deprenyl in Parkinson's disease. Lancet 1977;2:791–795.
41. Presthus J, Hajba A. Deprenyl (selegiline) combined with levodopa and a decarboxylase inhibitor in the treatment of Parkinson's disease. Acta Neurol Scand Suppl 1983;95:127–133.
42. Csanda E, Tarczy M. Clinical evaluation of deprenyl (selegiline) in the treatment of Parkinson's disease. Acta Neurol Scand Suppl 1983;95:117–122.
43. LeWitt P, Oakes D, Cui L. The need for levodopa as an end point of Parkinson's disease progression in a clinical trial of selegiline and alpha-tocopherol. Parkinson Study Group. Mov Disord 1997;12:183–189.
44. Parkinson Study Group. Effect of deprenyl on the progression of disability in early Parkinson's disease. N Engl J Med 1989;321:1364–1371.
45. Parkinson Study Group. Effects of tocopherol and deprenyl on the progression of disability in early Parkinson's disease. N Engl J Med 1993;328:176–183.
46. Parkinson Study Group. Impact of deprenyl and tocopherol treatment on Parkinson's disease in DATATOP subjects not requiring levodopa. Ann Neurol 1996;39:29–36.
47. Parkinson Study Group. Impact of deprenyl and tocopherol treatment on Parkinson's disease in DATATOP patients requiring levodopa. Ann Neurol 1996;39:37–45.
48. Palhagen S, Heinonen EH, Hagglund J, et al. Selegiline delays the onset of disability in de novo parkinsonian patients. Swedish Parkinson Study Group. Neurology 1998;51:520–525.
49. Olanow CW, Hauser RA, Gauger L, et al. The effect of deprenyl and levodopa on the progression of Parkinson's disease. Ann Neurol 1995;38:771–777.
50. Parkinson's Disease Research Group in the United Kingdom. Comparisons of therapeutic effects of levodopa, levodopa and selegiline, and bromocriptine in patients with early, mild Parkinson's disease: three year interim report. BMJ 1993;307:469–472.
51. Olanow CW, Fahn S, Langston JW, Godbold J. Selegiline and mortality in Parkinson's disease. Ann Neurol 1996;40:841–845.
52. Churchyard A, Mathias CJ, Boonkongchuen P, Lees AJ. Autonomic effects of selegiline: possible cardiovascular toxicity in Parkinson's disease. J Neurol Neurosurg Psychiatry 1997;63:228–234.
53. Turkka J, Suominen K, Tolonen U, et al. Selegiline diminishes cardiovascular autonomic responses in Parkinson's disease. Neurology 1997;48:662–667.
54. Olanow CW, Myllyla VV, Sotaniemi KA, et al. Effect of selegiline on mortality in patients with Parkinson's disease: a meta-analysis. Neurology 1998;51:825–830.
55. Parkinson Study Group. Mortality in DATATOP: a multicenter trial in early Parkinson's disease. Ann Neurol 1998;43:318–325.

Clinical Trials in Parkinson's Disease    195

56. Ben-Shlomo Y, Head J, Lees AJ. Mortality in DATATOP. Ann Neurol 1999;45:138–139.

57. Rinne UK. Early combination of bromocriptine and levodopa in the treatment of Parkinson's disease: a 5-year follow-up. Neurology 1987;37:826–828.

58. Rinne UK, Bracco F, Chouza C, et al. Early treatment of Parkinson's disease with cabergoline delays the onset of motor complications. Results of a double-blind levodopa controlled trial. The PKDS009 Study Group. Drugs 1998;55(Suppl 1):23–30.

59. Poewe W. Adjuncts to levodopa therapy: dopamine agonists. Neurology 1998;50:S23–S26.

60. Weiner WJ, Factor SA, Sanchez-Ramos JR, et al. Early combination therapy (bromocriptine and levodopa) does not prevent motor fluctuations in Parkinson's disease. Neurology 1993;43:21–27.

61. Grimes JD, King DB, Kofman OS, et al. Bromocriptine in the management of end of dose deterioration in Parkinson's disease. Can J Neurol Sci 1984;11:452–456.

62. Teychenne PF, Leigh PN, Reid JL, et al. Idiopathic parkinsonism treated with bromocriptine. Lancet 1975;2:473–476.

63. Kartzinel R, Teychenne P, Gillespie MM, et al. Bromocriptine and levodopa (with or without carbidopa) in parkinsonism. Lancet 1976;2:272–275.

64. Hely MA, Morris JG, Rail D, et al. The Sydney Multicentre Study of Parkinson's disease: a report on the first 3 years. J Neurol Neurosurg Psychiatry 1989;52:324–328.

65. Przuntek H, Welzel D, Gerlach M, et al. Early institution of bromocriptine in Parkinson's disease inhibits the emergence of levodopa-associated motor side effects. Long-term results of the PRADO study. J Neural Transm Gen Sect 1996;103:699–715.

66. Mannen T, Mizuno Y, Iwata M, et al. A multi-center, double-blind study on slow-release bromocriptine in the treatment of Parkinson's disease. Neurology 1991;41:1598–1602.

67. Sage JI, Duvoisin RC. Pergolide therapy in Parkinson's disease: a double-blind, placebo-controlled study. Clin Neuropharmacol 1985;8:260–265.

68. Ahlskog JE, Muenter MD. Treatment of Parkinson's disease with pergolide: a double-blind study. Mayo Clin Proc 1988;63:969–978.

69. Olanow CW, Fahn S, Muenter M, et al. A multicenter double-blind placebo-controlled trial of pergolide as an adjunct to Sinemet in Parkinson's disease. Mov Disord 1994;9:40–47.

70. Ahlskog JE, Muenter MD. Pergolide: long-term use in Parkinson's disease. Mayo Clin Proc 1988;63:979–987.

71. LeWitt PA, Ward CD, Larsen TA, et al. Comparison of pergolide and bromocriptine therapy in parkinsonism. Neurology 1983;33:1009–1014.

72. Goetz CG, Shannon KM, Tanner CM, et al. Agonist substitution in advanced Parkinson's disease. Neurology 1989;39:1121–1122.

73. Factor SA, Sanchez-Ramos JR, Weiner WJ. Parkinson's disease: an open label trial of pergolide in patients failing bromocriptine therapy. J Neurol Neurosurg Psychiatry 1988;51:529–533.

74. Safety and efficacy of pramipexole in early Parkinson disease. A randomized dose-ranging study. Parkinson Study Group. JAMA 1997;278:125–130.

75. Shannon KM, Bennett JP Jr, Friedman JH. Efficacy of pramipexole, a novel dopamine agonist, as monotherapy in mild to moderate Parkinson's disease. The Pramipexole Study Group [published erratum in Neurology 1998 Mar;50(3):838]. Neurology 1997;49:724–728.

76. Lieberman A, Ranhosky A, Korts D. Clinical evaluation of pramipexole in advanced Parkinson's disease: results of a double-blind, placebo-controlled, parallel-group study. Neurology 1997;49:162–168.

77. Adler CH, Sethi KD, Hauser RA, et al. Ropinirole for the treatment of early Parkinson's disease. The Ropinirole Study Group. Neurology 1997;49:393–399.

78. Brooks DJ, Abbott RJ, Lees AJ, et al. A placebo-controlled evaluation of ropinirole, a novel D2 agonist, as sole dopaminergic therapy in Parkinson's disease. Clin Neuropharmacol 1998;21:101–107.

79. Rascol O, Brooks DJ, Brunt ER, et al. Ropinirole in the treatment of early Parkinson's disease: a 6-month interim report of a 5-year levodopa-controlled study. 056 Study Group. Mov Disord 1998;13:39–45.

80. Korczyn AD, Brooks DJ, Brunt ER, et al. Ropinirole versus bromocriptine in the treatment of early Parkinson's disease: a 6-month interim report of a 3-year study. 053 Study Group. Mov Disord 1998;13:46–51.

81. Rascol O, Lees AJ, Senard JM, et al. Ropinirole in the treatment of levodopa-induced motor fluctuations in patients with Parkinson's disease. Clin Neuropharmacol 1996;19:234–245.

# 196    *Clinical Trials in Neurologic Practice*

82. Rascol O, Brooks DJ, Korczyn AD, et al. A five-year study of the incidence of dyskinesia in patients with early Parkinson's disease who were treated with ropinirole or levodopa. 056 Study Group. N Engl J Med 2000;342:1484–1491.

83. Rinne UK, Bracco F, Chouza C, et al. Cabergoline in the treatment of early Parkinson's disease: results of the first year of treatment in a double-blind comparison of cabergoline and levodopa. The PKDS009 Collaborative Study Group. Neurology 1997;48:363–368.

84. Lera G, Vaamonde J, Rodriguez M, Obeso JA. Cabergoline in Parkinson's disease: long-term follow-up. Neurology 1993;43:2587–2590.

85. Geminiani G, Fetoni V, Genitrini S, et al. Cabergoline in Parkinson's disease complicated by motor fluctuations. Mov Disord 1996;11:495–500.

86. Rabey JM, Nissipeanu P, Inzelberg R, Korczyn AD. Beneficial effect of cabergoline, new long-lasting D2 agonist in the treatment of Parkinson's disease. Clin Neuropharmacol 1994;17:286–293.

87. Inzelberg R, Nisipeanu P, Rabey MJ, Korczyn AD. Long-term tolerability and efficacy of cabergoline, a new long-acting dopamine agonist, in Parkinson's disease. Mov Disord 1995;10:604–607.

88. Hutton JT, Koller WC, Ahlskog JE, et al. Multicenter, placebo-controlled trial of cabergoline taken once daily in the treatment of Parkinson's disease. Neurology 1996;46:1062–1065.

89. Ahlskog JE, Wright KF, Muenter MD, Adler CH. Adjunctive cabergoline therapy of Parkinson's disease: comparison with placebo and assessment of dose responses and duration of effect. Clin Neuropharmacol 1996;19:202–212.

90. Inzelberg R, Nisipeanu P, Rabey JM, et al. Double-blind comparison of cabergoline and bromocriptine in Parkinson's disease patients with motor fluctuations. Neurology 1996;47:785–788.

91. Frucht S, Rogers JD, Greene PE. Falling asleep at the wheel: motor vehicle mishaps in persons taking pramipexole and ropinirole. Neurology 1999;52:1908–1910.

92. Ferreira JJ, Galitzky M, Montastruc JL. Sleep attacks and Parkinson's disease treatment (letter). Lancet 2000;355(9212):1333–1334.

93. Dewey RB Jr., Maraganore DM, Ahlskog JE, et al. A double-blind, placebo-controlled study of intranasal apomorphine spray as a rescue agent for off-states in Parkinson's disease. Movement Disorders 1998;13:782–787.

94. Brannan T, Prikhojan A, Yahr MD. Peripheral and central inhibitors of catechol-O-methyl transferase: effects on liver and brain COMT activity and L-DOPA metabolism. J Neural Transm (Budapest) 1997;104:77–87.

95. Nutt JG. Effects of catechol-O-methyltransferase (COMT) inhibition on the pharmacokinetics of L-DOPA. Adv Neurol 1996;69:493–496.

96. Jorga KM, Sedek G. Effect of the novel COMT-inhibitor TC on L-dopa pharmacokinetics when combined with different Sinemet formulations. Neurology 1995;45:291.

97. Kaakkola S, Gordin A, Mannisto PT. General properties and clinical possibilities of new selective inhibitors of catechol O-methyltransferase. Gen Pharmacol 1994;25:813–824.

98. Baas H, Beiske AG, Ghika J, et al. Catechol-O-methyltransferase inhibition with tolcapone reduces the "wearing off" phenomenon and levodopa requirements in fluctuating parkinsonian patients. Neurology 1998;50:S46–S53.

99. Ruottinen HM, Rinne UK. Entacapone prolongs levodopa response in a one month double blind study in parkinsonian patients with levodopa related fluctuations. J Neurol Neurosurg Psychiatry 1996;60:36–40.

100. Dingemanse J, Jorga K, Zurcher G, et al. Pharmacokinetic-pharmacodynamic interaction between the COMT inhibitor tolcapone and single-dose levodopa. Br J Clin Pharmacol 1995;40:253–262.

101. Dingemanse J, Jorga K, Zurcher G, et al. Multiple-dose clinical pharmacology of the catechol-O-methyl-transferase inhibitor tolcapone in elderly subjects. Eur J Clin Pharmacol 1996;50:47–55.

102. Kurth MC, Adler CH, Hilaire MS, et al. Tolcapone improves motor function and reduces levodopa requirement in patients with Parkinson's disease experiencing motor fluctuations: a multicenter, double-blind, randomized, placebo-controlled trial. Tolcapone Fluctuator Study Group I. Neurology 1997;48:81–87.

103. Waters CH, Kurth M, Bailey P, et al. Tolcapone in stable Parkinson's disease: efficacy and safety of long-term treatment. The Tolcapone Stable Study Group. Neurology 1997;49:665–671.

104. Tolcapone Study Group. Efficacy and tolerability of tolcapone compared with bromocriptine in levo-dopa treated parkinsonian patients. Mov Disord 1999;14:38–44.

105. Ruottinen HM, Rinne UK. A double-blind pharmacokinetic and clinical dose-response study of entacapone as an adjuvant to levodopa therapy in advanced Parkinson's disease. Clin Neuropharmacol 1996;19:283–296.
106. Entacapone improves motor fluctuations in levodopa-treated Parkinson's disease patients. Parkinson Study Group. Ann Neurol 1997;42:747–755.
107. Ahtila S, Kaakkola S, Gordin A, et al. Effect of entacapone, a COMT inhibitor, on the pharmacokinetics and metabolism of levodopa after administration of controlled-release levodopa-carbidopa in volunteers. Clin Neuropharmacol 1995;18:46–57.
108. Speelman JD, Bosch DA. Resurgence of functional neurosurgery for Parkinson's disease: a historical perspective. Mov Disord 1998;13:582–588.
109. Fox MW, Ahlskog JE, Kelly PJ. Stereotactic ventrolateralis thalamotomy for medically refractory tremor in post-levodopa era Parkinson's disease patients. J Neurosurg 1991;75:723–730.
110. Nagaseki Y, Shibazaki T, Hirai T, et al. Long-term follow-up results of selective VIM-thalamotomy. J Neurosurg 1986;65:296–302.
111. Matsumoto K, Shichijo F, Fukami T. Long-term follow-up review of cases of Parkinson's disease after unilateral or bilateral thalamotomy. J Neurosurg 1984;60:1033–1044.
112. Diederich N, Goetz CG, Stebbins GT, et al. Blinded evaluation confirms long-term asymmetric effect of unilateral thalamotomy or subthalamotomy on tremor in Parkinson's disease. Neurology 1992;42:1311–1314.
113. Duma CM, Jacques DB, Kopyov OV, et al. Gamma knife radiosurgery for thalamotomy in parkinsonian tremor: a five-year experience. J Neurosurg 1998;88:1044–1049.
114. Young RF, Shumway-Cook A, Vermeulen SS, et al. Gamma knife radiosurgery as a lesioning technique in movement disorder surgery. J Neurosurg 1998;89:183–193.
115. Benabid AL, Pollak P, Gao D, et al. Chronic electrical stimulation of the ventralis intermedius nucleus of the thalamus as a treatment of movement disorders. J Neurosurg 1996;84:203–214.
116. Koller W, Pahwa R, Busenbark K, et al. High-frequency unilateral thalamic stimulation in the treatment of essential and parkinsonian tremor. Ann Neurol 1997;42:292–299.
117. Hubble JP, Busenbark KL, Wilkinson S, et al. Effects of thalamic deep brain stimulation based on tremor type and diagnosis. Mov Disord 1997;12:337–341.
118. Tasker RR. Deep brain stimulation is preferable to thalamotomy for tremor suppression. Surg Neurol 1998;49:145–153;discussion 153–154.
119. Caparros-Lefebvre D, Blond S, Vermersch P, et al. Chronic thalamic stimulation improves tremor and levodopa induced dyskinesias in Parkinson's disease. J Neurol Neurosurg Psychiatry 1993;56:268–273.
120. Lozano AM, Lang AE. Pallidotomy for Parkinson's disease. Neurosurgery Clinics of North America 1998;9:325–336.
121. Laitinen LV, Bergenheim AT, Hariz MI. Leksell's posteroventral pallidotomy in the treatment of Parkinson's disease. J Neurosurg 1992;76:53–61.
122. Dogali M, Fazzini E, Kolodny E, et al. Stereotactic ventral pallidotomy for Parkinson's disease. Neurology 1995;45:753–761.
123. Fazzini E, Dogali M, Sterio D, et al. Stereotactic pallidotomy for Parkinson's disease: a long-term follow-up of unilateral pallidotomy. Neurology 1997;48:1273–1277.
124. Lozano AM, Lang AE, Galvez-Jimenez N, et al. Effect of GPi pallidotomy on motor function in Parkinson's disease. Lancet 1995;346:1383–1387.
125. Ondo WG, Jankovic J, Lai EC, et al. Assessment of motor function after stereotactic pallidotomy. Neurology 1998;50:266–270.
126. Lang AE, Lozano AM, Montgomery E, et al. Posteroventral medial pallidotomy in advanced Parkinson's disease. N Engl J Med 1997;337:1036–1042.
127. Baron MS, Vitek JL, Bakay RA, et al. Treatment of advanced Parkinson's disease by posterior GPi pallidotomy: 1-year results of a pilot study. Ann Neurol 1996;40:355–366.
128. Uitti RJ, Wharen RE Jr, Turk MF, et al. Unilateral pallidotomy for Parkinson's disease: comparison of outcome in younger versus elderly patients. Neurology 1997;49:1072–1077.
129. Desaloms JM, Krauss JK, Lai EC, et al. Posteroventral medial pallidotomy for treatment of Parkinson's disease: preoperative magnetic resonance imaging features and clinical outcome. J Neurosurg 1998;89:194–199.
130. Krauss JK, Desaloms JM, Lai EC, et al. Microelectrode-guided posteroventral pallidotomy for treatment of Parkinson's disease: postoperative magnetic resonance imaging analysis. J Neurosurg 1997;87:358–367.

## 198   *Clinical Trials in Neurologic Practice*

131. Kishore A, Turnbull IM, Snow BJ, et al. Efficacy, stability and predictors of outcome of pallidotomy for Parkinson's disease. Six-month follow-up with additional 1-year observations. Brain 1997;120:729–737.
132. Giller CA, Dewey RB, Ginsburg MI, et al. Stereotactic pallidotomy and thalamotomy using individual variations of anatomic landmarks for localization. Neurosurgery 1998;42:56–62;discussion 62–65.
133. Trepanier LL, Saint-Cyr JA, Lozano AM, Lang AE. Neuropsychological consequences of posteroventral pallidotomy for the treatment of Parkinson's disease. Neurology 1998;51:207–215.
134. Scott R, Gregory R, Hines N, et al. Neuropsychological, neurological and functional outcome following pallidotomy for Parkinson's disease. A consecutive series of eight simultaneous bilateral and twelve unilateral procedures. Brain 1998;121:659–675.
135. Vitek JL, Bakay RA, Hashimoto T, et al. Microelectrode-guided pallidotomy: technical approach and its application in medically intractable Parkinson's disease. J Neurosurg 1998;88:1027–1043.
136. Laitinen LV. Pallidotomy for Parkinson's disease. Neurosurg Clin N Am 1995;6:105–112.
137. Krauss JK, Jankovic J, Lai EC, et al. Posteroventral medial pallidotomy in levodopa-unresponsive parkinsonism. Arch Neurol 1997;54:1026–1029.
138. Rand RW, Jacques DB, Melbye RW, et al. Gamma knife thalamotomy and pallidotomy in patients with movement disorders: preliminary results. Stereotact Funct Neurosurg 1993;61(Suppl 1):65–92.
139. Friedman JH, Epstein M, Sanes JN, et al. Gamma knife pallidotomy in advanced Parkinson's disease. Ann Neurol 1996;39:535–538.
140. Gross C, Rougier A, Guehl D, et al. High-frequency stimulation of the globus pallidus internalis in Parkinson's disease: a study of seven cases. J Neurosurg 1997;87:491–498.
141. Pahwa R, Wilkinson S, Smith D, et al. High-frequency stimulation of the globus pallidus for the treatment of Parkinson's disease. Neurology 1997;49:249–253.
142. Siegfried J, Lippitz B. Bilateral chronic electrostimulation of ventroposterolateral pallidum: a new therapeutic approach for alleviating all parkinsonian symptoms. Neurosurgery 1994;35:1126–1129;discussion 1129–1133.
143. Troster AI, Fields JA, Wilkinson SB, et al. Unilateral pallidal stimulation for Parkinson's disease: neurobehavioral functioning before and 3 months after electrode implantation. Neurology 1997;49:1078–1083.
144. Merello M, Nouzeilles MI, Kuzis G, et al. Unilateral radiofrequency lesion versus electrostimulation of posteroventral pallidum: A prospective randomized comparison. Mov Disord 1999;14:50–56.
145. Galvez-Jimenez N, Lozano A, et al. Pallidal stimulation in Parkinson's disease patients with a prior unilateral pallidotomy. Can J Neurol Sci 1998;25:300–305.
146. Limousin P, Krack P, Pollak P, et al. Electrical stimulation of the subthalamic nucleus in advanced Parkinson's disease. N Engl J Med 1998;339:1105–1111.
147. Kumar R, Lozano AM, Kim YJ, et al. Double-blind evaluation of subthalamic nucleus deep brain stimulation in advanced Parkinson's disease. Neurology 1998;51:850–855.
148. Krack P, Pollak P, Limousin P, et al. Subthalamic nucleus or internal pallidal stimulation in young onset Parkinson's disease. Brain 1998;121:451–457.
149. Kumar R, Lozano AM, Montgomery E, Lang AE. Pallidotomy and deep brain stimulation of the pallidum and subthalamic nucleus in advanced Parkinson's disease. Mov Disord 1998;13(Suppl 1):73–82.
150. Lindvall O, Backlund EO, Farde L, et al. Transplantation in Parkinson's disease: two cases of adrenal medullary grafts to the putamen. Ann Neurol 1987;22:457–468.
151. Madrazo I, Drucker-Colin R, Diaz V, et al. Open microsurgical autograft of adrenal medulla to the right caudate nucleus in two patients with intractable Parkinson's disease. N Engl J Med 1987;316:831–834.
152. Goetz CG, Stebbins GT III, Klawans HL, et al. United Parkinson Foundation Neurotransplantation Registry on adrenal medullary transplants: presurgical, and 1- and 2-year follow-up. Neurology 1991;41:1719–1722.
153. Lindvall O, Sawle G, Widner H, et al. Evidence for long-term survival and function of dopaminergic grafts in progressive Parkinson's disease. Ann Neurol 1994;35:172–180.
154. Widner H, Tetrud J, Rehncrona S, et al. Bilateral fetal mesencephalic grafting in two patients with parkinsonism induced by 1-methyl-4-phenyl-1,2,3,6-tetrahydropyridine (MPTP). N Engl J Med 1992;327:1556–1563.
155. Freed CR, Breeze RE, Rosenberg NL, et al. Survival of implanted fetal dopamine cells and neurologic improvement 12 to 46 months after transplantation for Parkinson's disease. N Engl J Med 1992;327:1549–1555.

*Clinical Trials in Parkinson's Disease*   199

156. Freeman TB, Olanow CW, Hauser RA, et al. Bilateral fetal nigral transplantation into the postcommissural putamen in Parkinson's disease. Ann Neurol 1995;38:379–388.
157. Hauser RA, Freeman TB, Snow BJ, et al. Long-term evaluation of bilateral fetal nigral transplantation in Parkinson disease. Arch Neurol 1999;56:179–187.
158. Freeman TB, Olanow CW, Hauser RA, et al. Human Fetal Tissue Transplantation. In IM Germano (ed), Neurosurgical Treatment of Movement Disorders. American Association of Neurological Surgeons, 1998:177–192.
159. Kordower JH, Freeman TB, Snow BJ, et al. Neuropathological evidence of graft survival and striatal reinnervation after the transplantation of fetal mesencephalic tissue in a patient with Parkinson's disease. N Engl J Med 1995;332:1118–1124.
160. Kordower JH, Rosenstein JM, Collier TJ, et al. Functional fetal nigral grafts in a patient with Parkinson's disease: chemoanatomic, ultrastructural, and metabolic studies. J Comp Neurol 1996; 370:203–230.
161. Kordower JH, Freeman TB, Chen EY, et al. Fetal nigral grafts survive and mediate clinical benefit in a patient with Parkinson's disease. Mov Disord 1998;13:383–393.
162. Deacon T, Schumacher J, Dinsmore J, et al. Histological evidence of fetal pig neural cell survival after transplantation into a patient with Parkinson's disease. Nat Med 1997;3:350–353.
163. Fahn S. Double-blind controlled trial of embryonic dopaminergic tissue transplants in advanced Parkinson's disease. Mov Disord 2000;15(Suppl 3):7–8.

# 10
# Hyperkinetic Movement Disorders
Anna H. Hristova and William C. Koller

Because it is routine, humans often do not appreciate their gift of movement. Knowledge about movement disorders has grown rapidly. However, an important question remains: How reliable and reproducible is the constantly increasing amount of published data, which clinicians rely on for everyday clinical care? This chapter provides information about the reliability of the data and criteria that should be used when evaluating clinical trials performed in the hyperkinetic movement disorder field.

## TREMOR

Fifty-seven double-blind placebo-controlled clinical trials on tremor were identified during 1966–1998. The majority was based on results of open-label studies or anecdotal reports of benefit.[1–3] Sometimes, controlled and open-label studies can report opposite findings. For instance, two open-label studies on methazolamide have documented its efficacy in reducing hand, head, and voice tremor in patients with essential tremor (ET). However, two consecutive double-blind placebo-controlled trials assessed the drug effect on voice and hand tremor and reported no statistical difference when compared with placebo.[3,4] On the other hand, controlled studies on clonidine or flunarizine and ET have confirmed the previously reported benefit from open-label studies.

The inclusion criteria in tremor trials are specific. The homogeneity of the selected patients is important. Some of the trials on tremor have recruited only Parkinson's disease (PD) patients; others, only ET patients; and some, a mixture of patients with both diseases.[3,5,6] A study on ondansetron for cerebellar tremor included patients with multiple sclerosis, cerebellar degeneration, and drug-induced tremor.[7] The reported results were negative. The temptation to test one drug on different types of tremor in one clinical trial can lead to a type-2 error, as the study power decreases with the increasing numbers of disease groups.

202    *Clinical Trials in Neurologic Practice*

The disease diagnosis is essential. A study on gabapentin and tremor recruited 19 patients with advanced PD from PD support groups.[5] This resulted in exclusion of five patients after the recruitment; one of them, who was self-referred, was later diagnosed with ET. To solve this problem, experts have formulated definitions for definite, possible, and probable ET and PD.[8] However, some of the clinically "definitive" PD patients diagnosed by experts turned out to have multiple system atrophy on pathologic examination. On the other hand, some authors apply too strict criteria. A study on theophylline and ET required an absence of tremor at rest as an inclusion criterion, which does not reflect the natural disease spectrum in the patient population.[9] An absence of a tremor at rest is not included as a necessary criterion in the expert's definition of definite ET.[8]

Another important issue is tremor duration. A very short tremor duration increases the risk of diagnosis change over time. Chronic disease can cause irreversible damage of the tremor pathways with loss of possible positive drug-induced influence on the disease mechanisms in its earlier stages.

It is advisable to include patients of both genders, unless the disease itself has male or female predominance. Some studies, such as those for nadolol or clonidine for ET, have included only male patients,[10,11] whereas the botulinum toxin for head tremor study included predominantly female patients.[2] Both approaches neglect the natural disease expression.

Are drug-naïve or drug-treated patients better candidates for recruitment? It has been shown that L-dopa–naïve patients with PD do not respond in the same manner as patients who have been previously treated with L-dopa. This criterion could be significant in some clinical trials. Another important issue is the time of tremor presence. It is well known that the daily presence of tremor varies between patients and within the same patient. This makes the recording and reliable assessment of tremor difficult. Continuous presence of tremor appears to be a mandatory inclusion criterion. Not all trials on tremor consider this fact.

The drug and placebo side effects can be a major problem in clinical trials. A study on clonazepam and ET started with 15 patients but ended with only six patients entering the double-blind phase of the trial.[12] Nine patients dropped out because of intolerable drowsiness. Five of six recruited patients aged older than 70 years developed mild confusion, and three male patients complained of erectile failure. The study concludes no significant tremor reduction, but one can question the study's power. However, even when proved effective, the drug's pronounced side effects could overwhelm the potential benefits.

Test conditions to consider in a tremor trial are meal, alcohol, caffeine, and other substrates that can affect tremor presence. Drug dose is also of great importance. Single-dose and long-term drug administration studies have been conducted on tremor. The significance of dosage choice is illustrated by a study with theophylline and ET. A statistically significant tremor reduction is reported only after the second week of theophylline administration.[9] On the other hand, a single propranolol dose was reported to be as efficacious as prolonged drug administration in ET.[13–16] Therefore, individual hypotheses may need to be tested in different conditions. Another question is that of which hand to test—the most severely affected hand or both? And, are the results being divided by two? This becomes important when one of the hands has no tremor at all.

A question of importance remains: How do you record tremor? Most studies prefer an objective method, such as an accelerometer, electromyography, isoelectric transducing devices, or computer analyzers, combined with clinical scales (tremor scales, the United Parkinson's Disease Rating Scale [tremor part]), videotaping, or a subjective method, such as patient self-assessment.[17,18] A few studies have used only one criterion, as did the study on clozapine and parkinsonian tremor, which used only the tremor part of the United Parkinson's Disease Rating Scale to record the results.[1] The criteria to report the significance of the results are of crucial importance. What magnitude of amplitude decrement should be considered significant? This single fact could affect the results and percentage of patients reported to have benefit. The investigators from the study on clozapine and parkinsonian tremor chose to accept a tremor amplitude reduction of more than 50% as significant.[1] Other studies have chosen 15% tremor amplitude decrement as significant. Another study compares the difference in the amplitude reduction between placebo and the study drug and its statistical significance.[13] The study on postural tremor and PD provides us with another example of how to assess results.[6] The placebo group demonstrated up to 30% reduction in the tremor compared to baseline. Therefore, the investigators suggest a criterion of improvement at a level of greater than 30% benefit. The dose-related improvement as reported in many propranolol studies supports the presence of a true drug benefit.[19]

The results of the 57 double-blind placebo-controlled clinical trials on tremor, as well as other tremor studies performed in the last 32 years, have shed light on beta-adrenergic receptor antagonists, primidone, and ethanol, among other drugs.

## Beta-Adrenergic Receptor Antagonists

The beta-adrenergic receptor antagonists are well-established drugs of choice for ET treatment (level I evidence, grade A strength of recommendation). Fifty percent to 75% of patients benefit from this treatment. Most benefit incompletely.[20,21] The nonselective beta blockers, such as propranolol, timolol, and sotalol, were reported to have higher efficacy on ET control compared to $beta_1$-adrenoreceptor selective antagonists, such as metoprolol.[22] The selective $beta_2$-adrenergic receptor blocking drug ICI 118551 has shown equal potency to propranolol in reducing the magnitude of the tremor.[23,24] These results suggest that $beta_2$-receptor blockade plays a greater role than $beta_1$-receptor blockade in tremor suppression. The studies on sotalol, arotinol, LI 32-468, and hydrophilic drugs that have poor penetration of the central nervous system have shown that they are similar to propranolol efficacy on tremor reduction, suggesting a peripheral rather than a central mechanism of drug action.[25–27] Apart from ET, some PD patients with insufficient tremor response to L-dopa treatment could benefit from treatment with beta-adrenergic antagonists.[28] The membrane-stabilizing effect of propranolol, and its intrinsic sympathomimetic effects, did not seem to be related to tremor reduction. Supporting this hypothesis are studies on sotalol, LI 32-468, and buferolol—drugs that have little or no membrane-stabilizing effect compared to propranolol but have similar potency in ET reduction.[25,27,29] On the other hand, a D-isomer of propranolol, a drug with similar membrane-stabilizing activity but significantly lower beta-blocking activity, was reported to be ineffective in ET.[30] Pindolol, a drug with a high intrinsic sympathomimetic activity and less beta-blocking activity than pro-

204    *Clinical Trials in Neurologic Practice*

pranolol, did not show significant tremor reduction.[31] There is no correlation between propranolol plasma concentration and its tremorlytic effect.[32]

## Primidone

Primidone is another mainstream drug in the treatment of ET (level I evidence, grade A strength of recommendation).[33] The drug's action on tremor is mediated by a mechanism that is not well understood. Controlled studies of primidone and phenobarbital on ET showed statistically significant tremor improvement with primidone and no difference between placebo and phenobarbital.[34,35] These results suggest that phenobarbital, a major primidone metabolite, is not responsible for the tremor reduction. However, other controlled trials have reported opposite results, with equal potency of both drugs when compared to placebo.[15,36] One study of phenobarbitone on ET reported drug benefit versus placebo.[37] A controlled study on another metabolite of primidone, phenylethylmalonamide, failed to show efficacy.[38] These contradictory results are a good illustration of how important it is to be meticulous when performing controlled trials. Phenobarbital has not gained widespread use in practice. One-third of the patients with ET do not respond to primidone treatment or develop intolerable side effects.[39] Is primidone acting on tremor through peripherally or centrally mediated mechanisms? Administered orally, primidone quickly penetrates the central nervous system. It was reported that primidone limits the sustained high-frequency repetitive firing of mouse neurons in culture, especially in combination with phenobarbital, suggesting some potentiation of the drug and its metabolite and possible suppressive action on a central tremor pacemaker.[40]

## Ethanol

The majority of ET patients respond to ethanol.[41] Although some of the patients consume small amounts of ethanol to suppress their tremor, this type of treatment is not widely recommended. Studies on ethanol have reported tremor amplitude reduction only in ET, not in parkinsonian or cerebellar tremor.[42] The potential for ethanol abuse has not been proved.[43,44] The pathogenic mechanism of ethanol action remains unknown. It is possibly mediated by a nonselective beta-adrenergic blockade. A possible antianxiety central mechanism of ethanol action has also been tested in a controlled study with methylpentynol, an alcohol with antianxiety action, and ET. The results did not show tremor improvement as compared to placebo.[45]

## Other Drugs with Reported Effect on Tremor

### Clozapine

Clozapine, an atypical neuroleptic used to control L-dopa–induced hallucinations in PD patients and patients with psychiatric disorders, was assessed in a controlled trial and showed moderate to marked tremor reduction in 15 of 17 patients with PD.[1]

## Adenosine Antagonists

A controlled study on theophylline reported similar efficacy to propranolol for ET.[9] The effect reached significance only after the second week of theophylline administration, suggesting chronic upregulation of the adenosine receptors.

## Benzodiazepines

A controlled study of alprazolam, a minimally sedating triazolam analogue of the benzodiazepine class, showed significant improvement for head and hand ET.[46] Important drug side effects are the potential risk of addiction and the severe withdrawal reaction with abrupt discontinuation. It is recommended mainly for intermittent use on ET-affected patients who did not respond to treatment with beta blockers or primidone.

## Botulinum Toxin Type A

Botulinum toxin type A has been reported to be effective treatment for hand tremor in controlled trials.[47] A possible blockage of gamma-afferent loops on the spinal level has been suggested as a mechanism of its action. A controlled trial of botulinum toxin injections for essential head tremor control reported possible usefulness.[2]

## Calcium Channel Blockers

Trials on nimodipine and flunarizine reported positive effect of both drugs on ET.[48,49] Thirteen of 15 patients on flunarizine and eight of 15 patients on nimodipine showed benefit.

## Isoniazid

Several controlled trials for treatment of a cerebellar tremor using isoniazid, an antituberculous drug, reported it to have a definite but limited therapeutic role. The mechanism of action is unknown.[19] A controlled trial assessing the efficacy of propranolol, isoniazid, and ethyl alcohol failed to show statistically significant improvement on cerebellar tremor compared to placebo. Ondansetron, a 5-HT$_3$ antagonist administered in a single dose, showed a statistically significant improvement in cerebellar tremor, which suggests the possible importance of serotonin in tremor pathophysiology.[7]

206    *Clinical Trials in Neurologic Practice*

Ritanserin

Trials on drug-induced parkinsonism have been performed using ritanserin, a 5-HT$_2$ antagonist, and showed a statistically significant benefit on this type of tremor.[50] This fact supports the hypothesis of possible serotonin influence on the extrapyramidal physiology.

## Surgical Treatment of Tremor

There has been a flourish of operative tremor treatment. Surgery performed on the thalamic nucleus ventralis intermedius demonstrated good results for tremor control.[51] The thalamic surgery is performed mainly on patients with essential tremor or on patients with a tremor-dominant form of PD and unsatisfactory L-dopa response [51] The effect on tremor suppression is excellent with immediate results after the start of stimulation.[51,52] The question of which operation is better, thalamotomy or high-frequency thalamic stimulation, has no simple answer. Both types of surgical techniques have significant effects on tremor control but report a mortality rate of 1% and a complication rate of 2–6%, with complications, such as stroke, infection, and seizures.[53,54] In addition, thalamotomy causes irreversible neuronal cell death in the place of the lesion compared to the thalamic stimulator neuron-sparing effect. Another advantage of thalamic stimulators is the possibility for stimulation parameter adjustment, making this type of treatment more suitable to individual needs. Disadvantages of this procedure are the high cost and the necessity of battery change approximately every 3–5 years. Otherwise, both procedures have demonstrated high efficacy and relative safety.[51,52] The immediate effect of the thalamic stimulation on tremor suggests that the thalamus is a possible central tremor pacemaker or an important tremor circuit output. When the thalamic nuclei are stimulated intraoperatively with a frequency of 4–8 Hz (similar to that recorded peripherally), tremor can be induced. It has been found that frequency of more than 60 Hz should be used in an attempt to functionally disrupt the neuronal circuits responsible for the tremor production. During procedures of stimulator insertion in ventral internal pallidal nucleus, the so-called tremor cells have been discovered, firing spontaneously with frequency of 4–8 Hz, similar to that recorded peripherally.[55] A further subpopulation of neurons has been identified with micrographic techniques, but tremor synchronous cells were recognized only in some of the patients.[56] In conclusion, if a patient with ET does not respond to beta blockers or primidone therapy, the previously mentioned less successful drugs for tremor control can be tried. Patients with ET, and some patients with a tremor-dominant form of PD who do not respond to medication, are good candidates for surgical treatment.

## Treatments with No Tremor Effect Reported in Controlled Trials

Methazolamide, a carbonic anhydrase inhibitor, failed to show improvement in controlled trials on essential voice or hand tremor, although two previous open-label studies reported beneficial effect.[3,4] Progabide, a gamma-aminobutyric acid (GABA) receptor agonist, and gabapentin, an anticonvulsant with unknown effect, failed to show statistically significant improvement on ET, suggesting that GABA neurotransmission may not be involved in ET pathobiology.[5] Clonidine, a central alpha-adrenergic stimulant, failed to show ET improvement, suggesting these types of receptors are unimportant in tremor genesis.[11] Clonazepam, a potent antiepileptic benzodiazepine derivative, was reported to be ineffective in a controlled study on ET. However, a good response was found in kinetic tremor and orthostatic truncal tremor, with mechanism of action that is not well understood.[57,58] The efficacy of long-acting propranolol on neuroleptic-induced parkinsonism has been assessed with lack of tremor attenuation, suggesting a different tremorlytic mechanism for this type of tremor.[14]

One of the most important results of controlled clinical trials and other trials is the insight they provide on disease pathobiology. Some of the hypotheses have already been described. All tremor responders to beta$_2$ blockade have shown reduction of tremor magnitude but no change in a tremor frequency.[13] The records from limb extensor and flexor muscles have shown predominantly co-contraction of the agonists/antagonists in ET and predominantly consecutive contraction of the agonists/antagonists in parkinsonian tremor recording. A tremor frequency of 4–8 Hz for tremor at rest has been reported for both ET and parkinsonian tremor. A slight difference in tremor frequency has been noticed between rest and postural tremor, with a mean postural tremor frequency of 6–12 Hz. A tendency toward tremor frequency reduction and amplitude increment has been noticed with essential tremor disease progression.[13] It is known that apart from rest and postural tremor, PD patients can have action tremor, which is sometimes pronounced. A large parkinsonian family with an identified genetic defect has been reported, in which some affected subjects have phenotypically expressed pure ET with genotype identical to that of the parkinsonian members.[59] These facts suggest the possibility of a disease continuum with overlapping between PD and ET. Another idea is the possible existence of a central tremor pacemaker, which acts through central neuronal circuits and affects the peripheral spinal loops. Studies assessing central circuit influence on peripheral spinal loops have been performed.[60] The idea may be that a disinhibition of the cortical inhibition of the reciprocal spinal cord inhibition, directed more strongly from extensor toward flexor muscles, and less strongly from flexor toward extensor muscles exists. Damage to the central circuits enhances the peripheral reciprocal inhibition of the Ia fibers on a spinal cord level. This suggests possible peripheral ways to manipulate the tremor arc. The clinical significance of these observations is still under investigation.

## CHOREA

Twenty double-blind, placebo-controlled trials on chorea were identified between 1966 and 1998. Chorea is less well understood than tremor. That is why there are many trials in this field that report negative results. The majority of trials on chorea has been based on open-label and animal studies. The efficacy of deanol on chorea has been studied in animal models with positive results but has not been confirmed on subsequent open-label and controlled trials.[61] However, some patients had good results, suggesting a possible responsive patient subpopulation. Controlled trials

208   *Clinical Trials in Neurologic Practice*

on clozapine or cannabidiol and chorea did not confirm the previous positive results suggested by open-label trials.[62] On the other hand, an open-label study on clonazepam and chorea, supported by a subsequent controlled study on 158 patients with tardive dyskinesias (TDs), reported an 83% dyskinesia reduction but with less magnitude of benefit.[63] There is not a specific pattern predicting which open-label study's results will be confirmed with controlled trials, which is why we have no better tool to test a scientific hypothesis than performing double-blind, placebo-controlled, randomized clinical trials. In consideration of patient recruitment and diagnosis, most of the chorea studies were performed on Huntington's chorea (HC) patients and a few on TD patients, mainly because HC is a nontreatable disease and TDs are frequent neuroleptic treatment complications. Other choreas, such as chorea gravidarum, Sydenham's chorea, senile chorea, and the normal maturation chorea, are usually benign and self-limited diseases. Chorea related to a well-distinguished etiology, such as tumor, trauma, and infection, has not been the subject of clinical trials. Most of the studies were conducted purely on HC patients in stages 1–4 of the disease. It is important to keep in mind that the other features of HC, such as dementia and behavioral problems, are major limiting factors for recruitment. A few studies have used patients with various types of choreas, such as the study on tetrabenazine, which recruited six patients with Meige disease, two with static dyskinesias, four with tardive dyskinesias, and three with adult-onset dystonias. The only improvement reported was in four of six Meige patients, and accordingly, the study's power was significantly reduced.[64] It does not seem advisable to perform trials on mixed groups of choreatic patients, unless each group has sufficient power by itself.

The diagnosis of HC is of great importance. Most studies have used clinically typical HC patients and the autosomal dominant disease inheritance as sufficient diagnostic criteria. However, other controlled trials have strengthened the diagnosis with caudate nuclei atrophy proven with computed tomography or magnetic resonance.[65] A double-blind controlled trial on clozapine and chorea has confirmed the diagnosis with genetic tests.[62] It may seem overly meticulous to use such an inclusion criterion because the genetic studies are expensive. However, this is done because there are no data on how many false-positive or false-negative diagnoses of HC are made when the diagnosis is based only on disease clinical features and pattern of inheritance.

The importance of recruiting drug-naïve versus drug-treated chorea patients is not less than that for tremor. A controlled trial on clozapine and chorea did not show statistically significant chorea improvement unless results were calculated separately for drug-naïve and drug-treated patients. Only the drug-naïve group has reached significance in clozapine efficacy.[62] Because no treatment has proved to be efficacious on chorea reduction, the drug dose remains of even greater importance. A dose of 150-mg clozapine per day in a controlled trial on 33 patients with HC reported six dropouts due to intolerable side effects; in eight patients, the dose was reduced. This is approximately 50% of the recruited patients.[62] A few trials on different drugs and chorea have proven efficacy only with high drug dose, which suggests a remote drug effect on chorea pathways. A study on tiapride and chorea showed mild efficacy when a dose of 3 g per day was given, when the drug's usual dose was 0.3–0.6 g per day.[66]

Chorea has no predictable pattern of appearance. To solve this problem, experts agreed on the Unified Huntington's Disease Rating Scale, which proved to be an efficacious tool in assessing chorea in controlled trials and in clinical practice.[67] Other chorea scales used in controlled trials are abnormal involuntary movement scales and Marsden and Fahn's functional disability scale.[68] For tardive dyskinesias, the Simpson tardive dyskinesias rating scale is available.[61] Chorea is assessed frequently at rest, at maximum presence, or during a continuous observation. Most of the studies have used tasks from the patient's everyday life, such as screwing a nut onto a bolt, putting on a jacket, fastening buttons, putting on and taking off a shirt or socks, drinking out of a glass, and pouring water from a bottle into a glass. Subjective methods, such as patient diaries, nurse opinion, and partner questionnaires, have also been used.[69] The most objective method for chorea assessment is a video recording reviewed by a blinded rater. Most studies have used scales for behavioral, mood, or cognitive assessment as part of HC symptom monitoring as well. The study on apomorphine and chorea has reported repeated yawning in all patients on actual drug and only in a few of the placebo controls.[65]

The results of these 20 double-blind placebo-controlled clinical trials on chorea and other studies performed in the last 32 years suggest there is still not a highly efficacious treatment for chorea (level I evidence). Neuroleptic treatment is partially efficacious but has frequent side effects, such as production of parkinsonian symptoms (level I evidence, strength A of recommendation). Studies also strongly suggest the existence of chorea patient subpopulations, such as patients with predominantly dystonic movements and patients with predominantly choreoathetoid movements, or subpopulations related to the different types or subtypes of receptors, such as dopamine (D), GABA receptors, and $N$-methyl-D-aspartate (NMDA) receptors. Are the $D_1$, $D_2$, $D_3$, $D_4$, or $D_5$ receptors responsible for the chorea production? A selective loss of the medium-sized spiny striatal neurons has been reported on pathologic observation on the brains of patients who died with HC.[70] There are two subpopulations of medium spiny neurons. One subpopulation expresses $D_1$ receptors related to substance P and gives GABA efferents to globus pallidum internum (GPi). The other subpopulation expresses $D_2$-receptors related to enkephalin and has GABA projections to globus pallidum externum (GPe). The pathologically documented neuronal loss in GPe is larger than that in GPi.[71] When the cell loss in GPe is larger than that in Gpi, an akinetic-rigid syndrome is expressed. When GPi loss is larger, a mainly dystonic picture is clinically observed. When both parts of pallidum are equally affected, the symptoms are mixed.[72] Furthermore, there is greater substantia nigra pars reticulata than substantia nigra pars compacta neuronal loss that cannot be fully explained by the medium spiny striatal neuron reduction.

Studies on relatively selective dopamine receptor's agonists on chorea have been performed. A trial involving clozapine, a weak $D_2$-receptor agonist, conducted on 33 patients with Huntington's disease and chorea reported negative results when the effect was calculated for drug-naïve and drug-treated patients together. The study concludes that the results are probably negative because of the weak clozapine affinity to $D_2$-receptors.[62] Apomorphine, a $D_4$-receptor high-affinity agonist, was administered in controlled trials on nine patients with HC. A 38.54% reduction of chorea score has been documented with an apomorphine dose of 1.5 mg per day, and a 30.41% score reduction has been reported with apomorphine, 3 mg per day, with no change compared to baseline in controls receiving placebo.[65] It is difficult to

210  *Clinical Trials in Neurologic Practice*

interpret the D-receptor involvement in the HC pathogenesis because apomorphine has an intermediate affinity to $D_2$- and $D_3$-receptors and low affinity to the $D_1$- and $D_5$-receptors. The $D_2$ antagonist tiapride has been evaluated in a controlled trial on 23 HC patients. Tiapride was reported to significantly improve choreatic movements and motor skills when a dosage as high as 3 g per day was used.[66]

A nonspecific monoamine-depleting agent, tetrabenazine, which affects the storage and functional pool of dopamine, norepinephrine, and serotonin equally, has shown improvement in some patients with various chorea disorders.[64] The hypothesis of basal ganglia GABA reduction importance in chorea genesis has been tested with several GABA-ergic drugs. A study on large-dose isoniazid-treated animals showed GABA brain level increment due to inhibition of the first enzyme (aminotransferase) of GABA degradation pathway.[73] A controlled trial on human subjects with isoniazid reported minimal therapeutic improvement (but not substantial clinical improvement) in six of eight HC patients who completed the trial.[74] Cerebrospinal fluid (CSF) GABA elevation was reported, suggesting that the drop in the global brain GABA levels is not directly related to the chorea pathogenesis, and that this is probably a remote way to influence chorea. Clonazepam, another GABA-ergic drug, has been tested in 12 patients with TD.[63] A 41.5% reduction of the dystonic movements and a 26.5% reduction of the choreoathetoid movements has been reported, which points to the existence of a patient subpopulation. When compared to baseline, no change was reported in placebo controls. This suggests some significance of the GABA pathways in chorea generation.[63] On the other hand, piracetam, a metabolic enhancer in the brain, documented worsening of chorea in 11 HC patients.[75] This fact does not pinpoint the pathophysiologic defect, but rather suggests excitement-suppression disbalance. The reduced GABA stimulation from $D_2$ striatal neurons to GPe produces enhanced suppression of subthalamic nucleus and reduced glutamatergic stimulation of GPi, which is believed to contribute to dyskinesia generation. Remacemide, a noncompetitive NMDA receptor antagonist, was tested in a controlled trial on 31 patients with HC. Two hundred- and 600-mg daily drug doses were compared to placebo. The study was phase I, safety profile, and documented a good tolerability of the drug, but not significant efficacy.[76] However, there was a tendency for chorea reduction in patients with severe chorea; this, again, suggests existence of a patient subpopulation or a remote effect on chorea production. Another glutamate receptor agonist and glycine prodrug, milacemide, did not show statistically significant chorea reduction in seven patients with HC.[77] This suggests that glycine possibly has a specific modulatory effect on the NMDA subtype of glutamate receptors rather than on the alpha-amino-3-hydroxy-5-methyl-4-isoxazole-propionic acid subtype, which may be predominant in the target subthalamic nucleus (STN) neurons. This fact is a possible explanation for the reported negative results.

The role of oxidative stress in chorea genesis is also being explored. Proton magnetic imaging spectroscopy studies have documented increased lactate-pyruvate ratio in CSF of 18 patients with HC.[78] A treatment with coenzyme $Q_{10}$ ($CoQ_{10}$) significantly decreases the lactate cortical concentration, suggesting general energy defect as a part of the HC pathways. The investigators are working on the hypothesis of a defect in the mitochondrial energy metabolism in HC. The defect makes the striatal neurons more susceptible to excitotoxin-mediated damage. Lesions produced by inhibitors of mitochondrial energy metabolism in the HC striatum mimic neuropathology of HC. The neuronal damage can be prevented by NMDA-receptor antagonist administration.[79] Complex II and III from the mitochondrial oxidation chains are mainly affected. $CoQ_{10}$, or ubiquinone, is an electron carrier from complex I and II to complex III.[80,81] An open-label pilot study has been performed on $CoQ_{10}$ with 6-months' duration and daily dose of 600–1,200 mg on 10 patients with HC.[82] The study was designed as phase I safety and tolerability, which reported positive results. The study power was evaluated as insufficient for efficacy assessment. The study duration is probably too short, as the process of low metabolic energy level and subsequent free-radical cell damage needs time. The results did not reach statistical significance, but a tendency toward slowing of the total functional capacity decline was noticed. Controlled studies of $CoQ_{10}$ and chorea are being performed.

There are anecdotal reports of chorea improvement with cannabidiol. Cannabidiol is a major nonpsychotropic constituent of cannabis. A controlled trial reported that cannabidiol is neither symptomatically beneficial nor toxic to HC patients, suggesting opioid receptors are unimportant in chorea genesis.[83] There is a general hypothesis that the pathways of akinetic-rigid syndrome generation are opposite to that of hyperkinesia. There is a definite loss of dopaminergic neurons in substantia nigra in PD patients' brains, and the equilibrium between acetylcholine and dopamine in the striatum is shifted toward acetylcholine.[84] A controlled trial on deanol, a precursor of acetylcholine, in five patients with tardive dyskinesia and three patients with HC showed no significant effect on dyskinesias.[61] A trial on lithium, which may induce parkinsonian symptoms, failed to show improvement in six patients with HC.[85] When only some patients show improvement but no statistical significant difference of the drug benefit is reached, the possibility of a drug-responsive subpopulation remains. This fact suggests that performing controlled trials on carefully chosen subpopulations could be more successful. A combination of therapies, proven to have some efficacy in chorea reduction, may be of use in clinical practice.

What is the insight on the pathobiology of chorea brought about from controlled trials and other trials? It is well known that HC is a genetic disease with 100% penetrance. Cytosine-adenine-guanine (CAG) repeat expansions on the short arm of chromosome four have been identified as an underlying genetic defect related to the disease.[86] CAG repeat mutation gene evokes gain, rather than loss, of function. More than 38 CAG repeats are related to phenotypic disease expression.[87] The gene has been named *IT-15* and its product named *huntingtin*. Despite the hopes that this protein will have disease-specific tissue expression, huntingtin is widely expressed in neuronal and non-neuronal tissues.[88] A protein named *huntingtin-associated protein*, (*HAP-1*), was found to have similar heterogeneity of cellular-level expression when compared to huntingtin.[89] Both proteins have a subcellular distribution and a role in intracellular transport. HAP-1 is expressed predominantly in the brain.[90] However, HAP-1 is not present in the neuron aggregates containing fragments of mutant huntingtin in HC brains.[91] The size of huntingtin is directly proportional to the CAG repeats' length. The binding capacity of HAP-1 to huntingtin is enhanced with CAG repeats' length increment.[92]

212    *Clinical Trials in Neurologic Practice*

## TICS

Twenty double-blind placebo-controlled clinical trials on tics have been identified between 1966 and 1998. Almost all trials on tics are performed on Gilles de la Tourette (GTS) patients; this is probably because it is a life-long condition and the most disabling disorder when compared with other tic disorders. There are specific items that must be mentioned in these particular types of clinical trials. A definition of GTS is given by the Tourette Syndrome Classification Study Group.[93] Because the disease usually starts in childhood or adolescence, the majority of recruits for clinical trials are children or adolescents. This fact requires informed consent signed by the parents and assent consent signed by the subject. The compliance is more difficult to secure with children and needs objective confirmation. A study on clonidine and GTS has monitored the drug plasma levels and the pill number for this reason.[94]

The monitoring and the assessment of tics are equally as difficult as any other movement disorder symptom monitoring. There are many clinical scales available for tic assessment. Research tools are the Yale Global Tic Severity Scale, Tourette's Syndrome Severity Scale, Clinical Global Impression Scale, and Hopkins Motion and Vocal Scale.[95] These are the scales most widely used in controlled trials on tics. Again, the percentage of improvement taken as a positive tic response is important for the overall results. A study using prolactin monitoring of haloperidol and pimozide treatment in children with GTS has chosen a 50% or greater decrease in total Tourette Symptom Global Scale Score (TSGS) from baseline as a positive response to treatment.[96] This requirement will lower the level of the false-positive improvement but will also raise the level of the false-negative cases. The drug dose is usually calculated per kilogram, as most of the subjects are children. When two drugs are compared, an equivalent potency dose should be used for accuracy of the results. The above-mentioned study on GTS, haloperidol, and pimozide has used pimozide ($3.4 \pm 1.6$ mg/day) versus haloperidol ($3.5 \pm 2.2$ mg/day) as equivalent dose.[96] Because GTS is three times more frequent in men, male predominance in recruited subject numbers is acceptable.

The 20 double-blind and placebo-controlled clinical trials on GTS demonstrate the following:

1. It is highly advisable not to start treatment unless functional disability is present. A score of more than 20 on TSGS is suggested as a marker for a sufficient symptom severity to start treatment.
2. Family and patient education and participation in support groups are useful tools for delaying treatment.
3. The $\alpha_2$-receptor antagonist clonidine is suggested as one of the first drugs of choice. A controlled study on 47 GTS patients has confirmed its effectiveness versus placebo.[94] Clonidine has similar and sometimes superior effects on tics compared to neuroleptics and has a better side effect profile. The hypothetical action of clonidine is mediated via $\alpha_2$-receptors that modulate the neuron firing rates and the release of norepinephrine from the central norepinephrine neurons. Also, norepinephrine neurons regulate the firing rate of the dopamine neurons in the central tegmental area.
4. Neuroleptics are well-established drugs of choice for tic suppression, but have significant extrapyramidal side effects (EPS). One study has identified an

85% incidence of TD in children treated with haloperidol.[97] Apart from haloperidol, pimozide is the second most used neuroleptic for tic suppression. Both drugs can produce parkinsonian side effects, which may create a "zombie like" appearance in children. Haloperidol probably produces tardive syndrome through upregulation of $D_2$-receptors with chronic treatment, whereas pimozide downregulates the same receptors. Haloperidol is much more sedative than pimozide, but the latter drug can prolong the PQ cardiac interval, which can be hazardous for the patient. Two double-blind placebo-controlled studies were independently performed, comparing the efficacy of both drugs versus placebo on tic control. Both studies have documented efficacy of haloperidol and pimozide.[98,99] The main pathogenic mechanism of tic production is believed to be $D_2$-receptor upregulation. $D_2$-receptor blockage is likely to be a major way through which the neuroleptics reduce tics and produce EPS. In the search for a marker that can predict this side effect, a study using prolactin monitoring of haloperidol and pimozide response in 26 GTS patients has been performed.[96] Prolactin is a lactotroph and partial $D_2$-receptor antagonist and is expected to be elevated in the blood of patients chronically treated with neuroleptics because neuroleptics block the $D_2$-receptors. An elevated level of prolactin has been found only in the pimozide responders. The pimozide nonresponders, the patients treated with haloperidol, and the placebo controls did not show elevated levels of prolactin.[96] This finding was not related to the frequency of EPS appearance, but can be used to separate a well-defined patient subpopulation. A prolactin level of less than 10 ng/ml was related to a 90% EPS-free children and adolescent population, all of whom were on chronic haloperidol treatment. A study on haloperidol found that patient gender, rather than family history, predicts successful treatment outcome.[100]

5. The use of the calcium channel blockers flunarizine and nifedipine has been studied in seven patients with chronic tic disorders.[101] Flunarizine is a piperazine derivative with a mild $D_2$-receptor–blocking property. A single dose of nifedipine did not show statistically significant tic suppression. Despite the fact that calcium channel blocker effect is much milder compared to that of the neuroleptics, it is worth pointing out that 26.6% of the GTS patients experienced migraine, which makes this class of drugs a useful adjunct to tic therapy.

6. GTS is expressed three times more often in men. This fact raises the hypothesis that possible factors provoke the disease in men or suppress it in women. A controlled study on flutamide efficacy, a nonsteroidal androgen receptor–blocking agent with neither androgenic nor estrogenic effect, was performed on two patients in an open-label trial, and on one patient in a controlled trial, for 5 weeks.[102] A 45–60% reduction of tic severity was recorded. However, the one female patient developed severe side effects after the initial improvement, and one of the male patients subsequently lost the initial benefit. The second male patient used the drug after the end of the trial on an intermittent basis and has preserved its effectiveness. This trial shows the tendency to combine open-label and controlled trials using a small sample of patients with a goal of a maximum variety of test conditions, so that the results can be used as a base for further, more extended controlled trials.

7. Open-label trials on nicotine, risperidone, and clonazepam have demonstrated some efficacy on tic control.[103–105] In addition, a controlled trial with methylphenidate or dextroamphetamine in patients with GTS has shown that a

214    *Clinical Trials in Neurologic Practice*

substantial minority of patients worsen with stimulant treatment.[106] However, all the treated patients showed improvement in attention deficit hyperactivity disorder, which occurs in approximately 50% of GTS patients.

What insight did these trials bring to the understanding of the biology of symptom production? A CSF study on seven GTS patients found an increased level of dynorphin, suggesting that endogenous opioids are involved in the pathobiology of GTS and related disorders.[107] Contradictory data of reduced cyclic adenosine monophosphate in GTS patients' brains have been reported, suggesting possible abnormality in the second messenger systems as part of the disease biology.[108] Only four of 20 patients demonstrated significantly elevated $D_2$-receptors on positron emission tomography scan, suggesting a GTS patient subgroup.[109] A segregation analysis suggests GTS susceptibility conveyed by a major locus in combination with a multifactorial background. Only 2.2% of the men and 0.3% of the women who are homozygous for the major disease locus express the disease phenotypically.[110] Significant stress and frequent vomiting during the first trimester of pregnancy have been linked to increased tic severity in the offspring.[111] The disease is believed to be autosomal dominant with incomplete and sex-specific gene penetrance.[112] Various phenotypic expression, such as pure GTS, pure obsessive-compulsive disorder, a combination of both, or as a chronic tic disorder, may occur.[112] The clinical significance of the above-mentioned facts is still under investigation.

## MYOCLONUS, DYSTONIA, ATHETOSIS, RESTLESS LEG SYNDROME, PAINFUL LEGS, MOVING TOES, AKATHISIA, HYPEREXPLEXIA, AND OTHER MOVEMENT DISORDER SYMPTOMS

Not many clinical trials have been performed on movement disorder symptoms, such as myoclonus and dystonia. Myoclonus can be part of many diseases, which makes it difficult to devote clinical trials to myoclonus alone. In addition, myoclonus can be produced at different levels of the nervous system, such as the spinal cord, the brainstem, and the cortex. Two controlled trials on progressive myoclonic epilepsy have been performed in an attempt to assess the efficacy of piracetam, a neurotropic agent, and L-tryptophan, a serotonin precursor, on myoclonus suppression.[113,114] Both drugs demonstrated efficacy versus placebo. Piracetam, at a dose of 24 g per day, showed the highest efficacy. Another study on piracetam has documented a 22% rating scale improvement in 21 patients with disabling spontaneous or action myoclonus.[115]

The assessment of generalized myoclonus is very difficult. Usually, a six-component scale is used in assessing myoclonus: stimulus sensitivity, motor impairment, functional disability, and handwriting and global assessment by investigator and patient.[115]

Botulinum toxin injections have become a gold standard in the treatment of blepharospasm, hemifacial spasm, and torticollis, with proved efficacy by controlled trials and clinical practice.[116–118] Asterixis has been assessed in double-blind controlled trials mainly as a part of chronic hepatic encephalopathy, stereotypy as a

*Hyperkinetic Movement Disorders* 215

part of mental retardation syndrome, and akathisia as a part of schizophrenia.[119–121] The population of individuals with restless leg syndrome, painful legs, and moving toes is too small, which makes the planning of clinical trials difficult.

Hyperkinetic movement disorders are difficult to assess because of their clinical variability over time and because their pathogenesis is not fully understood. Future trials in the field are necessary to fill the blank spots in our present knowledge.

## REFERENCES

1. Bonuccelli U, Ceravolo R, Salvetti S, et al. Clozapine in Parkinson's disease tremor. Effects of acute and chronic administration. Neurology 1997;49(6):1587–1590.
2. Pahwa R, Busenbark K, Swansan-Hyland EF. Botulinum toxin treatment of essential head tremor. Neurology 1995;45:822–824.
3. Busenbark K, Pahwa R, Hubble J, et al. Double-blind controlled study on methazolamide in the treatment of essential tremor. Neurology 1993;43:1045–1047.
4. Busenbark K, Ramig L, Dromey C, Koller W. Methazolamide for essential voice tremor. Neurology 1996;47:1331–1332.
5. Olson WL, Gruenthal M, Mueller ME, Olson WH. Gabapentin for parkinsonism: a double-blind, placebo-controlled, crossover trial. Am J Med 1997;102(1):60–66.
6. Henderson JM, Jiannikas C, Morris JG, et al. Postural tremor of Parkinson's disease. Clin Neuropharmacol 1994;17(3):277–285.
7. Rice GP, Lesaux J, Vandervoort P, et al. Ondansetron, a 5-HT3 antagonist, improved cerebellar tremor. J Neurol Neurosurg Psychiatry 1997;62(3):282–284.
8. Findley LY, Koller WC, DeWitt P, et al. Classification and definition of tremor. In Lord Walton of Detchant (ed), Indications for and Clinical Implications of Botulinum Toxin Therapy. London: Royal Society of Medicine, 1993;22–23.
9. Mally J, Stone TW. Efficacy of adenosine antagonist, theophylline in essential tremor: comparison with placebo and phenobarbital. J Neurol Sci 1995;132(2):129–132.
10. Koller WC. Nadolol in essential tremor. Neurology 1983;33:1076–1077.
11. Koller WC, Herbster G, Cone S. Clonidine in the treatment of essential tremor. Mov Disord 1986;1(4):235–237.
12. Thompson C, Lang A, Parkes JD, Marsden CD. A double-blind trial of clonazepam in benign essential tremor. Clin Neuropharmacol 1984;7(1):83–88.
13. Calzetti S, Findley LY, Gresty MA, et al. Effect of a single oral dose of propranolol on essential tremor: a double-blind controlled study. Ann Neurol 1983;13:165–171.
14. Metzer WS, Paige SR, Newton JE. Inefficacy of propranolol in attenuation of drug-induced parkinsonian tremor. Mov Disord 1993;8(1):43–46.
15. Gorman WP, Cooper R, Pocock P, Campbell MJ. A comparison of primidone, propranolol and placebo in essential tremor, using quantitative analysis. J Neurol Neurosurg Psychiatry 1986;49:64–68.
16. Teravainen H, Larsen A, Fogelholm R. Comparison between the effects of pindolol and propranolol on essential tremor. Neurology 1977;27:439–442.
17. Koller WC, Busenbark KL. Essential Tremor. In RL Watts, WC Koller (eds), Movement Disorders. Neurologic Principles and Practice. McGraw-Hill, 1997;374–375.
18. Paulson HL, Stem MB. Clinical manifestations of Parkinson's disease. In RL Watts, WC Koller (eds), Movement Disorders. Neurologic Principles and Practice. McGraw-Hill, 1997;193–197.
19. Hallett M, Lindsey JN, Adelstein BD, Riley PO. Controlled trial of isoniazid therapy for severe postural cerebellar tremor in multiple sclerosis. Neurology 1985;35:1374–1377.
20. Teravainen H, Fogelholm R, Larsen A. Effect of propranolol on essential tremor. Neurology 1976;26:27–30.
21. Koller WC, Biary N. Metoprolol compared with propranolol in the treatment of essential tremor. Arch Neurol 1984;41:171–172.
22. Calzetti S, Findley LJ, Gresty MA, et al. Metoprolol and propranolol in essential tremor: a double-blind controlled study. J Neurol Neurosurg Psychiatry 1981;44(9):814–819.
23. Teravainen H, Huttunen J, Larsen TA. Selective adrenergic beta-2-receptor blocking drug, ICI-118.551, is effective in essential tremor. Acta Neurol Scand 1986;74:34–37.

216   *Clinical Trials in Neurologic Practice*

24. Jefferson D, Wharrad HJ, Birmingham AT, Patrick JM. The comparative effect of ICI 118551 and propranolol on essential tremor. Br J Clin Pharmacol 1987;24(6):729–734.
25. Jefferson D, Jenner P, Marsden CD. Beta-adrenoreceptor antagonists in essential tremor. J Neurol Neurosurg Psychiatry 1979;42:904–909.
26. Kuroda Y, Kakigi R, Shibasaki H. Treatment of essential tremor with arotinolol. Neurology 1988;38:650–652.
27. Cleeves L, Findley LJ. Beta-adrenoreceptor mechanisms in essential tremor: a comparative single dose study of the effect of a non-selective and a beta-2 selective adrenoreceptor antagonists. J Neurol Neurosurg Psychiatry 1984;47:976–982.
28. Foster NL, Newman RP, LeWitt PA, et al. Peripheral beta-adrenergic blockade treatment of parkinsonian tremor. Ann Neurol 1984;16:505–508.
29. Ogawa N, Takayama H, Yamamoto M. Comparative studies on the effect of beta-adrenergic blockade treatment in essential tremor. J Neurol 1987;235:31–33.
30. Calzetti S, Findley LJ. D,l-propranolol and d-propranolol in essential tremor. In LJ Findley, R Calpidea (eds), Movement Disorders: Tremor. New York: Oxford University Press, 1984;261–269.
31. Teravainen H, Larsen A, Fogelholm R. Comparison between the effects of pindolol and propranolol on essential tremor. Neurology 1997;27(5):439–442.
32. Jefferson D, Jenner P, Marsden CD. Relationship between plasma propranolol concentration and relief of essential tremor. J Neurol Neurosurg Psychiatry 1979;42:831–837.
33. Findley LJ, Cleeves L, Calzetti S. Primidone in essential tremor of the hands and head: a double blind controlled clinical study. J Neurol Neurosurg and Psychiatry 1985;48:911–915.
34. Sasso E, Perucca E, Fava R, Calzetti S. Quantitative comparison of barbiturates in essential hand and head tremor. Mov Disord 1991;6(1):65–68.
35. Sasso E, Emilio P, Calzetti S. Double-blind comparison of primidone and phenobarbital in essential tremor. Neurology 1988;38:808–810.
36. Baruzzi A, Procaccianti G, Martinelli P, et al. Phenobarbital and propranolol in essential tremor: a double-blind controlled clinical trial. Neurology 1983;33:296–300.
37. Findley LJ, Cleeves L. Phenobarbitone in essential tremor. Neurology 1985;35:1784–1787.
38. Calzetti S, Findley LJ, Pisani F, Richens A. Phenylethylmalonamide in essential tremor. A double-blind controlled study. J Neurol Neurosurg Psychiatry 1981;44(10):932–934.
39. Findley LJ. The pharmacological management of essential tremor. Clin Neuropharamacol 1986;9(Suppl 2):S61–S75.
40. McDonald RL, McLeod MJ. Anticonvulsant drugs; mechanism of action. Adv Neurol 1986; 44:713–736.
41. Koller WC, Biary N. Effect of alcohol on tremor: Comparison to propranolol. Neurology 1984; 34:221–222.
42. Rajput AH, Jamieson H, Hrish S, Quraishi A. Relative efficacy of alcohol and propranolol in action tremor. Can J Neurol Sci 1975;2:31–35.
43. Koller WC. Alcoholism in essential tremor. Neurology 1983;33:1074–1076.
44. Routakorpi I, Martila RJ, Rinne UK. Alcohol consumption of patients with essential tremor. Acta Neurol Scand. 1983;68:177–179.
45. Teravainen H, Huttunen J, Lewitt P. Ineffective treatment of essential tremor with an alcohol methylpentynol. J Neurol Neurosurg Psychiatry 1986;49:198–199.
46. Huber SJ, Paulson GW. Efficacy of alprazolam for essential tremor. Neurology 1988;38(2):241–243.
47. Jancovic J, Schwartz K, Clemenee W, et al. A randomized, double-blind, placebo-controlled study to evaluate botulinum toxin type A in essential hand tremor. Mov Disord 1996;11(3):250–256.
48. Biary N, Bahou J, Sofi M, et al. The effect of nimodipine on essential tremor. Neurology 1995;45:1523–1525.
49. Biary N, Al Deeb SM, Langerberg P. The effect of flunarizine on essential tremor. Neurology 1991;41:311–312.
50. Bersani G, Grispini A, Marini S. 5H$_2$ Antagonist ritanserin in neuroleptic-induced parkinsonism: a double-blind comparison with orphenadrine and placebo. Clin Neuropharmacol 1990;13(6):500–506.
51. Koller WC, Hristova AH. Efficacy and safety of stereotaxic surgical treatment of tremor disorders. Eur J Neurol 1996;3:507–514.
52. Koller WC, Wilkinson S, Pahwa R, Miyawaki K. Surgical treatment options in Parkinson's disease. Neurosurg Clin N Am 1998;9(2):295–306.
53. Obeso JA, Rodriguez MC, Gorospe A, et al. Surgical treatment of Parkinson's disease. Baillieres Clin Neurol. 1997;6(1):125–145.
54. Koller WC, Pahwa R, Busabark K, et al. High-frequency unilateral thalamic stimulation in the treatment of essential and parkinsonian tremor. Ann Neurol 1997;42(3):292–299.

## Hyperkinetic Movement Disorders    217

55. Hutchinson WP, Lozano AM, Tasker RR, et al. Identification and characterization of neurons with tremor-frequency activity in human globus pallidus. Exp Brain Res 1997;113(3):557–563.
56. Taha JM, Favre J, Baumann TK, Burchiel KJ. Tremor control after pallidotomy in patients with Parkinson's disease: correlation with microrecording findings. J Neurosurg 1997;86(4):642–647.
57. Biary N, Koller WC. Kinetic predominant tremor: effect of clonazepam. Neurology 1987;37:471–474.
58. Heiman KM. Orthostatic tremor. Arch Neurol 1984;4:880–881.
59. Conneally PM. Genetics of Parkinson's disease. Mov Disord 1998;13(Suppl 2):3.
60. Sabatino M, Sardo P, Ferraro G, et al. Bilateral reciprocal organisation in man: focus on IA interneuron. J Neural Transm Gen Sect 1994;96(1):31–39.
61. Tarsy D, Bralower M. Deanol acetamidobenzoate treatment in choreiform movement disorders. Arch Neurol 1977;34(12):756–758.
62. Van Vugt JP, Siesling S, Vergeer M, et al. Clozapine versus placebo in Huntington's disease a double-blind randomized comparative study. J Neurol Neurosurg Psychiatry 1997;63(1):35–39.
63. Thaker GK, Nguyen JA, Strauss ME, et al. Clonazepam treatment of tardive dyskinesia: a practical GABA mimetic strategy. Am J Psychiatry 1990;147(4):445–451.
64. Jancovic J. Treatment of hyperkinetic movement disorders with tetrabenazine: a double-blind crossover study. Ann Neurol 1982;11:41–47.
65. Albanese A, Cassetta E, Carretta D, et al. Acute challenge with apomorphine in Huntington's Disease: a double-blind study. Clin Neuropharmacol 1995;18(5):427–434.
66. Deroover J, Baro F, Bouguignon RP, Smets P. Tiapride versus placebo: a double-blind comparative study in the management of Huntington's chorea. Curr Med Res Opin 1984;9:329.
67. Huntington Study Group: Unified Huntington's Disease Rating Scale: reliability and consistency. Mov Disord 1996;11:136–142.
68. Shoulson I, Fahn S. Huntington's disease: clinical care and evaluation. Neurology 1979;29:1–3.
69. Aminoff MJ, Marchall J. Treatment of Huntington's chorea with lithium carbonate. Lancet 1974;1(7848):107–109.
70. Lange H, Thorner G, Hopt A, Schroder K. Morphometric studies of the neuropathological changes in choreatic diseases. J Neurol Sci 1976;23:401–425.
71. Reiner A, Albin RL, Anderson KP, et al. Differential loss of striatal projection neurons in Huntington's disease. Proc Natl Acad Sci U S A 1988;85(15):5733–5737.
72. Bucher SF, Seelos KC, Dodel RC, et al. Pallidal lesions. Structural and functional magnetic resonance imaging. Arch Neurol 1996;53(7):682–686.
73. Perry TL, Uruqhart N, Hansen S, Kennedy J. γ-Amino butyric acid: drug-induced elevation in monkey brains. J Neurochem 1974;23:443–445.
74. Manyam BV, Katz L, Hare TA, et al. Isoniazid-induced elevation of CSF GABA levels and effects on chorea in Huntington's disease. Ann Neurol 1981;10:35–37.
75. Mateo D, Gimenez-Roldan S. The effect of piracetam on involuntary movements in Huntington's disease. A double-blind, placebo-controlled study. Neurologia 1996;11(1):16–19.
76. Kieburtz K, Feigin A, McDermoff M, et al. A controlled trial on Remacemide hydrochloride in Huntington's Disease. Mov Disord 1996;11(3):273–277.
77. Giffra E, Mouradian M, Chase TN. Milacemide glutamatergic therapy of Huntington's chorea. Clin Neuropharmacol 1992;15(2):148–151.
78. Koroshetz WJ, Jenkins BG, Rosen BG, Beal MF. Energy metabolism defects in Huntington's disease and effects of coenzyme $Q_{10}$. Ann Neurol 1997;41(2):160–165.
79. Beal MF. Does impairment of energy metabolism result in excitotoxic neuronal death in neurodegenerative illnesses? Ann Neurol 1992;31(2):119–130.
80. Shapira AH. Mitochondrial dysfunction in neurodegenerative disorders. Biochim Biophys Acta 1998;1366:225–233.
81. Browne SE, Bowling AC, MacGarvey U, et al. Oxidative damage and metabolic dysfunction in Huntington's disease: selective vulnerability of the basal ganglia. Ann Neurol 1997;41(5):646–653.
82. Feigin A, Kieburtz K, Coup et al. Assessment of Coenzyme $Q_{10}$ tolerability in Huntington's disease. Mov Disord 1996;11(3):321–323.
83. Consroe P, Laguna J, Allender J, et al. Controlled clinical trials of cannabidiol in Huntington's disease. Pharmacol Biochem Behav 1991;40(3):701–708.
84. Wooten GF. Neurochemistry and Neuropharmacology of Parkinson's Disease. In RL Watts, WC Koller (eds), Movement Disorders. Neurologic Principle and Practice. McGraw-Hill, 1997;153–160.
85. Vestergaard P, Baastrup PC, Peterson H. Lithium treatment of Huntington's chorea a placebo controlled clinical trial. Acta Psychiat Scand 1977;56:183–188.

218  *Clinical Trials in Neurologic Practice*

86. Gusella JF, MacDonald E. Genetics and Molecular Biology of Huntington's Disease. In RL Watts RL, WC Koller (eds), Movement Disorders. Neurologic Principles and Practice. McGraw-Hill, 1997;477–491.
87. Culjkovic B, Ruzdijic S, Ranic L, Romac S. Improved polymerase chain reaction conditions for quick diagnostics of Huntington's disease. Brain Res Brain Res Protoc 1997;2(1):44–46.
88. Kosinski CM, Cha JH, Young AB, et al. Huntingtin immunoreactivity in the rat neostriatum: differential accumulation in projection and interneurons. Exp Neurol 1997;144(2):232–247.
89. Bloch-Balarza J, Chase KO, Sapp E, et al. Fast transport and retrograde movement of huntingtin and HAP-1 in axons. Neuroreport 1997;8(9–10):2247–2251.
90. Nasir J, Duan K, Nichol K, et al. Gene structure and map location of the murine homolog of the Huntington-associated protein, HAP 1. Mamm Genome 1998;9(7):567–570.
91. Gutekunst CA, Li SH, Yi H, et al. The cellular and subcellular localization of huntingtin-associated protein 1 (HAP 1): Comparison with huntingtin in rat and human. J Neurosci 1998;18(19):7674–7686.
92. Li HJ, Li SH, Sharp AH, et al. A huntingtin-associated protein enriched in brain with implications for pathology. Nature 1995;378(6555):398–402.
93. Tourette Syndrome Classification Study Group. Definition and classification of tic disorders. Arch Neurol 1993;50:1013–1016.
94. Leckman JF, Hardin MT, Riddle MA, et al. Clonidine treatment of Gilles de la Tourette's Syndrome. Arch Gen Psychiatry 1991;48(4):324–328.
95. Leckman JF, Riddle MA, Hardin MT, et al. The Yale Global Tic Severity Scale: initial testing of a clinician-rated scale of tic severity. J Am Acad Child Adolesc Psychiatry 1989;28(4):566–573.
96. Sallee FR, Dougherty D, Sethuraman G, Vrindavanam N. Prolactin monitoring of haloperidol and pimozide treatment in children with Tourette's Syndrome. Biol Psychiatry 1996;40:1044–1050.
97. Campbell M, Adams P, Perry R, et al. Tardive and withdrawal dyskinesia in autistic children: a prospective study. Psychopharmacol Bull 1988;24:251–255.
98. Sallee RF, Pharm LN, Pharm CJ, et al. Relative efficacy of haloperidol and pimozide in children and adolescents with Tourette's Disorder. Am J Psychiatry 1997;154:1057–1062.
99. Shapiro E, Shapiro A, Fulop G, et al. Controlled study on haloperidol, pimozide and placebo for the treatment of Gilles de la Tourette's Syndrome. Arch Gen Psychiatry 1989;46:722–730.
100. Schwabe MJ, Konkol RJ. Treating Tourette syndrome with haloperidol: predictors of success. Wis Med J 1989;88(10):23–27.
101. Micheli F, Gatto M, Lekluniec E, et al. Treatment of Tourette's syndrome with calcium antagonists. Clin Neuropharmacol 1990;13(1):77–83.
102. Peterson DS, Leckman JK, Scahill L, et al. Steroid hormones and Tourette's syndrome. Early Experience with Antiandrogen Therapy. J Clin Psychopharmacol 1994;14(2):131–135.
103. Dursun SM, Revelrey MA. Differential effects of transdermal nicotine on microstructured analysis of tics in Tourette's syndrome: an open study. Psychol Med 1991;27(2):483–487.
104. Bruun RD, Budman CL. Risperidone as a treatment for Tourette's syndrome. J Clin Psychiatry 1996;57(1):29–31.
105. Gonce M, Barbeau A. Seven cases of Gilles de la Tourette's syndrome: partial relief with Clonazepam: a pilot study. Can J Neurol Sci 1977;4(4):279–283.
106. Castellanos FX, Giedd JN, Elia J. Controlled stimulant treatment of ADHD and comorbid Tourette's syndrome: effects of stimulant and dose. J Am Acad Child Adolesc Psychiatry 1997;36(5):589–596.
107. Leckman JF, Riddle MA, Berrettini WH, et al. Elevated CSF dynorphin A [1-8] in Tourette's syndrome. Life Sci 1988;43(24):2015–2023.
108. Singer HS, Dickinson J, Martinic D, Levine M. Second messenger systems in Tourette's syndrome. J Neurol Sci 1995;128(1):78–83.
109. Wong DF, Singer HS, Brandt J, et al. $D_2$-like dopamine receptor density in Tourette syndrome measured by PET. J Nucl Med 1997;38(8):1243–1247.
110. Walkup JT, LaBuda MC, Singer HS, et al. Family study and segregation analysis of Tourette syndrome: evidence for a mixed model of inheritance. Am J Hum Genet 1996;59(3):684–693.
111. Leckman JF, Dolnasky ES, Hardin MT, et al. Perinatal factors in the expression of Tourette's syndrome: an exploratory study. J Am Acad Child Adolesc Psychiatry 1990;29(2):220–226.
112. Paul DL, Leckman JF. The inheritance of Gilles de la Tourette's syndrome and associated behaviours: evidence for autosomal dominant transmission. N Engl J Med 1986;315:993–997.
113. Koskiniemi M, Van-Vleymen B, Hakamies L, et al. Piracetam relieves symptoms in progressive myoclonus epilepsy: a multicentre, randomised, double-blind, crossover study comparing the efficacy and safety of three dosages of oral piracetam with placebo. J Neurol Neurosurg Psychiatry 1998;64(3):344–348.

## Hyperkinetic Movement Disorders    219

114. Koskiniemi M, Hyyppa M, Sainio K, et al. Transient effect of L-tryptophan in progressive myoclonus epilepsy without Lafora bodies. Epilepsia 1980;21(4):351–357.
115. Brown P, Steiger MJ, Thompson PD, et al. Effectiveness of piracetam in cortical myoclonus. Mov Disord 1993;8(1):63–68.
116. Park YC, Lim JK, Lee DK, Yi SD. Botulinum A toxin treatment of hemifacial spasm and blepharospasm. J Korean Med Sci 1993;8(5):334–340.
117. Ransmayr G, Kleedorfer B, Dierckx RA, et al. Pharmacological study in Meige's syndrome with predominant blepharospasm. Clin Neuropharmacol 1988;11(1):68–76.
118. Jankovic J, Oram J. Botulinum A toxin for cranial-cervical dystonia; a double blind, placebo-controlled study. Neurology 1987;37(4):616–623.
119. Riggio O, Ariosto F, Meril M, et al. Short-term oral zinc supplementation does not improve chronic hepatic encephalopathy, results of a double-blind, crossover trial. Dig Dis Sci 1991;36(9):1204–1208.
120. Lewis MH, Bredfish JW, Powell SB, Golden RN. Clomipramine treatment for stereotype and related repetitive movement disorders associated with mental retardation. Am J Ment Retard 1995;100(3):299–312.
121. Small JG, Hirsch SR, Arvanitis LA, et al. Quetiapine in patients with schizophrenia. A high and low dose double-blind comparison with placebo. Seroquel Study Group. Arch Gen Psychiatry 1997;54(6):549–557.

# 11
## Multiple Sclerosis
Myriam Schluep and Julien Bogousslavsky

Multiple sclerosis (MS) is an inflammatory demyelinating disease of the central nervous system that has variable and unpredictable courses. The evaluation of the effect and efficacy of therapies in MS has thus always been a difficult task. The presumed but unspecified immune-mediated cause of MS has led to an attempt to develop therapies that can modify the immune response. The design of the clinical trials conducted in MS has usually included a group of patients receiving placebo, looking for differences in behavior between the various groups of patients tested using several outcome measures. The standard methods used to assess MS activity, and therefore to judge the potential therapeutic efficacy of new components, are commonly the Kurtzke Expanded Disability Status Scale (EDSS),[1] a measure of the neurologic handicap, the exacerbation rate, and magnetic resonance imaging (MRI). MRI studies are complementary to clinical assessments because serial MRI studies of the brain have proven that frequent asymptomatic disease activity occurs in relapsing-remitting MS, and in MS in general.[2] This observation reflects that there are many more active lesions in the brain than clinical relapses (15:1 ratio[2]). Consequently, the clinical measure of MS poorly reflects MS activity, although the desired efficacy of developing treatments deals mostly with the possibility of interfering with the progression of neurologic handicap. The therapeutic strategies used, developed, and tested in clinical trials in MS generally deal with three different objects: (1) the treatment of acute relapses, (2) the prevention of acute relapses, and (3) the prevention of disease progression, measured using MRI techniques and the assessment of the neurologic handicap (EDSS).

Placebo-controlled double-blind clinical trials are designed to demonstrate whether a specific substance has any pharmacologic and dose-responsive effects on MS course and/or activity. These kinds of trials are more appropriate for this purpose than other types of clinical studies, such as the ones that use historical controls. The patients receiving placebo should behave as they would in the natural course of the disease. However, some inevitable biases are usually encountered, such as the effect of trial selection, the different care received by patients during any trial (in comparison to that received in the absence of trial), and of

222    *Clinical Trials in Neurologic Practice*

the placebo itself, which has less negative effect than no intervention. These effects may influence the analysis of the results, because of the behavior of the placebo-control group, and also because of the possible placebo effect of the drug tested.

Clinical trials have largely been conducted, or are still in progress, in relapsing-remitting MS, secondary progressive MS, and clinically probable MS (inclusion of the patients shortly after first relapse). However, few clinical trials have been conducted in primary progressive MS. Clinical studies usually look for an effect of the tested substance on the relapse rate, the progression of disability (EDSS), and on MRI lesion load and activity.

Because there is an incomplete understanding of the pathogenesis of MS, treatments that aim to interfere with MS course are empirically based, and their testing encounters some major obstacles to progress: the highly variable course of MS, the long-term nature of the most important clinical outcome measures, and the lack of objective markers of treatment effect (particularly in the short-term). However, the development of objective outcome measures based on MRI and the knowledge of the many pitfalls of clinical trials have led to improved trial methods and a better interpretation of the results.

## CLINICAL TRIALS EVALUATING THE MANAGEMENT OF ACUTE RELAPSE

Both corticosteroids and adrenocorticotropic hormone (ACTH) were demonstrated to accelerate the recovery[3,4] of acute relapses, and since then steroids have become an established treatment of acute exacerbations in MS. High-dose intravenous methylprednisolone (IVMP) and ACTH were shown to have similar influence on the rate of recovery and the final outcome of acute exacerbations,[3] and equivalent high doses of oral MP and IVMP were shown to have identical efficacy.[5] It is important for the care of individual patients that such trials demonstrate that high doses of IVMP can significantly decrease clinical disability scores at short-term after the beginning of the treatment of relapse (at 1 and 4 weeks) in comparison with the absence of therapy. These trials did not, however, prevent the development of further relapse or progression of the disease.[4] However, the documentation that the treatment of acute optic neuritis, which may be the first clinical manifestation of MS, without probable or definite MS and with high doses of IVMP followed by oral prednisone delayed the development of definite MS[6] and had some practical implications in the care of such patients. Thus, this effect was mostly seen in patients with multiple focal brain MRI abnormalities, and the clinical benefit of IVMP lasted for 2 years, with lack of difference between treatment groups at 4 years. One study has compared commonly used courses of oral versus intravenous steroids,[7] without finding any significant difference in the clinical outcome or efficacy of the two treatment groups. Although only a restricted number of patients were included, this study raises the open question of the most adequate route of administration, and possibly doses, for steroids in the treatment of acute MS exacerbations. The need to answer this question is emphasized by the difference in the cost between the treatment regimens and by the rare, but possible, serious complications of IVMP.

*Multiple Sclerosis* 223

In addition to its administration in acute relapses, pulse IVMP was attempted in secondary progressive MS.[8] MS patients were receiving high- or low-dose IVMP every other month in a phase II study. No treatment effect was evident for the primary outcome, a comparison of the proportions of patients in each treatment group who after 2 years experienced sustained progression of disability. However, a relative treatment effect was detected in the high-dose regimen when time to onset of sustained progression of disability was analyzed.

The beneficial effect of IVMP is not completely understood, but is probably correlated to both nonimmunomodulatory and immunomodulatory properties of steroids. IVMP acts on the blood–brain barrier. Blood–brain barrier breakdown, in association with inflammation, is an early or even preceding event in the appearance of acute demyelinating lesions in MS.[9] Blood–brain barrier disruption is the earliest sign detected in the development of new MS lesions, and is temporarily reduced by IVMP. MRI studies showed that IVMP rapidly reduces blood–brain barrier abnormalities in 96% of gadolinium diethylenetriamine pentaacetic acid (Gd-DTPA)–enhancing lesions. However, Gd-DTPA re-enhancement of many lesions was observed within a few days after stopping IVMP, and new MS lesions appeared within a few days after stopping treatment but were more frequently identified after 1 month.[10] The suppression of Gd-DTPA enhancement by IVMP is correlated with concomitant clinical improvement[11] and was shown to be accompanied by a decrease in myelin breakdown, as assessed by measurement of myelin basic protein level in cerebrospinal fluid.[12] Corticosteroids also have immunoregulatory effects, including cytokine production inhibition,[13,14] such as interleukin (IL) IL-1$\alpha$, IL-2, IL-4, IL-6, IL-10, interferon-$\gamma$, and tumor necrosis factor–$\alpha$.

This lack of a complete understanding of corticosteroid biologic effects in MS may partly explain why there is no clear consensus as to which agent to use, the dosage, or the duration of treatment.[15] Thus, the incomplete data obtained from the trials already conducted may warrant some further larger trials. However, any type of corticosteroid has limited effect on the overall course of MS, and there is no evidence that corticosteroids affect relapse frequency or the long-term risk for disability. The development of more effective treatments for acute relapse, as well as therapies to reduce the frequency of relapse, is an important goal to pursue.

## Clinical Studies Evaluating Interferon-$\beta$

Three randomized double-blind, placebo-controlled clinical trials have been conducted to evaluate the efficacy of interferon-$\beta$ (IFN-$\beta$) in relapsing-remitting MS. One trial assessed IFN-$\beta$ 1b[16,17] and two trials assessed IFN-$\beta$ 1a,[18–20] using different outcomes measures (Table 11.1). One further comparable trial evaluated the effect of IFN-$\beta$ 1b in secondary progressive MS.[21] The parameters used (see Table 11.1) aim to evaluate the effect of IFN-$\beta$ on the course of MS in the different groups of patients considered within each study. However, these parameters may be of limited value in evaluating the responsiveness of individual patients because they may fluctuate unpredictably and be difficult to measure because they are too infrequent (e.g., relapse rate) or have too low a sensitivity for detecting mild changes (e.g., EDSS). Furthermore, MRI activity and lesion

## 224   *Clinical Trials in Neurologic Practice*

*Table 11.1*   Outcome measures used in multiple sclerosis (MS) clinical trials as potential markers of interferon-β responsiveness and efficacy*

| | |
|---|---|
| **Clinical assessment** | Relapse rate |
| | Percentage of patients relapse-free |
| | Number of moderate to severe relapses |
| | Number of steroid courses and hospitalizations |
| | Time to confirmed progression in disability |
| | Integrated disability status scale |
| **MRI assessment** | Burden of disease (total lesion load; T2) |
| | Active, new, or enlarging lesions (T2; Gd-DTPA enhancement) |

MRI = magnetic resonance imaging.

*Relapse definition: appearance of a new symptom or worsening of an old symptom over at least 24 hours, that could be attributed to MS activity and that was preceded by stability or improvement for at least 30 days.

load are not accepted as being as important as MS clinical activity, and have only a restricted correlation with the clinical outcome measures used in clinical trials (see Table 11.1).

IFN-β 1b (Betaferon), a recombinant molecule produced in *Escherichia coli* that differs from human IFN-β by the absence of glycosylation, the substitution of a serine for cysteine at position 17, and the lack of N-terminal methionine, was the first IFN-β to demonstrate its efficacy in relapsing-remitting MS.[16,17] Three hundred seventy-two patients (EDSS score, 0–5.5) received subcutaneously every other day 1.8 MIU, 8 MIU of IFN-β 1b, or placebo. Primary outcome measures were annual exacerbation rate and proportion of exacerbation-free patients. The following results were reported for the high-dosage group in comparison to the placebo cohort:

1. Approximately one-third reduction in the frequency of exacerbations (0.84 versus 1.27 at 2 years; 0.84 versus 1.21 at 3 years)
2. A 50% reduction in moderate and severe exacerbations
3. A prolongation of the time to first or second relapse
4. An increase in the number of patients exacerbation-free after 2 years. (This increase disappeared after 3 years.)
5. A mean increase in MRI lesion area of 17.1% in the placebo group
6. A mean decrease of 6.2% in the 8 MIU group at 3 years
7. A median reduction of 83% in the rate of active lesions compared with the placebo group for a subgroup of patients having MRI scans performed at 6-week intervals

There was a trend, without statistical significance, for a slower progression of disability (progression in disability defined as a persistent and confirmed increase of one or more points in the EDSS score) in the 8 MIU group.[22] As a consequence of the above effects on MS course assessed clinically and by MRI, IFN-β 1b was approved for use in selected patients with MS.[23] However, the observation that the development of neutralizing antibodies (NAB) that block its activity in 31% of treated patients at 1 year and 38% at 3 years (for the 8 MIU cohort, with comparable frequency in the 1.6 MIU–treated group, suggesting that it was not dose dependent)[22,24] may limit its use in some groups of patients.[25] Indeed, the development of NAB was associated with an increase in the rate of acute exacerbations per year, which was similar to the placebo group at 18 months. NAB development was also associated with a greater number of enlarging lesions and new lesions in MRI when compared to patients without antibodies against IFN-β 1b.[24] However, when up to 5 years' data from the same trial were analyzed in a longitudinal way (to evaluate whether the change from NAB-negative to NAB-positive in individual patients was associated with a lower clinical efficacy), different conclusions were reached regarding the effects of NAB on drug efficacy. A statistically significant increase in the annual exacerbation rate was observed in patients developing NAB only in the low-dose arm, but not in the 8 MIU group; only a nonsignificant trend of increased relapse rate was noted in the 8 MIU group. Furthermore, a change from NAB-negative to NAB-positive status was associated with a statistically suggestive improvement in the percentage change in MRI lesion burden for the 8 MIU group. Thus, conclusions reached after analysis of these same data using different approaches have not consistently indicated that changing from NAB-negative to NAB-positive status correlates with a diminished clinical efficacy.[26]

On this basis, IFN-β 1b prescription was assessed to be indicated in patients with relapsing-remitting MS and also to be sensible in patients with relapsing-progressive MS showing signs of active disease.[27] Probable disease activity could be indicated by the occurrence of relapses during the 2 previous years, as well as by the presence of Gd-DTPA–enhanced lesions on MRI.

IFN-β 1a, a recombinant glycosylated molecule produced in Chinese hamster ovary cells and similar to human IFN-β, was evaluated in patients presenting with relapsing MS using 6 MIU (30 μg) intramuscular weekly injections (Avonex) in a randomized double-blind placebo-controlled study, including 301 patients with an EDSS of 1.0–3.5.[18,19] IFN-β 1a:

1. Decreased the annual exacerbation rate in IFN-β 1a treated patients (0.61 with IFN-β 1a versus 0.90 with placebo)
2. Lengthened the time to sustained progression in EDSS score (increase of at least 1 point; primary end point)
3. Slowed the accumulation of neurologic disability with progression by the end of 104 weeks in 34.9% of the patients in the placebo group and 21.9% of patients in the IFN-β 1a treated group
4. Diminished the number and volume of Gd-DTPA–enhanced MRI lesions, although IFN-1β 1a did not have an effect on T2 lesion volume.

Although there was a significant delay in 6-month–confirmed progression by 1 point in the lower part of the EDSS, which essentially measures impairment and not disability, the clinical significance of these results is not completely clear because of the small numbers of patients (172 patients at 2 years, 31 patients at 3 years) and the premature termination of the trial. The occurrence of NAB against IFN-β 1a (14–22% of the patients) was associated with the following: a trend for reduced benefits of IFN-β 1a on MRI activity (patients were considered positive with a single positive titer), and positive patients displaying suggestively more contrast-enhancing brain lesions on MRI at the end of the second year than antibody-negative patients. No correlation with relapse rate or disability progression could be found after 2 years.[18,19,28]

226    *Clinical Trials in Neurologic Practice*

A third study, which tested IFN-β 1a (Rebif), investigated the optimum dose and degree of clinical benefit with IFN-β 1a in relapsing-remitting MS.[20] Five hundred and sixty patients with an EDSS score ranging from 0 to 5 were investigated in a randomized double-blind placebo-controlled trial. They received 22 μg (6 MIU), 44 μg (12 MIU), or placebo subcutaneously three times weekly for 2 years; 502 patients (90%) completed the study and were analyzed. The major outcome parameters studied were relapse rate, disability, disease activity, and burden of disease shown by MRI. The primary outcome measure was the relapse count over the course of the study. Other outcome measures included the times to develop the first and second relapse, the proportion of relapse-free patients, the progression in disability, the ambulation index, the arm-function index, the need for steroid therapy, hospital admissions, disease activity evaluated with MRI and burden of disease, and the integrated disability status scale (IDSS; area under a time/EDSS curve). The relapse rate was significantly lower at 1 and 2 years with a risk reduction of 27% and 33%, respectively, for the 22-μg and 44-μg groups, compared to placebo (mean number of relapses per patient: 2.56 for placebo, 1.82 for 22 μg, and 1.73 for 44 μg); the time to develop the first relapse was prolonged by 3 and 5 months in the 22-μg and 44-μg groups, respectively, and the proportion of relapse-free patients was significantly increased; the mean number of moderate and severe relapses during the 2-year follow-up period was lower in both IFN-β 1a groups than in the placebo group (placebo, mean 0.99; 22 μg, 0.71; 44 μg, 0.62); IFN-β 1a delayed the progression of disability (defined as an increase in EDSS of at least 1 point sustained over at least 3 months), and decreased accumulated disability during the study. The time in months to confirmed progression in disability for all included patients was 11.9 in the placebo group, 18.5 with 22 μg, and 21.3 with 44 μg. The time in months for patients with a baseline EDSS greater than 3.5 was 7.3 with placebo, 7.5 with 22 μg (not significant), and 21.3 with 44 μg. The evaluation of IDSS, a summary measure of disability occurring during the study period, demonstrated that it did not increase during the study in IFN-β 1a therapy groups, but the placebo group had an increase of 0.4 IDSS steps per year. The accumulation of burden of disease (T2 MRI; progressive median increase of 10.9% in placebo-treated patients, median decrease of 1.2% with 22 μg, and of 3.8% with 44 μg, in comparison with placebo) and the number of T2-active lesions on MRI were lower in both treatment groups than in the placebo group. Dose effects were demonstrated for most clinical outcome measures including relapse rates and severity, and were even more pronounced for MRI outcomes. Also, in the subgroup of patients likely to develop progressive MS (EDSS >3.5), the 44-μg dose delayed progression of disability significantly better than 22 μg or placebo. The use of IDSS allowed quantification of temporary and unremitting disability during the study period, and, therefore, has several advantages and may be complementary to the standard measure of time to confirmed progression. At 2 years, NAB occurred in 23.8% of the patients receiving 22 μg, and in 12.5% receiving 44 μg. The presence of NAB did not affect the mean relapse count.

IFN-β 1b (Betaferon) was also tested in secondary progressive MS,[21] in a double-blind, randomized, placebo-controlled trial, including 718 patients with an EDSS score of 3.0–6.5. Patients received either 8 MIU IFN-β 1b subcutaneously every other day or placebo for 2–3 years. (The study was stopped after interim analysis because of some evidence for efficacy; analysis of 531 patients.) The cohort studied included patients who were progressing with or without superimposed relapses following an initial relapsing-remitting phase.[29] Patients were in the early stage of progression, beginning approximately 10 years after the initial diagnosis of MS, and had active disease during the 2 years before their entry in the study. The primary outcome was the time to develop confirmed progression in disability as measured by a 1 point increase in the EDSS, sustained for at least 3 months, or a 0.5 point increase if the baseline EDSS was 6.0 or 6.5. IFN-β 1b significantly delayed the time to onset of sustained progression of disability (range of delay, 9–12 months, with a probability of 65% and 60% to remain progression-free; study period of 2–3 years) in patients with superimposed relapses and in patients who had only progressive deterioration without relapses; 49.7% of patients had confirmed progression in the placebo group, compared to 38.9% in the IFN-β 1b group. IFN-β 1b also significantly increased the time to become wheelchair-bound (delay of up to 9 months longer in the treatment group in comparison with placebo) and reduced the following: relapse rate and severity, the number of steroid treatments and hospital admissions, the number of newly active MRI lesions (diminution of 65–78% compared to placebo), and the progression of total T2-weighted lesion load (increase by approximately 8% in the placebo group of the mean T2-lesion volume; decrease of 5% in the IFN-β 1b group). NAB were detected in 27.8% patients (with some of the patients [37 of 100] remaining negative in subsequent tests); positive NAB patients had a significant decrease of the therapeutic effect for the relapse rate but not for changes on the EDSS.

Because the EDSS is poorly sensitive at certain levels, particularly between 6.0 and 7.0, 0.5 point steps were counted as full steps from a baseline EDSS of 6.0 or 6.5[30] in this last clinical trial. Thus, the length of time spent at these EDSS levels are frequently prolonged in comparison to other points on the EDSS scale, reflecting the usually more extended period of deterioration leading to the loss of the ability to walk. In secondary progressive MS, two different mechanisms of deterioration occur: incomplete recovery from relapses and slow insidious progression. Relapses, corresponding to acute inflammation phases, are likely to induce and be associated with demyelination and axonal loss. Disease progression may be associated with continuous damage due to low-grade inflammatory activity or to a degenerative process. Two potential modes of action may then be hypothesized for an effect of IFN-β 1b on disability progression in secondary progressive MS: the suppression of low-grade inflammation or eventually a protective effect on myelin and axons. These results on disease progression may justify expanding the indications for IFN-β 1b to patients with secondary progressive MS, possibly even if they do not present with superimposed relapses. This attitude may, however, have to be modulated in the future: some yet unpublished data (preliminary oral communications) from two recently terminated double-blind, placebo-controlled trials testing, respectively, IFN-β 1a (Rebif; $3 \times 22$ mg or $3 \times 44$ mg per week) or IFN-β 1b (Betaferon; 8 MIU every other day) against placebo in secondary progressive MS did not seem to confirm the results of the above study.[21] Complementary results are awaited.

Although the grouped data of the different above-mentioned clinical trials show a consistent therapeutic effect of IFN-β on the reduction in relapse rate, the time to develop disability, the percentage of patients progressing, and on several different MRI measures, there are few data to guide the neurologist in determin-

228    *Clinical Trials in Neurologic Practice*

ing whether a given patient will obtain a clinical benefit from IFN-β therapy. There are no tools available to follow individual clinical responses easily or to know whether a patient is no longer responding to IFN-β. The use of frequent Gd-DTPA–enhanced MRI could provide an MRI definition for identifying responders and nonresponders, but its cost and absence of clear clinical correlation are against its usefulness in neurologic practice. The development of NAB, although initially thought to be a predictor for the loss of IFN-β biologic activity, does not emerge, used solely, as a reliable indicator for evaluating responsiveness, and may, furthermore, be only a transient phenomenon.

It has been shown, in a large population-based natural history study,[31] that a high-relapse frequency early in MS correlates with the 10-year disability outcome. However, whether the decrease in relapses induced by IFN-β leads to a reduction in long-term disability still remains to be shown. Disability in MS may result from two distinct but often overlapping mechanisms: the failure to recover from relapses (incomplete remission) and a slow continuous progression. These mechanisms may have different underlying pathologies.[32] Secondary progressive MS is the phase of the disease in which major irreversible disabilities most often appear. The goal of treatments in MS is to prevent relapses as well as progressive worsening of the disease. The decision to initiate IFN-β therapy in individual MS patients should be based on the course of the patient's disease and on the probability, in each case, of developing severe disabling disease before neurologic deficits persist and become fixed. IFN-β treatment should be optimally considered early in the course of MS for patients with an unfavorable prognosis.

Side effects associated with IFN-β 1a[20] included injection-site reactions; influenza-like symptoms; fatigue; significant asymptomatic decreases in white cells, neutrophils, and lymphocytes; thrombocytopenia; and elevated liver aminotransferase values (more pronounced in the higher dose, 44 µg IFN-β 1a). Side effects associated with IFN-β 1b[21] were comparable and included flu-like symptoms, injection site necrosis, muscle hypertonia, hypertension, leukopenia, and abnormal values of liver enzymes.

## Therapeutic Approaches with Interferon-β from Clinical Trial Results

Clinical trials conducted with different IFN-βs provide some evidence for a dose-response phenomenon for clinical and MRI responses, which was also documented in another double-blind study including 293 patients presenting with relapsing-remitting MS (EDSS, 0–5.0) testing weekly subcutaneous injection of 22 µg or 44 µg of IFN-β 1a (Rebif), or placebo.[33] For 48 weeks, results showed a dose effect for IFN-β 1a on relapse frequency, and on MRI parameters including disease activity and burden of disease. But, no significant clinical effect was demonstrated. These results point out the necessity for a better delineation of the factors that may influence individual patients' response to IFN-β (e.g., relapse rate during the 2 years preceding therapy; EDSS score; MRI spectroscopy studies to detect reduced *N*-acetyl aspartate, a hallmark for axonal changes and degeneration) or other similar therapies. The early initiation of such treatments that reduce inflammation may also potentially emphasize their effect on disease progression because axonal transection, an irreversible step that may be the pathologic correlate of irreversible neurologic impairment, already occurs in central nervous system areas of active demyelination and inflammation.[34]

The different clinical trials testing IFN-β 1a and IFN-β 1b all tended to demonstrate, to some extent, the same positive effects on MS course. This observation reinforced the results obtained in the various studies that were differently powered to show changes in chosen parameters (e.g., disability [EDSS], relapse frequency). The fact that up to 5-years' data confirmed the positive effects obtained after 3 years[22] (e.g., absence of significant increase in MRI lesion burden, and sustained decrease of approximately 30% of the relapse frequency in patients included for a median time of approximately 4 years) demonstrates a persistence of treatment efficacy and also sustains the results already obtained.

What is the relevance of NAB?[35] Antibodies produced against injected proteins do not all have the same impact. Some antibodies may only bind to the concerned protein, whereas others may neutralize its action(s). Because the mechanisms of action of IFN-β are not exactly known, no in vitro assay of effective neutralizing antibodies exists; there are only surrogate assays. Existing assays are based on different biologic effects of IFN, and the assays being used include the cytopathic effect assays and myxovirus resistance gene assays, as well as antiproliferative neutralization assays. It is open to debate whether these assays are all equivalent, and whether viral inhibition (cytopathic effect; assay used in Betaferon, Avonex, Rebif studies) confers the beneficial effect of IFN-β in MS is speculative. On the other hand, it must be assessed whether antibodies directed against a drug are always detrimental. There is some evidence of no (or only partial) alteration of the functions of the concerned protein after antibody binding has been shown: the binding of antibodies may potentially have a positive effect by acting as carriers for cytokines and prolonging their half-life for biologic activity.[34] Other issues are as follows: (1) the possibility, once induced, that NAB may be transient and not permanent; and (2) the unknown long-term effects of NAB, with the assumption that IFN-β NAB have the potential to diminish patients' defenses against viruses and possibly cancer as well. What are the consequences of all the above-mentioned controversies and the unanswered questions for the practicing neurologist? Decisions for discontinuing IFN-β or changing therapies are best made on a clinical basis. The presence of NAB may add support to a decision to alter therapy, but such decisions should not be based solely on the presence of NAB. For example, if an individual patient still continues to have relapses of the same severity and frequency after a period of treatment with IFN-β at 6 or more months as before, a switch to another agent may be advisable. This is particularly true if high titers of NAB are persistently present, with the restriction that the patient was receiving an appropriate dosage of IFN-β (with reference to the type of MS and to the patient's EDSS score) and was not underdosed. There is, however, not enough information regarding the interpretations of the results of already existing IFN-β NAB assays to warrant routine NAB testing.[36]

## CLINICAL TRIALS EVALUATING GLATIRAMER ACETATE (COPOLYMER 1)

Glatiramer acetate (Copaxone) is a random synthetic amino acid copolymer, composed of L-alanine, L-glutamic acid, L-lysine, and L-tyrosine, and is immu-

230 *Clinical Trials in Neurologic Practice*

nologically cross-reactive with myelin basic protein. A double-blind, randomized, placebo-controlled trial including 251 patients with relapsing-remitting MS (EDSS score, 0–5) tested daily administration of 20-mg glatiramer acetate injected subcutaneously for 2 years[37] (215 patients were analyzed). The primary end point was the mean number of relapses occurring during the study. Glatiramer acetate induced, in comparison with placebo, a 29% reduction of the exacerbation rate[37,38] (mean relapse rate of 1.19 for placebo, and 1.68 for glatiramer acetate), with a trend for a more pronounced effect on relapses in patients presenting with low EDSS scores. Furthermore, the benefit diminished with the increase of disability at entry in the study.[37] Although glatiramer acetate also demonstrated a trend for efficacy on the progression of neurologic disability,[37] there was no significant difference between the two groups of patients for the proportion of relapse-free patients, the time to first relapse, or for the progression of disability (defined as an increase of at least 1 point on the EDSS, persistent for at least 3 months). A further extension of the glatiramer acetate trial[39] of 1–11 months revealed a 32% reduction in relapse rate (mean relapse rate, 1.34 for placebo and 1.98 for glatiramer acetate), but still no significant effect on sustained progression was detected (total blinded treatment–period of 35 months). However, a trend for more pronounced progression was noted in the placebo group (29.4%) compared to the glatiramer acetate group (23.2%; not significant). Thus, a complementary approach evaluating EDSS changes of at least 1.5 points in patients that were not experiencing a relapse led to the observation that 41.5% of placebo patients worsened, whereas only 21.2% of those receiving glatiramer acetate deteriorated. The effect of glatiramer acetate was thus comparable to IFN-β, although no extensive dose-finding data are available. Side effects were mostly characterized by injection site reactions, flushing, chest tightness, palpitations, dyspnea, and anxiety. The use of glatiramer acetate may be an alternative to IFN-β, and is indicated mostly in relapsing-remitting MS with low neurologic disability.

## CLINICAL TRIALS EVALUATING INTRAVENOUS IMMUNOGLOBULIN

A placebo-controlled 2-year study was performed in relapsing-remitting MS,[40] including 148 patients (EDSS score, 1–6) that were randomly assigned to monthly intravenous immunoglobulin (IVIG; 0.15-0.20 g/kg body weight) or to placebo. IVIG is suspected to act through immunomodulatory mechanisms and to promote remyelination in MS. IVIG reduced the annual relapse frequency by 59% in comparison with placebo, and there was a higher proportion of relapse-free patients in the IVIG group. Disease progression was 0.35 of a point less in the IVIG group than in the placebo group, but this result was based on a final unconfirmed EDSS score (assessed as 1 point or more improvement on the EDSS). The improvement of clinical disability occurred during the first 6 months of treatment, and was sustained during the next 18 months. IVIG was well tolerated, and adverse events included cutaneous reactions.

Another randomized double-blind, placebo-controlled trial tested IVIG administered with a loading dose (0.4 g/kg body weight per day for 5 consecutive days)

*Multiple Sclerosis* 231

followed by single boosters (0.4 g/kg body weight) every 2 months for 2 years, versus placebo in 40 patients presenting with relapsing-remitting MS (EDSS score, 0–6).[41] Primary outcome measures included change in the yearly exacerbation rate, the percentage of exacerbation-free patients, and the time until the first exacerbation appears. Secondary outcome measures included neurologic disability, severity of exacerbations, and changes in MRI total lesion area. Relapse rate was reduced by 36.8% in favor of the IVIG group, with a decrease in IVIG patients from 1.85 to 0.75 at 1 year, and 0.42 at 2 years (versus from 1.55 to 1.80 at 1 year, and 1.4 at 2 years in the placebo group). IVIG significantly delayed the median time to the development of the first relapse, and increased the proportion of exacerbation-free patients in comparison with placebo. Other outcome measures did not reveal any significant change between IVIG and placebo.

## CLINICAL TRIALS EVALUATING IMMUNOSUPPRESSIVE TREATMENTS

Different immunosuppressive drugs have been tested in MS, which have shown modest efficacy. *Azathioprine* was evaluated in several clinical trials,[42–44] and a meta-analysis[45] of all published blind, randomized, controlled trials (793 patients included in five double-blind and two single-blind studies) demonstrated a mild beneficial effect of azathioprine on EDSS progression after 2 and 3 years (reduction of EDSS progression by 0.24 points), as well as a reduced risk to develop relapses since the first year of treatment. However, the interpretation of the latter analysis may be biased by the fact that patients with both relapsing-remitting and progressive MS were included, and no study tested the effect of azathioprine on MRI activity. *Mitoxantrone*, an anthracenedione which intercalates into DNA and has antiproliferative and immunomodulating properties, efficacy, and tolerance, was mostly studied in open trials.[46,47] There was no strong evidence for efficacy in progressive MS,[46] but the combined use of mitoxantrone and methylprednisolone (compared to methylprednisolone only) in relapsing-remitting and secondary progressive MS showed a positive effect on the appearance and the total number of new Gd-DTPA–enhancing lesions on brain MRI, as well as on EDSS and the number of exacerbations.[47] Although mitoxantrone seems to be effective in active MS, the design of the above-mentioned studies only gives indications on short-term efficacy of mitoxantrone on MS course. *Cyclophosphamide* was mostly evaluated in chronic progressive MS. Contradictory observations were reported: the use of a profound induction phase of immunosuppression with cyclophosphamide and ACTH, plus additional boosters of cyclophosphamide, slowed MS progression at 24 and 30 months when compared with patients who did not receive cyclophosphamide boosters,[48] although this effect was not seen in patients older than 40 years; other placebo-controlled trials testing cyclophosphamide alone,[49] or various regimens of cyclophosphamide plus prednisone and plasmapheresis,[50] failed to demonstrate any benefit for the use of cyclophosphamide. *Methotrexate* was assessed using weekly oral low doses in chronic progressive MS,[51,52] and showed a modest effect on disease progression, with a reduced clinical deterioration sustained mostly by tests of upper-extremity function. *Cladribine*,

232    *Clinical Trials in Neurologic Practice*

a specific antilymphocyte agent that induces lymphocytic apoptosis, was tested in chronic progressive MS[53,54] and revealed a significant positive effect on neurologic handicap (stabilization or improvement of EDSS), and on MRI total lesion volumes in comparison to placebo.

## COMPLETED AND ONGOING CLINICAL TRIALS EVALUATING OTHER IMMUNOMODULATORY TREATMENTS

*Linomide*, a quinoline-3-carboxamide that facilitates different T cell subset responses and increases natural killer cell activity, was tested in secondary progressive[55] and relapsing-remitting MS[56] in two double-blind trials that included a restricted numbers of patients. They both showed a decrease in MRI new, enlarged, and Gd-DTPA–enhanced lesions with Linomide, as well as a tendency toward clinical improvement, when compared to placebo. If confirmed by larger trials, Linomide could be an oral therapy for MS patients who could not benefit from other immunomodulatory treatments, although side effects such as pleuropericarditis, myalgia, diarrhea, and dyspnea have been recorded. A humanized mouse *monoclonal anti-TNF-α antibody (cA2)* was tested in two rapidly progressive MS patients in a phase I open safety trial. In spite of its beneficial effect in experimental autoimmune encephalomyelitis, an MS animal model, cA2 transiently increased the number of MRI Gd-enhancing lesions as well as cerebrospinal fluid leukocyte counts and immunoglobulin G index in both patients.[57] Other recent and preliminary clinical trials include immunization with T cell receptor peptides,[58,59] vaccination with attenuated autoimmune T cells,[60,61] and administration of humanized monoclonal antilymphocyte antibodies[62]; antibodies targeting adhesion molecules,[63] matrix metalloproteinase inhibitors,[64] and oral administration of copolymer 1[65] have proven their beneficial effect in experimental autoimmune encephalomyelitis, and are also potential therapeutic agents to be tested in MS.

## LIMITATIONS OF METHODOLOGIES USED IN CLINICAL TRIALS

In spite of documented problems of standardization, sensitivity, reliability, and rater-to-rater variability, the EDSS has been extensively used for assessing disability and its changes in nearly every therapeutic drug trial for MS, and it remains a useful tool for classifying MS patients by disease severity. With the introduction of new treatments that have a favorable impact on the course of MS, the use of placebo control groups in further therapeutic trials is questionable, both ethically and practically. Future randomized clinical trials may replace placebo groups by actively treated control groups for some forms of MS. This tendency may likely give rise to smaller differences between groups, and increase the required sample size and/or lengthen the duration of trials to achieve sufficient statistical power in the absence of more sensitive and responsive outcome measures. Thus, in the aim to define improved clinical outcome measures, the Clinical Outcomes Assessment Task Force[66] developed a composite measure encompassing the major clinical dimensions of arm function, leg function, ambulation, and cognitive function—the MS functional composite.

The evaluation of treatment effect will also depend on two further parameters: the behavior of the placebo groups and statistical methods. The behavior of control groups in large randomized clinical trials may contribute to an apparent lack of efficacy or to the modesty of some efficacy.[67] The rate of deterioration of the control groups subsequent to enrollment was observed to be generally much lower than the pre-enrollment rate of deterioration. New statistical methods may be much more powerful to demonstrate a therapeutic effect. These include repeated measures[37] and related methods using measurement of the area under the curve (e.g., area under a time/EDSS curve[20]). Using more powerful methods emphasizes valuable partial effects in small patient groups, but may also exaggerate the significance of some parameters.

Moreover, international consensus guidelines for the use of MRI in MS clinical trials were stated.[68] They proposed monthly T2-weighted and Gd-enhanced MRI as an adequate tool as the primary end point in short-term exploratory trials testing new agents in relapsing-remitting and secondary progressive MS. Failure to demonstrate a reduction in lesion activity avoids the development of larger clinical end point studies. However, because conventional MRI findings have only a limited correlation with disability, the primary end point of definite clinical trials should then be clinical, and serial MRI at 6–12 month intervals used as a secondary end point.

Another challenge for developing potent clinical trials with sensitive outcome measures is the evaluation of combinations of already licensed therapies. The existence of multiple therapies with moderate effect, acting through different immunologic mechanisms, raises the possibility of some synergistic or additive effects when these therapies are combined. Combination therapy approaches have been studied in only a few in vitro and in vivo models,[69,70] and no data suggest improved efficacy of combined treatments in humans in comparison to single agents (e.g., glatiramer acetate and IFN-β, oral myelin and IFN-β, azathioprine and IFN-β). The safety of combining different agents is also unknown. To compare the effect of a combination of two effective drugs with that of one, or both alone, would require larger groups of patients and more complex study design to be able to demonstrate the superiority of the combination, than would the evaluation of a single agent against a placebo group.

Although IFN-β, glatiramer acetate, and, to a certain extent, IVIG have proven that they can change or at least delay the clinical outcome of MS, there is now a need for trial designs that allow groups of patients to be followed for extended periods, possibly as very long-term crossover studies, to evaluate long-term treatment effects. The effect of the discussed treatments on the course of MS, especially the development of neurologic handicap, is moderate. Because these treatments do not interfere with the primary pathogenetic processes of MS, long-term therapy will be necessary for a sustained beneficial effect with the possible development of unknown delayed secondary effects.

234 *Clinical Trials in Neurologic Practice*

## REFERENCES

1. Kurtzke JF. Rating neurological impairment in multiple sclerosis: an expanded disability status scale (EDSS). Neurology 1983;33:1444–1452.
2. Thorpe JW, Kidd D, Moseley IF, et al. Serial gadolinium-enhanced MRI of the brain and spinal cord in early relapsing-remitting multiple sclerosis. Neurology 1996;46:373–378.
3. Thompson AJ, Kennard C, Swash M, et al. Relative efficacy of intravenous methylprednisolone and ACTH in the treatment of acute relapse in MS. Neurology 1989;39:969–971.
4. Milligan NM, Newcombe R, Compston DAS. A double-blind controlled trial of high dose methylprednisolone in patients with multiple sclerosis: 1. Clinical effects. J Neurol Neurosurg Psychiatry 1987;50:511–516.
5. Alam SM, Kyriakides T, Lawden M, Newman PK. Methylprednisolone in multiple sclerosis: a comparison of oral with intravenous therapy at equivalent high dose. J Neurol Neurosurg Psychiatry 1993;56:1219–1220.
6. Beck RW, Cleary PA, Trobe JD, et al. The effect of corticosteroids for acute optic neuritis on the subsequent development of multiple sclerosis. N Engl J Med 1993;329:1764–1769.
7. Barnes D, Hughes RAC, Morris RW, et al. Randomised trial of oral and intravenous methylprednisolone in acute relapses of multiple sclerosis. Lancet 1997;349:902–906.
8. Goodkin DE, Kindel RP, Weinstock-Guttman B, et al. A phase II study of IV methylprednisolone in secondary-progressive multiple sclerosis. Neurology 1998;51:239–245.
9. Kermode AG, Thompson AJ, Tofts PS, et al. Breakdown of the blood-brain barrier precedes symptoms and other MRI signs of new lesions in multiple sclerosis: pathogenetic and clinical implications. Brain 1990;113:1477–1489.
10. Miller DH, Thompson AJ, Morrissey SP, et al. High dose steroids in acute relapses of multiple sclerosis: MRI evidence for a possible mechanism of therapeutic effect. J Neurol Neurosurg Psychiatry 1992;55:450–453.
11. Burnham JA, Wright RR, Dreisbach J, Murray RS. The effect of high dose steroids on MRI gadolinium enhancement in acute demyelinating lesions. Neurology 1991;41:1349–1354.
12. Barkhof F, Frequin STFM, Hommes OR, et al. A correlative triad of gadolinium-DTPA MRI, EDSS, and CSF-MBP in relapsing multiple sclerosis patients treated with high-dose intravenous methylprednisolone. Neurology 1992;42:63–67.
13. Kunicka JE, Talle MA, Denhardt H, et al. Immunosuppression by glucocorticoids: inhibition of production of multiple lymphokines by in vivo administration of dexamethasone. Cell Immunol 1993;149:39–49.
14. Hardin J, McLeod S, Grigorieva I, et al. Interleukin-6 prevents dexamethasone-induced myeloma cell death. Blood 1994;84:3063–3070.
15. Tremlett HL, Luscombe DK, Wiles CM. Use of corticosteroids in multiple sclerosis in the United Kingdom. J Neurol Neurosurg Psychiatry 1998;65:362–365.
16. The IFNB Multiple Sclerosis Study Group. Interferon beta-1b is effective in relapsing-remitting multiple sclerosis. I. Clinical results of a multicenter, randomized, double-blind, placebo-controlled trial. Neurology 1993;43:655–661.
17. Paty DW, Li DKB, the UBC MS/MRI Study Group, the IFNB Multiple Sclerosis Study Group. Interferon beta-1b is effective in relapsing-remitting multiple sclerosis. II. MRI analysis results of a multicenter, randomized, double-blind, placebo-controlled trial. Neurology 1993;43:662–667.
18. Jacobs LD, Cookfair DL, Rudick RA, et al. Intramuscular interferon beta-1a for disease progression in relapsing multiple sclerosis. Ann Neurol 1996;39:285–294.
19. Rudick RA, Goodkin DE, Jacobs LD, et al. Impact of interferon beta-1a on neurologic disability in relapsing multiple sclerosis. Neurology 1997;49:358–363.
20. PRISMS (Prevention of Relapse and Disability by Interferon β-1a Subcutaneously in Multiple Sclerosis) Study Group. Randomised double-blind placebo-controlled study of interferon β-1a in relapsing-remitting multiple sclerosis. Lancet 1998;352:1498–1504.
21. European Study Group on interferon β-1b in secondary progressive MS. Placebo-controlled multicentre randomized trial on interferon β-1b in treatment of secondary progressive multiple sclerosis. Lancet 1998;352:1491–1497.
22. The IFNB Multiple Sclerosis Study Group, the University of British Columbia MS/MRI Analysis Group. Interferon beta-1b in the treatment of multiple sclerosis: final outcome of the randomized controlled trial. Neurology 1995;45:1277–1285.
23. Quality Standards Subcommittee of the American Academy of Neurology. Practice advisory on selection of patients with multiple sclerosis for treatment with Betaseron. Neurology 1994; 44: 1537–1540.

*Multiple Sclerosis*  235

24. The IFNB Multiple Sclerosis Study Group, the University of British Columbia MS/MRI Analysis Group. Neutralizing antibodies during treatment of multiple sclerosis with interferon beta-1b: Experience during the first three years. Neurology 1996;47:889–894.
25. Paty DW, Goodkin D, Thompson A, Rice G. Guidelines for physicians with patients on IFN-β 1b: The use of an assay for neuralizing antibodies (NAB). Neurology 1996;47:865–866.
26. Petkau J, White R. Neutralizing antibodies and the efficacy of interferon beta-1b in relapsing-remitting multiple sclerosis (abstr). Mult Scler 1997;3:402.
27. Lublin FD, Whitaker JN, Eidelman BH, et al. Management of patients receiving interferon beta-1b for multiple sclerosis: Report of a consensus conference. Neurology 1996;46:12–18.
28. Rudick RA, Simonian NA, Alam JA, et al. Incidence and significance of neutralizing antibodies to interferon beta-1a in multiple sclerosis. Neurology 1998;50:1266–1272.
29. Lublin FD, Reingold SC. Defining the clinical course of multiple sclerosis: results of an international survey. Neurology 1996;48:907–1011.
30. Weinshenker BG, Issa M, Baskerville J. Meta-analysis of the placebo-treated groups in clinical trials of progressive MS. Neurology 1996;46:1613–1619.
31. Weishenker BG, Bass B, Rice GPA, et al. The natural history of multiple sclerosis: a geographically based study - 2, predictive value of the early clinical course. Brain 1989;112:1419–1428.
32. Lucchinetti CF, Brück W, Rodriguez M, Lassmann H. Distinct patterns of multiple sclerosis pathology indicates heterogeneity in pathogenesis. Brain Pathol 1996;6:259–274.
33. The Once Weekly Interferon for MS Study Group (OWIMS). Evidence of interferon β-1a dose response in a relapsing-remitting MS. The OWIMS Study. Neurology 1999;53:679–686.
34. Trapp BD, Peterson J, Ransohoff RM, et al. Axonal transection in the lesions of multiple sclerosis. N Engl J Med 1998;338:278–285.
35. Cross AH, Antel JP. Antibodies to beta-interferons in multiple sclerosis. Can we neutralize the controversy? Neurology 1998;50:1206–1208.
36. Finkelman FD, Madden KB, Morris SC, et al. Anti-cytokine antibodies as carrier proteins. Prolongation of in vivo effects of exogenous cytokines by injection of cytokine-anticytokine antibody complexes. J Immunol 1993;151:1235–1244.
37. Johnson KP, Brooks BR, Cohen JA, et al. Copolymer 1 reduces relapse rate and improves disability in relapsing-remitting multiple sclerosis. Neurology 1995;45:1268–1276.
38. Johnson KP. A review of the clinical efficacy profile of copolymer 1: new U.S. phase III trial data. J Neurol 1996;243(Suppl 1):S3–S7.
39. Johnson KP, Brooks BR, Cohen JA, et al. Extended use of glatiramer acetate (Copaxone) is well tolerated and maintains its clinical effect on multiple sclerosis relapse rate and degree of disability. Neurology 1998;50:701–708.
40. Fazekas F, Deisenhammer F, Strasser-Fuchs S, et al. Randomised placebo-controlled trial of monthly intravenous immunoglobulin therapy in relapsing-remitting multiple sclerosis. Lancet 1997;349:589–593.
41. Achiron A, Gabbay U, Gilad R, et al. Intravenous immunoglobulin treatment in multiple sclerosis. Effect on relapses. Neurology 1998;50:398–402.
42. British and Dutch multiple sclerosis azathioprine trial group. Double-masked trial of azathioprine in multiple sclerosis. Lancet 1988;2:179–183.
43. Ellison GW, Myers LW, Mickey MR, et al. A placebo-controlled, randomized, double-masked, variable dosage, clinical trial of azathioprine with and without methylprednisolone in multiple sclerosis. Neurology 1989;39:1018–1026.
44. Goodkin DE, Bailly RC, Teetzen ML, et al. The efficacy of azathioprine in relapsing-remitting multiple sclerosis. Neurology 1991;41:20–25.
45. Yudkin PL, Ellison GW, Ghezzi A, et al. Overview of azathioprine treatment in multiple sclerosis. Lancet 1991;338:1051–1055.
46. Noseworthy JH, Hopkins MB, Vandervoort MK, et al. An open-trial evaluation of mitoxantrone in the treatment of progressive MS. Neurology 1993;43:1401–1406.
47. Edan G, Miller D, Clanet M, et al. Therapeutic effect of mitoxantrone combined with methylprednisolone in multiple sclerosis: a randomised multicentre study of active disease using MRI and clinical criteria. J Neurol Neurosurg Psychiatry 1997;62:112–118.
48. Weiner HL, Mackin GA, Oray EJ, et al. Intermittent cyclophosphamide pulse therapy in progressive multiple sclerosis: Final report of the Northeast Cooperative Multiple Sclerosis Treatment Group. Neurology 1993;43:910–918.
49. Likosky WH, Fireman B, Elmore R, et al. Intense immunosuppression in chronic progressive multiple sclerosis: the Kaiser study. J Neurol Neurosurg Psychiatry 1991;54:1055–1060.

## 236   *Clinical Trials in Neurologic Practice*

50. The Canadian Cooperative Multiple Sclerosis Study Group. The Canadian cooperative trail of cyclophosphamide and plasma exchange in progressive multiple sclerosis. Lancet 1991;337:441–446.

51. Goodkin DE, Rudick RA, VanderBrug Medendorp S, et al. Low-dose (7.5 mg) oral methotrexate reduces the rate of progression in chronic progressive multiple sclerosis. Ann Neurol 1995;37:30–40.

52. Goodkin DE, Rudick RA, VanderBrug Medendorp S, et al. Low-dose oral methotrexate in chronic progressive multiple sclerosis: Analyses of serial MRIs. Neurology 1996;47:1153–1157.

53. Sipe JC, Romine JS, Koziol JA, et al. Cladribine in treatment of chronic progressive multiple sclerosis. Lancet 1994;344:9–13.

54. Beutler E, Sipe JC, Romine JS, et al. The treatment of chronic progressive multiple sclerosis with cladribine. Proc Natl Acad Sci U S A 1996;93:1716–1720.

55. Karussis DM, Meiner Z, Lehmann D, et al. Treatment of secondary progressive multiple sclerosis with the immunomodulator linomide - A double blind, placebo-controlled pilot study with monthly magnetic resonance imaging evaluation. Neurology 1996;47:341–346.

56. Andersen O, Lycke J, Tollesson PO, et al. Linomide reduces the rate of active lesions in relapsing-remitting multiple sclerosis. Neurology 1996;47:895–900.

57. van Oosten BW, Barkhof F, Truyen L, et al. Increased MRI activity and immune activation in two multiple sclerosis patients treated with the monoclonal anti-tumor necrosis factor antibody cA2. Neurology 1996;47:1531–1534.

58. Vandenbark AA, Bourdette DN, Whitham R, et al. T-cell receptor peptide therapy in EAE and MS. Clin Exp Rheumatol 1993;11(Suppl 8):S51–S53.

59. Gold DP, Smith RA, Golding AB, et al. Results of a phase I clinical trial of a T-cell receptor vaccine in patients with multiple sclerosis. 2. Comparative analysis of TCR utilization in CSF T-cell populations before and after vaccination with TCRV-BETA-6 CDR2 peptide. J Neuroimmunol 1997;76:29–38.

60. Ben-Nun A, Cohen IR. Vaccination against autoimmune encephalomyelitis (EAE): attenuated autoimmune T lymphocytes confer resistance to induction of active EAE but not to EAE mediated by the intact T lymphocytes lines. Eur Neurol 1981;11:949–952.

61. Hafler DA, Cohen I, Benjamin DS, et al. T cell vaccination in multiple sclerosis: a preliminary report. Clin Immunol Immunopathol 1992;62:307–313.

62. Moreau T, Thorpe J, Miller D, et al. Preliminary evidence from magnetic resonance imaging for reduction in disease activity after lymphocyte depletion in multiple sclerosis. Lancet 1994;344: 298–301.

63. Cannella B, Cross AH, Raine CS. Anti-adhesion molecule therapy in experimental autoimmune encephalomyelitis. J Neuroimmunol 1993;46:43–56.

64. Liedtke W, Cannella B, Mazzaccaro RJ, et al. Effective treatment of models of multiple sclerosis by matrix metalloproteinase inhibitors. Ann Neurol 1998;44:35–46.

65. Teitelbaum D, Arnon R, Sela M. Immunomodulation of experimental autoimmune encephalomyelitis by oral administration of copolymer 1. Proc Natl Acad Sci U S A 1999;96:3842–3847.

66. Cutter GR, Baier ML, Rudick RA, et al. Development of a multiple sclerosis functional composite as a clinical trial outcome measure. Brain 1999;122:871–882.

67. Weinshenker BG, Issa M, Baskerville J. Meta-analysis of the placebo-treated groups in clinical trials of progressive MS. Neurology 1996;46:1613–1619.

68. Miller DH, Albert PS, Barkhof F, et al. Guidelines for the use of magnetic resonance techniques in monitoring the treatment of multiples sclerosis. Ann Neurol 1996;39:6–16.

69. Milo R, Panitch H. Additive effects of copolymer-1 and interferon β-1b on immune response to myelin basic protein. J Neuroimmunol 1995;61:85–193.

70. Al-Sabbagh A, Nelson PA, Weiner HL. Beta interferon enhances oral tolerance to MBP and PLP in experimental autoimmune encephalomyelitis. Neurology 1994;44(Suppl 2):A242.

# 12
## Clinical Trials in Central Nervous System Infections
Cynthia M. Hingtgen and Karen L. Roos

Our knowledge of the pathogenesis, diagnosis, and treatment of central nervous system (CNS) infectious diseases has increased tremendously over the last 10 years. New pathogenic organisms have been discovered, the development of the polymerase chain reaction (PCR) technique has improved the laboratory identification of the infecting organism, meningeal pathogens have developed resistance to traditional antimicrobial therapies, and the importance of the immune system in the pathophysiology of the neurologic complications of CNS infections is increasingly understood. Clinical trials have been instrumental in improving the treatment of bacterial meningitis, herpes simplex virus (HSV) encephalitis, and the CNS complications of human immunodeficiency virus (HIV) infection. The treatment of bacterial meningitis has been complicated by the emergence of organisms that are resistant to the commonly prescribed antimicrobial agents, necessitating continuous re-evaluation of recommended antimicrobial regimens. Clinical trials in bacterial meningitis have also been important in developing therapeutic modalities that attenuate the CNS inflammatory response to infection that is responsible for the neurologic complications. The clinical trials in HSV encephalitis demonstrated the efficacy of acyclovir over vidarabine in the treatment of this infection. Clinical trials on the CNS complications of HIV infection have decided therapies for opportunistic infections and HIV-associated dementia complex.

In this chapter, clinical trials in bacterial meningitis, HSV encephalitis, varicella-zoster virus infection, and the CNS complications of HIV infection are reviewed. Essential questions that await answers from ongoing clinical trials are addressed, as well as issues for future clinical trials.

238    *Clinical Trials in Neurologic Practice*

## BACTERIAL MENINGITIS

### Empiric Antimicrobial Therapy

Decisions on empiric antimicrobial therapy for bacterial meningitis are made before the results of cerebrospinal fluid (CSF) Gram's stain and culture, and antimicrobial susceptibility tests are known. The emergence of penicillin and cephalosporin-resistant pneumococcal organisms has resulted in a change in the recommendations for empiric therapy of community-acquired bacterial meningitis. Empiric therapy should include a third-generation cephalosporin, either ceftriaxone or cefotaxime, plus vancomycin.[1] In the elderly, very young, or immunocompromised patient for whom *Listeria monocytogenes* may be the meningeal pathogen, ampicillin should be added to the empiric regimen. Ceftazidime should be substituted for ceftriaxone or cefotaxime in the neurosurgical or neutropenic patient because *Pseudomonas aeruginosa* may be the infectious agent in this population.

There are a number of clinical trials demonstrating the efficacy of the third-generation cephalosporins, ceftriaxone and cefotaxime, in bacterial meningitis. These cephalosporins are used relatively interchangeably in the empiric therapy of bacterial meningitis for both children and adults. Both have undergone extensive investigation of safety and efficacy against the common meningeal pathogens. A prospective, randomized, multicenter clinical trial compared chloramphenicol (100 mg/kg per day in divided doses every 6 hours), ampicillin (250 mg/kg per day in divided doses every 6 hours, initially with chloramphenicol), cefotaxime (150 mg/kg per day in divided doses every 6 hours), and ceftriaxone (100 mg/kg per day) in 220 cases of bacterial meningitis in children.[2] *Haemophilus influenzae* type b (Hib) was the infecting organism in 73% of the cases. At 24 hours, the CSF was sterile in a greater number of children who were treated with the cephalosporins than in those treated with chloramphenicol and ampicillin. Time to sterilization of the CSF has been associated with both morbidity and mortality, and therefore it is an important variable to examine in clinical trials evaluating treatment for bacterial meningitis.

The efficacy and safety of ceftriaxone and cefotaxime were compared in a prospective, randomized, multicenter clinical trial.[3] Ninety-nine children between the ages of 6 weeks and 16 years were treated with cefotaxime (200 mg/kg per day in divided doses every 6 hours) or ceftriaxone (100 mg/kg per day on day 1, and then 75 mg/kg per day). *Neisseria meningitidis* was the meningeal pathogen in 50% of cases, *Streptococcus pneumoniae* in 20%, and Hib in 20%. The results of this clinical trial, and others like it, are important not only because they demonstrated that ceftriaxone and cefotaxime are equally efficacious and equally well tolerated in the treatment of bacterial meningitis, but also because the majority of patients in this trial was infected with an organism other than Hib. The number of cases of meningitis due to Hib has decreased since the licensure of the Hib conjugate vaccine in 1987.[4] Before this time, Hib was the most common cause of bacterial meningitis in children in the United States. The relevance of older clinical trials to therapeutic decisions has been diminished by the change in the predominant organisms causing meningitis.

It remains unclear if ceftriaxone should be given once a day or twice a day in bacterial meningitis. A clinical trial that evaluates the two dosing regimens in

*Clinical Trials in Central Nervous System Infections* 239

terms of length of time to sterilization of CSF, incidence of neurologic complications, and length of time to clinical recovery would be worthwhile.

## Vancomycin

The incidence of pneumococcal isolates with intermediate resistance to third-generation cephalosporins is as high as 20% in certain areas.[5] The prevalence of these organisms has resulted in the recommendation that vancomycin be added to the empiric regimen for bacterial meningitis. A dose of 60 mg/kg per day of vancomycin is recommended until the pathogen has been identified and the results of susceptibility tests are known. This recommendation is based on in vitro susceptibility profiles that demonstrate that all strains of *S. pneumoniae* are susceptible to vancomycin with a minimal inhibitory concentration of less than 1 µg/ml. In addition, vancomycin and ceftriaxone have shown synergistic antimicrobial properties in vitro and in animal models of experimental meningitis.[6,7] Rifampin is also active against penicillin-resistant pneumococci, but rifampin should never be used alone because strains resistant to rifampin can develop rapidly during therapy.[5]

There are a number of published reports on the penetration of vancomycin into the CSF, and the effect of dexamethasone on the penetration of this antibiotic. Early clinical trials examined the penetration of vancomycin into CSF in the absence of meningeal inflammation. Measurable drug could not be detected in the CSF of 11 adult volunteers 1–3 hours after a 500-mg intravenous dose of vancomycin.[8] In comparison, vancomycin concentrations in the CSF are frequently in the therapeutically effective range in patients with meningitis.[9,10] This led to a concern that the use of dexamethasone as an adjunctive agent would decrease the penetration of vancomycin into the CSF because it decreased meningeal inflammation. In experimental models of pneumococcal meningitis, dexamethasone reduced the penetration of vancomycin into the CSF.[11,12] In a prospective, randomized clinical trial of the bactericidal activity of vancomycin against cephalosporin-resistant pneumococci in CSF of children with acute bacterial meningitis, vancomycin in a dosage of 60 mg/kg per day penetrated reliably into the CSF when the children were treated concomitantly with dexamethasone (0.6 mg/kg per day, divided into four doses for 4 days).[13] The discrepancy between the results of this clinical trial and the observations in experimental models of meningitis may be explained by differences in the blood–CSF barrier between animals and children, and emphasizes the importance of both in vivo and in vitro studies.

Additional concern about the effect of dexamethasone on the efficacy of vancomycin in adults with pneumococcal meningitis was raised by a prospective study of 11 adults with community-acquired pneumococcal meningitis. The patients were treated with vancomycin at a dose of 15 mg/kg every 8 hours or 7.5 mg/kg every 6 hours.[10] Both of these doses of vancomycin are below the recommended daily dose of 60 mg/kg per day. Patients also received high doses of dexamethasone, phenytoin, and mannitol. Four of 11 patients were reported as therapeutic failures. Subtherapeutic doses of vancomycin were used, and this may have contributed to therapeutic failure. The results of this study should not be interpreted as evidence of a reduced efficacy of vancomycin when used con-

240    *Clinical Trials in Neurologic Practice*

comitantly with dexamethasone. The dose of an antibiotic used in a clinical trial is critical to the interpretation of the results. In the 1940s, low doses of intravenous penicillin were used to treat bacterial meningitis, requiring the addition of intrathecal penicillin for therapeutic success. When it was recognized that higher doses of parenteral penicillin were successful in eradicating the infection, the intrathecal administration of penicillin was no longer required.

A clinical trial that measures serum and CSF concentrations of vancomycin in children and adults with bacterial meningitis and correlates these concentrations with outcome measures would be very helpful. In such a trial, the timing of the administration of dexamethasone must be rigidly adhered to as maximum benefit is achieved when dexamethasone is administered before the first dose of antibiotic.

## Newer Antimicrobial Agents

It is always anticipated that the development of a new antibiotic will simplify the treatment of a disease by an extended broad-spectrum activity against traditional organisms as well as activity against resistant strains. The adverse effects of an antibiotic, especially its propensity to cause seizure activity, are important to determine before the drug is recommended for the treatment of CNS infections.

Meropenem is a carbapenem with similar in vitro antimicrobial activity to imipenem, but with reportedly less seizure proclivity.[14] This antibiotic is active against a broad range of gram-negative and gram-positive bacteria, and has several-fold greater activity than that of imipenem against Hib and *N. meningitidis*.[15,16] Imipenem is not recommended in the treatment of bacterial meningitis. Two multicenter clinical trials have been conducted to compare the efficacy of meropenem to cefotaxime and ceftriaxone.[16,17] In a prospective, randomized clinical trial of 139 children (3 months to 14 years of age) with bacterial meningitis, 75 children were treated with meropenem (40 mg/kg every 8 hours) and 64 children were treated with cefotaxime (75–100 mg/kg every 8 hours).[16] The meningeal pathogen was Hib in 66 cases, *N. meningitidis* in 50 cases, and *S. pneumoniae* in 21 cases. Three patients had cephalosporin-resistant pneumococcal meningitis. The time to sterilization of the CSF was measured, as well as hearing impairment and neurologic deficits. Ninety-seven percent of the 63 patients in the meropenem-treated group and 98% of the 58 patients in the cefotaxime-treated group, who had repeat lumbar punctures between 18 and 36 hours after antimicrobial therapy was initiated, had sterilization of CSF cultures. Four of 74 meropenem-treated patients and 2 of 81 cefotaxime-treated patients had neurologic sequelae. The severity of hearing impairment was similar in both groups. The number of patients with pneumococcal infection, the most common cause of bacterial meningitis, was too small to assess the efficacy of meropenem in the treatment of pneumococcal meningitis. An additional aspect of this study was assessing the propensity for meropenem to cause seizures. Five of 82 patients treated with meropenem (6.1%) and 1 of 86 patients treated with cefotaxime (1.1%) had seizures after the start of antibiotic therapy. These six patients had no history of seizures before antibiotic therapy was initiated. However, this compares favorably to treatment with imipenem-cilastatin, which was associated with the development of seizures in 39% of children who had no previous history of seizures. The investigators of the meropenem study

*Clinical Trials in Central Nervous System Infections* 241

are careful to point out that the number of patients in their study may not be sufficient to correctly assess the epileptogenic potential of the newer carbapenem.

Another prospective, randomized controlled trial was performed in adults with bacterial meningitis to compare the efficacy of meropenem with the third-generation cephalosporins.[17] Fifty-six patients were entered into the study, but 11 patients were subsequently disqualified because they had viral meningitis (two patients), cerebral abscess (four patients), or a noninfectious problem (one patient). Four patients received less than 48 hours of therapy and 20 patients had been pretreated with oral antibiotics. This left 23 meropenem-treated patients for evaluation. The meningeal pathogen could be identified in only 16 cases. There were five cases of meningitis due to *N. meningitidis*, six cases due to *S. pneumoniae*, and four cases due to rarer pathogens. The small numbers in each group preclude drawing conclusions from this study on the efficacy of meropenem in community-acquired meningitis. Before recommendations can be made about the use of this antibiotic in the treatment of patients with bacterial meningitis, larger numbers of patients must be enrolled in clinical trials and a significant number of cases caused by cephalosporin-resistant organisms must be evaluated.

Cefepime is a fourth-generation broad-spectrum cephalosporin with in vitro activity similar to that of cefotaxime or ceftriaxone against Hib, *S. pneumoniae*, and *N. meningitidis*, and demonstrates greater activity against *Enterobacter* species and *Pseudomonas aeruginosa*.[18,19] There has been one prospective, randomized clinical trial comparing the safety and efficacy of cefepime to cefotaxime for the treatment of bacterial meningitis in infants and children.[19] A total of 76 patients with culture-proven bacterial meningitis were evaluated. In 46 cases, the causative organism was Hib; in 14 cases, *N. meningitidis*; and in 10 cases, *S. pneumoniae*. There were no cases of meningitis due to *Enterobacter* species or *Pseudomonas aeruginosa*. All patients were also treated with dexamethasone. In this trial, cefepime was equivalent to cefotaxime in the treatment of bacterial meningitis due to the common meningeal pathogens in infants and children. The efficacy of this cephalosporin in meningitis caused by *Enterobacter* species and *Pseudomonas aeruginosa*, and as an "extended broad spectrum" cephalosporin awaits further clinical trials.

*Pseudomonas aeruginosa* causes meningitis in the elderly with chronic disease, the neurosurgical patient, and the neutropenic patient. Clinical trials to evaluate the efficacy of cefepime in bacterial meningitis caused by penicillin- and cephalosporin-resistant pneumococcal organisms, *Enterobacter* species, and *Pseudomonas aeruginosa* should examine time to sterilization of CSF, incidence and severity of neurologic and audiologic sequelae, case-fatality rates, antibiotic toxicity, and CSF penetration of cefepime when dexamethasone is used concomitantly. Cefepime cannot be recommended in the empiric therapy of bacterial meningitis.

## Adjuvant Anti-Inflammatory Therapy

The inflammatory cytokines, specifically tumor necrosis factor and interleukin-1, have a critical role in the pathophysiology of the neurologic complications of bacterial meningitis. The production of the inflammatory cytokines by monocytes, macrophages, and brain astrocytes and microglial cells (CNS macrophage–

242　*Clinical Trials in Neurologic Practice*

equivalent cells) is stimulated by the presence of bacterial cell wall components in the subarachnoid space. Interleukin-1 and tumor necrosis factor alter the permeability of the blood–brain barrier allowing for the exudation of serum proteins into the CSF, and recruitment of polymorphonuclear leukocytes from the bloodstream that contribute to the purulent exudate and obstruct the flow of CSF.[20] Treatment of bacterial meningitis with bactericidal antibiotics that release bacterial cell wall components contributes to and accentuates inflammation in the subarachnoid space and the pathophysiologic consequences.[21] This is supported by the observation that inflammatory changes in the subarachnoid space increase after antibiotic therapy is initiated.[22] Therapeutic agents that attenuate the inflammatory response have been investigated in experimental models of meningitis and in clinical trials. One such agent is dexamethasone, which inhibits the production of the inflammatory cytokines at the molecular level, decreases CSF outflow resistance, and stabilizes the blood–brain barrier.

There have been a number of clinical trials, dating back to 1950, that were designed to evaluate the efficacy of corticosteroids on mortality and morbidity in bacterial meningitis.[23] In the 1960s, methylprednisolone, hydrocortisone, and varying doses of dexamethasone were investigated with conflicting results.[24,25] Corticosteroid therapy for bacterial meningitis received renewed interest in the 1980s, and this interest was increased by the evidence that dexamethasone was more effective than methylprednisolone in reducing inflammation and its pathophysiologic consequences in experimental models of meningitis.[26]

In 1988, Lebel et al.[27] published the results of two prospective, double-blind, placebo-controlled trials involving 200 infants and children (aged 2 months old and older) on the efficacy of dexamethasone therapy in bacterial meningitis. The etiologic organism of the meningitis was Hib in 154 cases. The administration of dexamethasone caused an increase in the CSF glucose concentration and a decrease in the CSF protein concentration in the first 24 hours of therapy. Dexamethasone also significantly reduced the frequency of moderate, severe, or profound bilateral sensorineural hearing loss in children with Hib meningitis. Since then, there have been a number of additional clinical trials with dexamethasone as adjunctive therapy in bacterial meningitis.[28–37] The effect of dexamethasone on CSF leukocyte counts, protein and glucose concentrations (as a measure of CSF inflammation), the incidence of neurologic deficits, sensorineural hearing loss, and mortality were examined. A meta-analysis of the randomized, concurrently controlled trials of dexamethasone therapy in bacterial meningitis published from 1988 to 1996 confirmed benefit for Hib meningitis.[38] This analysis also suggested a benefit from dexamethasone treatment for pneumococcal meningitis in children if the steroid was administered at the same time or before intravenous antibiotics.

There are a number of variables in these clinical trials of dexamethasone. Timing of the first dose of dexamethasone differed greatly between studies. Dexamethasone was administered before antibiotic therapy by at least 20 minutes, as is currently recommended, in only two clinical trials; in both cases, dexamethasone was shown to be efficacious.[30,31] As stated, dexamethasone inhibits the production of inflammatory cytokines. Once bactericidal antibiotics have lysed bacteria and bacterial cell wall components are present in the subarachnoid space, the production of the inflammatory cytokines has begun. Maximum benefit from dexamethasone therapy is dependent on timing. In a placebo-controlled, double-blind trial of dexamethasone therapy in 101 infants and children with bacterial meningitis, dexamethasone was given 15–20 minutes before the first dose of antibiotic. There was a significant reduction in meningeal inflammation, and a significant increase in the Glasgow Coma Scale at 24 hours, in the patients treated with dexamethasone compared with the patients given placebo. After 12 hours of therapy, all indices of inflammation in the CSF (CSF lactate, leukocytes, glucose and protein concentrations) had improved with dexamethasone therapy, whereas they had uniformly worsened in the patients given placebo. Neurologic sequelae occurred significantly more often in the patients who were given placebo.[30] In another prospective, placebo-controlled, double-blind trial of dexamethasone therapy in 115 children with bacterial meningitis, dexamethasone therapy was started 10 minutes before the first dose of ceftriaxone and given every 12 hours for 2 days. Three of 60 (5%) of the dexamethasone recipients had one or more neurologic or audiologic sequelae compared with 9 of 55 (16%) placebo recipients at follow-up examination at 3, 9, and 15 months after hospital discharge.[31] To have an effect on the production of the inflammatory cytokines, dexamethasone must be given early. The results in the clinical trials where dexamethasone was given hours after antibiotic therapy was initiated were affected by the timing of the administration of dexamethasone.

A common criticism of the dexamethasone trials is that in the majority of cases, the causative organism of the meningitis was Hib. This is no longer one of the most common etiologic organisms of bacterial meningitis because of the success of the Hib conjugate vaccine. Another problem is, with the exception of the clinical trial by Girgis et al.,[29] the patients in the steroid trials have been mostly infants and children, not adults. Girgis et al. did demonstrate a reduction in mortality from pneumococcal meningitis in adults who were treated with dexamethasone therapy. This reduction in mortality is an important observation, and probably more so given the fact that this study used antibiotics (chloramphenicol and ampicillin), which are less efficacious than third-generation cephalosporins in treating bacterial meningitis.

The American Academy of Pediatrics recommends the use of dexamethasone (0.6 mg/kg per day in divided doses every 6 hours for 4 days) for bacterial meningitis in infants and children.[39] The first dose of dexamethasone should be given before the first dose of antibiotic. The results of studies in experimental models of meningitis, and the understanding of the molecular basis of the inflammatory response in bacterial meningitis, favor the use of dexamethasone in adults, but this has not been demonstrated in clinical trials. Clearly, the development of other adjunctive agents that can attenuate the inflammatory response in bacterial meningitis are needed. Clinical trials to investigate the efficacy of these agents are in progress.

## CHEMOPROPHYLAXIS

Chemoprophylaxis is used for the prevention of secondary cases once an index case of meningococcal or Hib meningitis has been identified. The risk of developing meningitis is highest immediately after contact with an index case, with the majority of secondary cases occurring within the first week after the index case.

244    *Clinical Trials in Neurologic Practice*

Asymptomatic nasopharyngeal carriage of meningococci is common in healthy individuals. A number of host factors are important in determining whether a newly infected individual becomes an asymptomatic carrier or develops meningitis. These include the presence of specific functional antibodies for opsonophagocytosis and bactericidal activity, an intact complement pathway, and a normal reticuloendothelial system. Close contacts of the index case should receive chemoprophylaxis as soon as the primary case is identified. *Close contacts* are defined as those individuals who have had contact with the patient's oral secretions. Rifampin is the recommended antimicrobial agent for chemoprophylaxis of meningococcal meningitis. The recommended dose is 600 mg every 12 hours for 2 days in adults, 10 mg/kg every 12 hours for 2 days in children older than 1 year of age, and 5 mg/kg every 12 hours for 2 days in children younger than 1 year of age. Rifampin should not be used during pregnancy. Ciprofloxacin has been effective in eradicating meningococci from the nasopharynx and has the advantage of being effective after a single oral dose. The dose is 750 mg. There is some concern about using ciprofloxacin in individuals less than 18 years of age because of a risk of arthropathy. It is unlikely, however, that a single dose would have any adverse effect on bone development. A single intramuscular injection of ceftriaxone (250 mg for adults, 125 mg for children) is also effective in eradicating the organism from the nasopharynx. Chemoprophylaxis should be given to the index patient before hospital discharge.

The American Academy of Pediatrics recommends rifampin prophylaxis (20 mg/kg per day orally for 4 days—maximum 600 mg/day) for all individuals in households with at least one child younger than 24 months or with a nonimmunized child 24–48 months of age when there has been a patient in the house with Hib meningitis. The risk of Hib meningitis in children that share the same class room with a child who has had Hib meningitis is similar to that for household contacts. Prophylaxis for the children and staff in daycare centers should be provided if the center has children under 2 years of age.

## HERPES SIMPLEX VIRUS ENCEPHALITIS AND VARICELLA INFECTIONS

Before the availability of antiviral therapy in the early 1980s, HSV encephalitis had a mortality rate of 70%, and survivors had devastating neurologic sequelae. Early clinical trials were designed to compare the efficacy of two antiviral agents, vidarabine and acyclovir, in the treatment of HSV encephalitis.[40,41] The diagnosis of HSV encephalitis was established by brain biopsy in these studies. The definitive diagnosis of HSV encephalitis by brain biopsy was critically important in establishing the reliability of the results. These are landmark clinical trials that demonstrated that acyclovir reduced mortality more than vidarabine, making acyclovir the drug of choice for HSV encephalitis. These clinical trials also demonstrated that for acyclovir or vidarabine to be beneficial, therapy must be initiated before a deterioration in the level of consciousness occurs.[41]

Brain biopsy has been the gold standard for the diagnosis of HSV encephalitis. The last decade has seen brain biopsy replaced by the PCR technique. The PCR technique can detect HSV DNA (HSV-1 and HSV-2) in CSF within 24–48

*Clinical Trials in Central Nervous System Infections* 245

hours of the onset of symptoms.[42,43] Retrospective analysis of CSF samples from France, Sweden, and the National Institute of Allergy and Infectious Diseases (NIAID) Collaborative Antiviral Study Group of therapeutic studies of HSV encephalitis suggested the PCR technique was highly sensitive and specific.[44-46] Clinical experience with this technique, however, has demonstrated some limitations of the PCR assay. The PCR assay includes both HSV-1 and HSV-2 primers. A commensal virus in the CNS in many adults, HSV-2, could reactivate in the setting of fever and encephalitis, and be detected by the PCR assay when it is not the causative agent of the encephalitis. False-negative PCR results can occur when red blood cells are present in the CSF. Contamination of the CSF sample can give a false-positive result. The PCR assay is most likely to be positive early in infection, and then it becomes increasingly harder to detect HSV DNA. By 10–14 days after the onset of symptoms, the PCR assay for HSV DNA may become negative. The HSV antibody assay is a complementary test to the PCR assay. Intrathecal antibody production is usually detectable between days 3 and 10 after the onset of symptoms and remains detectable for up to 30 days.[47] A ratio of serum to CSF titers of IgG antibodies to HSV of 20:1 or less is indicative of active infection.[48] These highly sensitive and specific tests may require weeks for completion by outside reference laboratories. As acyclovir has been shown to be a safe and effective treatment of HSV encephalitis, and the untreated rates of morbidity and mortality are high, it is reasonable to begin empiric treatment in probable HSV encephalitis based on clinical presentation, neuroimaging, electroencephalography, and CSF examination. A dose of 10 mg/kg of acyclovir intravenously every 8 hours is recommended and should be continued until the diagnosis of HSV encephalitis has been eliminated.

In 1986, the NIAID Collaborative Antiviral Study Group recommended acyclovir be given for at least 10 days for the treatment of HSV encephalitis.[41] Over the last several years, a number of case reports have appeared in the literature describing patients that initially improved with acyclovir and then relapsed, prompting the recommendation that a longer duration of therapy be considered.[44-53] A clinical trial that compared the standard 10-day course of therapy to a 14–21 day course of therapy would be helpful. The clinical course as well as CSF PCR for HSV DNA should be examined. Acyclovir-resistant HSV isolates have been identified as the cause of encephalitis in organ-transplant recipients and in HIV-infected individuals. Clinical trials are necessary to determine the best management of HSV encephalitis in these patients.

The varicella-zoster virus is a herpes virus that causes chicken pox, establishes latency in the CNS, and reactivates later in life or in the setting of immunosuppression to cause herpes zoster or shingles. Clinical trials on the antiviral therapy of herpes zoster have investigated the efficacy of various antiviral agents in reducing the length of time for healing of cutaneous lesions and on decreasing the incidence and severity of postherpetic neuralgia.

Valacyclovir is an oral antiviral agent that is converted to acyclovir by hepatic mechanisms.[54-56] When valacyclovir is administered orally, at a dose of 2,000 mg four times a day, the total serum concentration of acyclovir is equivalent to that measured with 10 mg/kg intravenous acyclovir administered three times a day. The tolerability and safety of lower doses of valacyclovir (up to 1,000 mg three times a day) are similar to acyclovir. Valacyclovir was compared to acyclovir in a clinical trial of 1,141 immunocompetent patients older than 50 years of

246    *Clinical Trials in Neurologic Practice*

age with herpes zoster. Valacyclovir (1,000 mg three times daily) and acyclovir (800 mg five times daily) were approximately equivalent in their ability to reduce the duration of virus shedding and accelerate cutaneous healing. The valacyclovir group had a shorter period of postherpetic pain.[57,58]

Another antiviral agent related to acyclovir is famciclovir.[59,60] This drug is converted to the active compound penciclovir after oral administration. Penciclovir and acyclovir have similar in vitro activity against the herpes viruses. In a trial comparing famciclovir (at doses of 250, 500, or 750 mg three times daily) with acyclovir (800 mg five times daily) in 544 immunocompetent adults with herpes zoster, famciclovir was equivalent to acyclovir in amount of time to healing of cutaneous lesions, resolution of acute pain, and safety and tolerance.[58,61]

Because these studies have shown that valacyclovir and famciclovir produce an improvement in the symptoms of herpes zoster, it is reasonable to speculate whether these oral prodrugs may aid in the treatment of HSV encephalitis. The inconvenience and expense related to prolonged intravenous acyclovir therapy makes an oral agent to complete therapy desirable. The efficacy of both valacyclovir and famciclovir against the HSV in genital infections has been investigated,[55,59,60] but there is no information on whether these drugs are effective in the treatment of HSV encephalitis. Initial studies to examine the CSF levels of these drugs after oral administration would be informative to assure sufficient CNS penetration. Clinical trials comparing the efficacy of high doses of oral valacyclovir or famciclovir to standard intravenous doses of acyclovir to complete the treatment of HSV encephalitis are needed. Frequent CSF sampling with measurements of HSV DNA by PCR and clinical markers of recovery should be used as end points.

## HUMAN IMMUNODEFICIENCY VIRUS

Clinical trials in HIV-1 infection of the CNS have focused both on primary HIV-associated disorders, such as dementia, and opportunistic infections including toxoplasmosis, cryptococcal meningitis, cytomegalovirus encephalitis (CMV), progressive multifocal leukoencephalopathy, and primary CNS lymphoma.

### HIV-Dementia

The syndrome of HIV-dementia is associated with clinical features of a subcortical dementia, including impairment of attention, concentration, and short-term memory; motor impairment with slowing of fine motor movements, tremor, balance difficulties and ataxia; and apathy, irritability and emotional lability.[62,63] The American Academy of Neurology's diagnostic criteria for HIV-dementia are: (1) HIV-1 seropositivity (Western blot confirmation); (2) history of progressive cognitive and behavioral decline from premorbid baseline; and (3) exclusion of CNS opportunistic infections by computed tomography (CT), magnetic resonance imaging (MRI), and CSF analysis.[64] The onset of dementia is uncommon before the occurrence of other acquired immunodeficiency syndrome (AIDS)-defining illnesses.[65] In the Multicenter AIDS Cohort Study, HIV-

*Clinical Trials in Central Nervous System Infections* 247

dementia was more common in individuals with CD4 lymphocyte counts of 200/mm[3] or less.[65,66] Cells of the monocyte/macrophage lineage are the predominant cell type infected by HIV. These are the same cells that express the CD4 receptor. In the brain, infection is more frequent in the diencephalic nuclei and the white matter than in other areas. Infection alone, however, appears to be insufficient for the full expression of the clinical deficit of HIV-dementia and additional immune-mediated mechanisms of tissue injury, such as the release of cytokines from activated macrophages, may compound tissue damage.[67,68]

Treatment of systemic HIV infection falls into three categories: (1) nucleoside analogues that act by inhibiting reverse transcriptase (zidovudine, dideoxyinosine, dideoxycytidine, stavudine, lamivudine); (2) non-nucleoside reverse transcriptase inhibitors (nevirapine); and (3) protease inhibitors (indinavir, saquinavir, ritonavir). The efficacy of zidovudine (azidothymidine or AZT) in the prevention and treatment of HIV-dementia has been evaluated in one placebo-controlled trial and several observational studies.[69–73] The results of these studies have suggested a therapeutic benefit of zidovudine in the treatment of HIV-dementia, but did not define the role of zidovudine in preventing cognitive dysfunction. After the introduction of zidovudine as part of the standard pharmacologic regimen for the treatment of HIV infection, a decrease in the incidence of HIV-dementia was observed by epidemiologic data.[65]

The optimal dose of zidovudine for the treatment of HIV-dementia has not been established. In a placebo-controlled trial of zidovudine in HIV-dementia, significant improvement in a battery of neuropsychological tests was demonstrated only in the group receiving 2,000 mg of zidovudine per day.[69] This dose of zidovudine is considerably higher than the 600-mg dose that is recommended to prevent systemic infections, may not be tolerated by all patients, and carries a significant risk of anemia. In addition, this was a small study with only nine patients in each group completing the trial. This small number of patients reduces the power of the study to detect differences that exist between the treatments; trends that are not statistically significant with a small number of subjects might reach statistical significance with a larger sample. In general, however, this study did show some positive effects of zidovudine therapy on cognitive function. The other studies that have reported some effect of zidovudine in HIV-dementia are observational.[70–73] These trials were designed to evaluate the actions of the antiviral agent on HIV infection in general, but retrospective analysis has been used to answer questions about HIV-dementia. In these trials, the doses of zidovudine used are in the usual range (500–600 mg/day), and there is a suggestion of improved cognitive function with zidovudine therapy.

Another nucleoside reverse transcriptase inhibitor used in the treatment of HIV is didanosine (ddI). Observations from a phase I–II study of this drug in HIV-infected children showed that some of the children had increased intelligence quotient (IQ) scores after treatment with ddI.[74] Improvement in IQ scores after treatment with ddI was observed in 2 of 11 children that had encephalopathy at the beginning of the trial, and in 4 of 14 children with baseline IQ scores in the normal range. These improvements in IQ score correlated with plasma concentrations of ddI. These children were not on zidovudine concurrently, secondary to intolerance or suspected resistance. A randomized, doubleblind trial of ddI in adults with symptomatic HIV infection who were intolerant of zidovudine failed to demonstrate a benefit in preventing HIV-dementia.[75]

248   *Clinical Trials in Neurologic Practice*

Fifty-eight patients were assigned to receive one of two doses of ddI. The percentage of patients who subsequently developed HIV-dementia was 14%, which is similar to the natural prevalence.

It has become the standard of care to use multidrug therapy in the treatment of HIV infection.[76,77] Combination therapy is more efficacious in suppressing HIV replication than single-drug therapy. In a double-blind controlled trial, 97 HIV-infected patients who had received zidovudine treatment for at least 6 months were randomly assigned to one of three treatments for up to 52 weeks: 800 mg of indinavir every 8 hours; 200 mg zidovudine every 8 hours combined with 150 mg of lamivudine twice daily; or, all three drugs.[76] The decrease in HIV ribonucleic acid over the first 24 weeks was greater in the three-drug group than in the other groups. The increase in CD4 lymphocyte counts over the first 24 weeks was greater in the two groups receiving indinavir than in the zidovudine-lamivudine group. The changes in the viral load and the CD4 cell count persisted for up to 52 weeks. In a clinical trial that recruited patients from 33 AIDS Clinical Trials Units and seven National Hemophilia Foundation sites in the United States and Puerto Rico, a total of 1,156 HIV-infected patients, who did not yet have AIDS, were randomly assigned to one of two daily regimens: 600 mg of zidovudine and 300 mg of lamivudine, or that regimen in addition to 2,400 mg of indinavir.[77] The primary end point was the time to the development of AIDS or death. This study demonstrated a superiority of the three-drug regimen containing indinavir over the two-drug regimen in slowing the progression of HIV disease.

Because of the effectiveness of multidrug therapy for HIV infection, it has become difficult to evaluate the efficacy of any one drug on any one HIV-related syndrome. Using monotherapy would be unethical. Only patients who are intolerant of multidrug therapy would be eligible for single-drug studies and this might represent a skewed population. For this reason, it is necessary to use observational studies to determine if certain antiviral combinations are more effective than others in reducing the incidence or severity of HIV-dementia.

To aid in evaluation of drug efficacy, a number of studies have attempted to demonstrate a correlation between CSF concentrations of surrogate markers, such as neopterin, quinolinic acid, $\beta$2-microglobulin, and HIV-dementia.[78–80] One study examined CSF from HIV-infected patients with various neurologic complications, neurologically normal HIV-infected individuals, and HIV-seronegative individuals.[78] The highest CSF concentrations of neopterin were observed in patients with CNS infections and primary CNS lymphoma. CSF concentrations of neopterin were also consistently elevated in patients with HIV-dementia. In a study that measured quinolinic acid concentrations in CSF in control subjects, nondemented HIV-infected individuals, and demented HIV-infected individuals, the highest concentrations of quinolinic acid were detected in the CSF of the HIV-infected individuals with dementia.[79] In an investigation of 78 patients with HIV-dementia, there was a high correlation between CSF $\beta$2-microglobulin concentrations and severity of HIV-dementia.[80] In contrast, a prospective study of 94 patients with HIV-dementia investigated the relationship between CSF HIV-1 p24 antigen and the severity of HIV-dementia and found no correlation which offers additional evidence that viral load itself is not the pathophysiologic basis for dementia.[81] The release of proinflammatory cytokines from activated macrophages and circulating neurotoxins, such as quinolinic acid, contribute to brain dysfunction. The ability to detect and measure these biologic markers in

CSF is helpful in developing adjunctive therapies to treat the pathophysiology and clinical symptomatology of HIV-dementia.

As with all clinical trials in chronic disease, patient compliance is a critical issue. This is especially important in HIV-dementia, as resistant mutations of virus may develop due to poor adherence to virologic suppression therapies. In addition, many of these patients are on multidrug regimens, increasing the risk of intolerable side effects. Confounding factors such as depression, metabolic abnormalities, and other infections must be identified to prevent misinterpretation of cognitive changes.

## Progressive Multifocal Leukoencephalopathy

Progressive multifocal leukoencephalopathy (PML) is a progressive demyelinating disease caused by the JC virus.[82] It occurs in individuals with a defect in cell-mediated immunity from organ transplantation, AIDS, cancer and cancer chemotherapy, sarcoidosis, and autoimmune diseases. The clinical manifestations include weakness, altered mental status, visual disturbances, and gait abnormalities. A presumptive diagnosis can be made with neuroimaging, but definitive diagnosis requires brain biopsy. The PCR technique can detect JC virus DNA in CSF, but the sensitivity and specificity of this test have not been well defined.

There is no proven therapy at the present time for PML. The average length of time from diagnosis to death is approximately 3 months. A small percentage of patients will survive for more than a year. Anecdotal experience suggests that combination antiretroviral therapy, which includes protease inhibitors, may improve survival. There are a number of case reports of clinical improvement and decrease in the demyelinative lesions on neuroimaging with zidovudine or cytarabine.[83–85] A randomized, multicenter, open-label trial involving 57 patients with HIV infection and biopsy-confirmed PML examined the efficacy of cytarabine.[86] The patients were randomized to receive intrathecal cytarabine (50 mg/week), intravenous cytarabine (4 mg/kg per day), or no cytarabine. All patients were on antiretroviral therapy with different combinations of zidovudine, ddI, zalcitabine, and saquinavir. There was no improvement in survival (the primary end point measurement used) in the cytarabine group, nor did high-dose antiretroviral therapy alone appear to improve survival over that reported in untreated patients. The study was concluded early because of lack of therapeutic effect and because of the significantly increased incidence of thrombocytopenia and anemia in the treatment groups receiving cytarabine. Case reports have suggested that the newer combinations of antiretroviral therapies may be effective against PML,[87–89] and additional clinical trials are in progress. No new antiviral agents yet have been demonstrated to be efficacious.

There are some basic methodologic problems in assessing the efficacy of a treatment for PML. First, the patients eligible are likely to be on different combinations of antiretroviral agents, and to be intolerant of certain antiretroviral agents. The same antiretroviral regimen should be established for all patients so that the results of a clinical trial can be interpreted. Second, patients with AIDS and PML may have or may develop additional opportunistic CNS infections, concomitant HIV encephalitis, or HIV-dementia during the treatment trial. Although stereotactic brain biopsy is the definitive test to make the diagnosis of

250 *Clinical Trials in Neurologic Practice*

PML, serial brain biopsies are impractical when additional white matter lesions develop on neuroimaging studies. The evaluation of CSF for JC virus DNA by PCR has a sensitivity of 43–82%, depending on the primer pair used.[90] Increasing experience with PCR should make PCR analysis of CSF the definitive test to evaluate the efficacy of treatment trials in patients with PML, which will alleviate some of these methodologic problems.

### Cryptococcal Meningitis

Cryptococcal meningitis is the most common life-threatening fungal infection in patients with AIDS.[91] The clinical presentation includes fever, headache, malaise, nausea, and vomiting. The most common abnormality on neuroimaging is meningeal enhancement; ring-enhancing lesions are rare. *Cryptococcus neoformans* can be demonstrated in smear and culture of the spinal fluid, and detected by the cryptococcal antigen test. The treatment of acute cryptococcal meningitis and maintenance therapy in persons with AIDS who have completed acute therapy are continually undergoing re-evaluation in clinical trials.

In a randomized multicenter trial conducted by the Mycosis Study Group (MSG) and the AIDS Clinical Trials Group (ACTG) of the NIAID, intravenous amphotericin B was compared with oral fluconazole (200 mg daily) as primary therapy for AIDS-associated acute cryptococcal meningitis.[92] The mean dosage of amphotericin B used in the study was 0.4 mg/kg per day. Forty percent (25 of 63) of patients treated with amphotericin B responded (defined as two negative cultures of CSF by 10 weeks of treatment) compared with 34% (44 of 131) of patients receiving fluconazole. There was no significant difference in mortality between the two treatment groups; however, mortality during the first 2 weeks of therapy was higher in the fluconazole group (15% versus 8%). Although the results of this study may suggest that fluconazole is effective in the initial therapy of cryptococcal meningitis, there was a major problem with the design of this study. The dose of amphotericin B used in these patients was relatively low (mean dose of 0.4–0.5 mg/kg per day), which may have significantly altered the apparent efficacy of fluconazole by reducing the efficacy of amphotericin B. The investigators of this study recognized this and suggested that a higher dose of amphotericin B (0.7 mg/ kg or greater) be used in the initial treatment of cryptococcal meningitis.

A subsequent multicenter trial by the MSG/ACTG looked at the efficacy of oral fluconazole or itraconazole in maintenance therapy of AIDS-associated cryptococcal meningitis after an initial 2 weeks of treatment with amphotericin B (0.7 mg/kg per day) with or without flucytosine.[93] Although this study had no placebo group, both oral agents seemed effective in maintaining good clinical response and sterilization of the CSF. The California Collaborative Treatment Group compared fluconazole with placebo for maintenance therapy in a controlled double-blind trial of patients who had been treated for acute cryptococcal meningitis with amphotericin B.[94] Four of 27 patients receiving placebo (15%) and none of 34 patients receiving fluconazole had meningeal recurrence. Six of 20 patients receiving placebo (30%) and one of 27 patients receiving fluconazole (4%) had a urinary recurrence.

The results of clinical trials in cryptococcal meningitis that is not associated with AIDS favor treatment with a combination of amphotericin B and flucytosine. In a randomized trial that compared a combination of amphotericin B (0.3 mg/kg per day) and flucytosine (150 mg/kg per day) for a 6-week course of therapy with amphotericin B alone (0.4 mg/kg per day for 42 days, followed by 0.8 mg/kg every other day for 28 days), the two-drug regimen was associated with a higher rate of recovery.[95] There were also fewer relapses, and sterilization of the CSF was more rapid when flucytosine was added. The use of flucytosine in the treatment of cryptococcal meningitis in AIDS patients has been evaluated more recently. In the 1997 MSG/ACTG trial, the addition of flucytosine was independently associated with a better outcome in the multivariate analysis, and was not associated with an increased incidence of toxic effects.[93] The results of a smaller study also demonstrated the efficacy of the combination of higher doses of amphotericin B with flucytosine in the primary therapy of AIDS-associated cryptococcal meningitis.[96]

The results of these clinical trials have led to recommendations that cryptococcal meningitis in patients with HIV infection be treated with a combination of amphotericin B (0.7 mg/kg per day) and flucytosine 100 mg/kg per day (in four divided doses) for 2–3 weeks followed by fluconazole (400 mg/day) to complete a 10-week course of therapy.[91] Fluconazole 200 mg per day is recommended for life-long maintenance therapy to prevent relapse. Fluconazole is preferred to itraconazole because of its superior penetration into the CSF.[94]

The administration of amphotericin B at the doses required to treat cryptococcal meningitis may lead to renal toxicity. Reduction of the daily dose of amphotericin B or fluconazole alone may not be effective to treat the infection. To address alternative therapy options, a prospective open-label clinical trial of a combination of fluconazole (400 mg daily) with flucytosine (150 mg daily) was conducted in 32 patients with AIDS-associated cryptococcal meningitis.[97] After 10 weeks of therapy, 22 patients had been successfully treated. This success rate of 63% would recommend combination therapy with fluconazole and flucytosine only for those patients unable to tolerate amphotericin B.

Multifactorial analysis of pretreatment factors has identified three significant predictors of a favorable response in the treatment of cryptococcal meningitis.[98] When a patient presents with headache, normal mental status, and a CSF white blood cell count greater than 20 cells/mm$^3$, the chance for a good treatment outcome is better. Similar prognostic factors appear important in AIDS-related cryptococcal meningitis with the most important predictor of early mortality the mental status of the patient at presentation.[91,92] In addition, other factors that are predictive of mortality during treatment include a CSF cryptococcal antigen titer of greater than 1:1,054, a low leukocyte count in CSF (less than 20 cells/mm$^3$), and age younger than 35 years. This information is important in the design of a clinical trial for the treatment of cryptococcal meningitis, as the severity of disease is an important determinant of outcome. The sicker the patients in the clinical trial, the poorer the outcome, regardless of the efficacy of the drug.

## Cytomegalovirus Encephalitis

CMV encephalitis, an important opportunistic infection in organ transplant recipients, is rare in immunocompetent individuals, and has dramatically declined in HIV-infected individuals with the advent of extremely potent antiret-

252    *Clinical Trials in Neurologic Practice*

roviral therapy. There are two clinically and neuropathologically distinct syndromes of CMV encephalitis in AIDS. The more common syndrome is a multifocal, diffusely scattered, micronodular encephalitis that resembles HIV encephalitis and presents with confusion, apathy, and psychomotor slowing. The less common syndrome is a ventriculoencephalitis that presents as a rapidly progressive delirium with cranial nerve deficits and progressive enlargement of the ventricles.[99] The detection of CMV DNA in CSF by PCR is a specific and sensitive test for the diagnosis of CMV infection in the CNS in AIDS patients, but the clinical use of CSF PCR has been limited by the observation that CMV DNA can be detected by PCR in CSF from patients with minimal disease, as well as those with clinically severe disease.[100,101]

Treatment of CMV encephalitis is based on the treatment of CMV retinitis and involves an induction phase with intravenous ganciclovir (5 mg/kg every 12 hours) or foscarnet (60 mg/kg every 8 hours) for a minimum of 2–3 weeks followed by maintenance therapy with ganciclovir (5 mg/kg per day) or foscarnet (100 mg/kg per day).[102,103] There have been no prospective clinical trials to evaluate the efficacy of these regimens in the treatment of CMV encephalitis.

### *Toxoplasma* Encephalitis and Primary Central Nervous System Lymphoma

The most common cause of focal brain lesions in HIV-infected patients is *Toxoplasma gondii* infection.[104] The lesions are a result of reactivation of latent infection because of immunosuppression. *Toxoplasma gondii* has a special predilection for the brain and causes a multifocal encephalitis when the CD4 lymphocyte count decreases (less than 100 cells/mm$^3$). Primary CNS lymphoma is the second most common cause of focal mass lesions in HIV-infected individuals and occurs in as many as 1–4% of HIV-infected persons.[105] When an HIV-positive individual presents with a focal brain lesion or lesions, it is critical to determine whether the disease is *Toxoplasma* encephalitis or primary CNS lymphoma so that appropriate therapy can begin. Because of the importance of differentiating these two entities, many investigators have examined a variety of diagnostic tests to aid in distinguishing *Toxoplasma* encephalitis from primary CNS lymphoma.

Separating cases of *Toxoplasma* encephalitis from primary CNS lymphoma on clinical grounds can be difficult.[104,105] Both complications occur in patients with more advanced disease, although lymphoma is unusual in patients with CD4 counts higher than 50 cells/mm$^3$ and *Toxoplasma* encephalitis can occur with CD4 counts higher than 100 cells/mm$^3$. Patients present with focal neurologic deficits, seizures, and encephalopathic changes in either syndrome. *Toxoplasma* encephalitis can present with fever and headache, but these symptoms are more common in patients who have a higher CD4 count and can still mount an immunologic response. Findings on neurologic examination are usually similar. Both lymphoma and toxoplasmosis can cause focal neurologic deficits and seizures. Thus, there are not any clinical features that can reliably differentiate *Toxoplasma* encephalitis from primary CNS lymphoma.

The advancements in neuroimaging techniques have allowed early identification of CNS lesions in patients with AIDS. Both lymphoma and toxoplasmosis can have ring-enhancing characteristics on contrast-enhanced CT or MRI.[104,105]

*Clinical Trials in Central Nervous System Infections*   253

The presence of a single lesion is much more likely to be lymphoma than *Toxoplasma* encephalitis,[106] but otherwise CT and MRI cannot help differentiate the two entities. Single-photon emission CT with thallium-201 was used to distinguish primary CNS lymphoma from nonlymphoma masses in 37 AIDS patients.[107] All 12 of the 37 patients who had increased focal thallium-201 uptake were later shown to have lymphoma on biopsy. Of the remaining 25 patients without increased uptake, 24 had biopsy-proven *Toxoplasma gondii* lesions and one patient had a tuberculosis abscess. Another study examined the use of positron emission tomography (PET) in differentiating *Toxoplasma gondii* from lymphoma.[108] Twenty AIDS patients with enhancing lesions on MRI of the head underwent PET scanning. All of the patients who were later diagnosed with *Toxoplasma* encephalitis (on the basis of clinical response to therapy or autopsy) had hypometabolic lesions on PET, whereas all of the cases of lymphoma had hypermetabolic lesions. Although these two studies suggest that the newer imaging techniques may be helpful in distinguishing lymphoma from *Toxoplasma* encephalitis, the cost and limited availability of this technology limit the clinical use of PET and single-photon emission CT at the present time.

Ancillary laboratory tests have been examined to aid in diagnostic differentiation.[109–114] Serum antitoxoplasma IgG antibodies are detected in 12–50% of HIV-infected individuals whether or not they have an active encephalitis.[104] A negative antibody titer would be highly unlikely, therefore, in a patient with multiple focal brain lesions from *Toxoplasma gondii*. Detection of *Toxoplasma gondii* in the CSF is possible using PCR techniques.[109] In one study of 88 HIV-infected patients with focal brain lesions, the sensitivity of this assay for *Toxoplasma* encephalitis was only 33.3%, whereas the specificity was 100%. Because of its low sensitivity, this test cannot be used alone to diagnose *Toxoplasma* encephalitis. Epstein-Barr virus (EBV) is frequently detected in HIV-associated primary CNS lymphoma.[110] The CSF can be examined for EBV DNA using PCR. When the CSF of 85 patients with HIV-related CNS abnormalities was examined, the sensitivity of CSF PCR for EBV DNA in lymphoma was 100%, and the specificity was 98.5% as compared with histologic studies at autopsy.[111] This suggests that PCR for EBV DNA provides valuable information in differentiating the etiology of focal brain lesions in HIV-infected individuals. It may not always be practical to obtain CSF, however, in patients with multiple brain lesions associated with mass effect.

The recommendation for differentiating *Toxoplasma* encephalitis from primary CNS lymphoma is a diagnostic treatment trial for *Toxoplasma* encephalitis when there is more than one enhancing brain lesion on neuroimaging and detectable serum antitoxoplasma IgG. If no clinical or radiologic improvement occurs within 14 days, consideration should be given to a brain biopsy.

Once a presumptive diagnosis of *Toxoplasma* encephalitis is made, standard treatment includes pyrimethamine (100–200 mg orally initially, followed by 75–100 mg orally each day), sulfadiazine (1.5–2.0 g orally four times a day), and folinic acid (10–50 mg orally each day) for 6 weeks. These should be followed by lower doses to suppress recurrence for the lifetime of the individual (pyrimethamine 25–50 mg orally each day; sulfadiazine 1 g orally 3 or 4 times a day; folinic acid 10–50 mg orally each day). This has a success rate of greater than 80%, but adverse reactions, including leukopenia, thrombocytopenia, fever, rash, or renal failure, make the therapy intolerable for approximately 20% of

254 *Clinical Trials in Neurologic Practice*

patients.[115,116] One alternative is to use clindamycin (600–900 mg orally four times a day for 6 weeks, followed by 300–450 mg orally three to four times a day for life) instead of sulfadiazine. A randomized trial of 84 patients with *Toxoplasma* encephalitis showed that pyrimethamine plus clindamycin was equally efficacious in the acute phase.[117] A larger European study with 299 patients also showed similar efficacy in the acute phase of treatment, but the clindamycin regimen was less effective in maintenance with a twofold higher relapse rate.[118] In both studies, clindamycin was associated with a significant number of serious hematologic or dermatologic adverse reactions, albeit a smaller number than in the sulfadiazine groups.[117,118]

Since both of the accepted therapeutic regimens have serious toxicities and because patients require life-long suppressive therapy, alternative therapies for the treatment of *Toxoplasma* encephalitis are being investigated. Three trials have looked at the efficacy of atovaquone.[119–121] All of the studies involved patients that were intolerant or resistant to therapy with pyrimethamine, sulfadiazine, or clindamycin. In the initial phase of therapy, 26% of patients receiving 750 mg of atovaquone orally four times a day showed improvement.[120] Improvement was associated with higher plasma levels of the drug. Seventy percent of patients who received atovaquone for maintenance therapy after an initial course of traditional therapy were alive a year after diagnosis.[121] All three studies showed atovaquone to be well tolerated.[119–121] These studies suggest that atovaquone is an effective alternative in those intolerant of traditional therapy. Whether this drug is more appropriate for maintenance therapy than the traditional regimen, or whether it is effective for resistant organisms, awaits future clinical trials.

In contrast to the largely effective treatment for *Toxoplasma* encephalitis, primary CNS lymphoma has been much harder to treat. Since primary CNS lymphoma in non-AIDS patients is sensitive to radiation therapy, this modality was evaluated in those with AIDS-related lymphoma. In an initial study of radiation therapy, 6 of 10 patients with biopsy-proven CNS lymphoma showed radiographic improvement in lesions after treatment.[122] Larger studies have shown that approximately 70% of patients with AIDS-related primary CNS lymphoma respond to radiation therapy.[123–125] The survival remains short, however, in the range of 3–6 months.

To improve survival, adjuvant chemotherapy options have been explored. Primary CNS lymphoma in the non-AIDS patient has been more successfully treated with methotrexate, cytarabine, and radiation therapy than with radiation therapy alone.[126] Various combinations of chemotherapy have been tried to enhance survival in patients with AIDS-related CNS lymphoma receiving radiation therapy.[127,128] Selected patients do appear to have improved survival but this is highly dependent on pretherapy characteristics such as stage of disease, CD4 lymphocyte count, Karnofsky score, and comorbid conditions and infections. Prospective clinical trials to examine the efficacy of chemotherapy in addition to radiation therapy are ongoing.

The problems with future clinical trials for *Toxoplasma* encephalitis and primary CNS lymphoma are similar. The first problem is rapid and accurate diagnosis and the second is offering alternative treatments in a randomized and blinded fashion. Current therapies have already been shown to be effective, and, therefore, new therapies are left for those patients who are intolerant to traditional therapy or who fail initial therapy. This is a skewed population. Last, the patient with AIDS has a

## Clinical Trials in Central Nervous System Infections    255

complicated course with many concomitant illnesses. Recovery from any one AIDS-related illness is related to the overall state of the patient. Using survival as an outcome measurement for treatment of any one entity is problematic. There has been great progress in the treatment of these infectious diseases of the CNS, and many more advances will be made in the years to come.

## REFERENCES

1. McCracken GH, Nelson JD, Kaplan SL, et al. Consensus report: antimicrobial therapy for bacterial meningitis in infants and children. Pediatr Infect Dis J 1987;6:501–505.
2. Peltola H, Anttila M, Renkonen O. Randomized comparison of chloramphenicol, ampicillin, cefotaxime, and ceftriaxone for childhood bacterial meningitis. Lancet 1989;i:1281–1287.
3. Scholz H, Hofmann T, Noack R, et al. Prospective comparison of ceftriaxone and cefotaxime for the short-term treatment of bacterial meningitis in children. Chemotherapy 1998;44:142–147.
4. Schoendorf KC, Adams WG, Kiely JL, Wenger JD. National trends in *Haemophilus influenzae* meningitis mortality and hospitalization among children, 1980 through 1991. Pediatrics 1994;93: 663–669.
5. American Academy of Pediatrics Committee on Infectious Diseases. Therapy for children with invasive pneumococcal infections. Pediatrics 1997;99:289–299.
6. Friedland IR, Paris M, Shelton S, McCracken GH. Time-kill studies of antibiotic combinations against penicillin-resistant and -susceptible *Streptococcus pneumoniae*. J Antimicrob Chemother 1994;34:231–237.
7. Friedland IR, Paris M, Ehrett S, et al. Evaluation of antimicrobial regimens for treatment of experimental penicillin- and cephalosporin-resistant pneumococcal meningitis. Antimicrob Agents Chemother 1993;37:1630–1636.
8. Ahmed A. A critical evaluation of vancomycin for treatment of bacterial meningitis. Pediatr Infect Dis J 1997;16:895–903.
9. Gump DW. Vancomycin for treatment of bacterial meningitis. Rev Infect Dis 1981;3(Suppl):S289–S292.
10. Viladrich PF, Gudiol F, Linares J, et al. Evaluation of vancomycin for therapy of adult pneumococcal meningitis. Antimicrob Agents Chemother 1991;35:2467–2472.
11. Paris MM, Hickey SM, Uscher MI, et al. Effect of dexamethasone on therapy of experimental penicillin- and cephalosporin-resistant pneumococcal meningitis. Antimicrob Agents Chemother 1994; 38:1320–1324.
12. Cabellos C, Martinez-Lacasa J, Martos A, et al. Influence of dexamethasone on efficacy of ceftriaxone and vancomycin therapy in experimental pneumococcal meningitis. Antimicrob Agents Chemother 1995;39:2158–2160.
13. Klugman KP, Friedland IR, Bradley JS. Bactericidal activity against cephalosporin-resistant *Streptococcus pneumoniae* in cerebrospinal fluid of children with acute bacterial meningitis. Antimicrob Agents Chemother 1995;39:1988–1992.
14. Patel JB, Giles RE. Meropenem: evidence of lack of proconvulsive tendency in mice. J Antimicrob Chemother 1989;24(Suppl A):307–309.
15. Catchpole CR, Wise R, Thornber D, Andrews JM. In vitro activity of L-627, a new carbapenem. Antimicrob Agents Chemother 1992;36:1928–1934.
16. Klugman KP, Dagan R. Randomized comparison of meropenem with cefotaxime for treatment of bacterial meningitis. Antimicrob Agents Chemother 1995;39:1140–1146.
17. Schmutzhard E, Williams KJ, Vukmirovits G, et al. A randomized comparison of meropenem with cefotaxime or ceftriaxone for the treatment of bacterial meningitis in adults. J Antimicrob Chemother 1995;36(Suppl A):85–97.
18. Sanders CC. Cefepime: the next generation? Clin Infect Dis 1993;17:369–379.
19. Sáez-Llorens X, Castaño E, García R, et al. Prospective randomized comparison of cefepime and cefotaxime for treatment of bacterial meningitis in infants and children. Antimicrob Agents Chemother 1995;39:937–940.
20. Roos KL. Bacterial meningitis. In KL Roos (ed), Central Nervous System Infectious Diseases and Therapy. New York: Marcel Dekker, Inc. 1997;99–126.

## 256    Clinical Trials in Neurologic Practice

21. Townsend GC, Scheld WM. Adjunctive therapy for meningitis: rationale for use, current status, and prospects for the future. Clin Infect Dis 1993;17(Suppl 2):S537–S549.
22. Tuomanen E. Adjunctive therapy of experimental meningitis: agents other than steroids. Antibiot Chemother 1992;45:184–191.
23. Lepper MH, Spies HW. Treatment of pneumococcic meningitis. AMA Arch Intern Med 1959; 104:253–259.
24. DeLemos RA, Haggerty RJ. Corticosteroids as an adjunct to treatment in bacterial meningitis. Pediatrics 1969;44:30–34.
25. Belsey MA, Hoffpauir CW, Smith MHD. Dexamethasone in the treatment of acute bacterial meningitis: the effect of study design on the interpretation of results. Pediatrics 1969;44:503–513.
26. Täuber MG, Khayam-Bashi H, Sande M. Effects of ampicillin and corticosteroids on brain water content, cerebrospinal fluid pressure, and cerebrospinal fluid lactate levels in experimental pneumococcal meningitis. J Infect Dis 1985;151:528–534.
27. Lebel MH, Freij B, Syrogiannopoulos GA, et al. Dexamethasone therapy for bacterial meningitis. N Engl J Med 1988;319:964–971.
28. Lebel MH, Hoyt MJ, Waagner DC, et al. Magnetic resonance imaging and dexamethasone therapy for bacterial meningitis. AJDC 1989;143:301–306.
29. Girgis NI, Farid Z, Mikhail IA, et al. Dexamethasone treatment for bacterial meningitis in children and adults. Pediatr Infect Dis J 1989;8:848–851.
30. Odio CM, Faingezicht I, Paris M, et al. The beneficial effects of early dexamethasone administration in infants and children with bacterial meningitis. N Engl J Med 1991;324:1525–1531.
31. Schaad UB, Lips U, Gnehm HE, et al. Dexamethasone therapy for bacterial meningitis in children. Lancet 1993;342:457–461.
32. King SM, Law B, Langley JM, et al. Dexamethasone therapy for bacterial meningitis: better never than late? Can J Infect Dis 1994;5:210–215.
33. Wald ER, Kaplan SL, Mason EO, et al. Dexamethasone therapy for children with bacterial meningitis. Pediatrics 1995;95:21–28.
34. Kilpi T, Peltola H, Jauhiainen T, Kallio MJ. Oral glycerol and intravenous dexamethasone in preventing neurologic and audiologic sequelae of childhood bacterial meningitis. Pediatr Infect Dis J 1995;14:270–278.
35. Ciana G, Antonio C, Pivetta S, et al. Effectiveness of adjunctive treatment with steroids in reducing short term mortality in a high-risk population of children with bacterial meningitis. J Trop Pediatr 1995;41:164–168.
36. Kanra GY, Özen H, Seçmeer G, et al. Beneficial effects of dexamethasone in children with pneumococcal meningitis. Pediatr Infect Dis J 1995;14:490–494.
37. Qazi S, Khan MA, Mughal N, et al. Dexamethasone and bacterial meningitis in Pakistan. Arch Dis Child 1996;75:482–488.
38. McIntyre PB, Berkey CS, King SM, et al. Dexamethasone as adjunctive therapy in bacterial meningitis. JAMA 1997;278:925–931.
39. American Academy of Pediatrics Committee on Infectious Diseases. Dexamethasone therapy for bacterial meningitis in infants and children. Pediatrics 1990;86:130–133.
40. Sköldenberg B, Forsgren M, Alestig K, et al. Acyclovir versus vidarabine in herpes simplex encephalitis. Lancet 1984;ii:707–711.
41. Whitley RJ, Alford CA, Hirsch MS, et al. Vidarabine versus acyclovir therapy in herpes simplex encephalitis. N Engl J Med 1986;314:144–149.
42. Rowley AH, Whitley RJ, Lakeman FD, Wolinsky SM. Rapid detection of herpes-simplex-virus DNA in cerebrospinal fluid of patients with herpes simplex encephalitis. Lancet 1990;335:440–441.
43. Aurelius E, Johansson B, Sköldenberg B, et al. Rapid diagnosis of herpes simplex encephalitis by nested polymerase chain reaction assay of cerebrospinal fluid. Lancet 1991;337:189–192.
44. Guffond T, Dewilde A, Lobert P-E, et al. Significance and clinical relevance of the detection of herpes simplex virus DNA by the polymerase chain reaction in cerebrospinal fluid from patients with presumed encephalitis. Clin Infect Dis 1994;18:744–749.
45. Aurelius E, Johansson B, Sköldenberg B, Forgren M. Encephalitis in immunocompetent patients due to herpes simplex virus type 1 or 2 as determined by type-specific polymerase chain reaction and antibody assays of cerebrospinal fluid. J Med Virol 1993;39:179–186.
46. Lakeman FD, Whitley RJ. Diagnosis of herpes simplex encephalitis: application of polymerase chain reaction to cerebrospinal fluid from brain-biopsied patients and correlation with disease. J Infect Dis 1995;171:857–863.

## Clinical Trials in Central Nervous System Infections    257

47. Nahmias AJ, Whitley RJ, Visintine AN, et al. Herpes simplex virus encephalitis: laboratory evaluations and their diagnostic significance. J Infect Dis 1982;145:829–836.
48. Levine DP, Lauter CB, Lerner AM. Simultaneous serum and CSF antibodies in herpes simplex virus encephalitis. JAMA 1978;240:356–360.
49. Knezevic W, Carroll WM. Relapse of herpes simplex encephalitis after acyclovir therapy. Aust N Z J Med 1983;13:625–626.
50. Barthez MA, Billard C, Santini JJ. Relapse of herpes simplex encephalitis. Neuropediatrics 1987; 18:3–7.
51. Van Landingham KE, Marsteller HB, Ross GW, Hayden FG. Relapse of herpes simplex encephalitis after conventional acyclovir therapy. JAMA 1988;259:1051–1053.
52. Kimura H, Aso K, Kuzushima K, et al. Relapse of herpes simplex encephalitis in children. Pediatrics 1992;89:891–894.
53. Nicolaidou P, Iacovidou N, Youroukos S, et al. Relapse of herpes simplex encephalitis after acyclovir therapy. Eur J Pediatr 1993;152:737–738.
54. Acosta EP, Fletcher CV. Valacyclovir. Ann Pharmacother 1997;31:185–191.
55. Perry CM, Faulds D. Valacyclovir. Drugs 1996;52:754–772.
56. The Medical Letter. Valacyclovir. Med Lett 1996;38:3–4.
57. Beutner KR, Friedman DJ, Forszpaniak C, et al. Valacyclovir compared with acyclovir for improved therapy for herpes zoster in immunocompetent adults. Antimicrob Agents Chemother 1995;39:1546–1553.
58. Gnann JW. New antivirals with activity against varicella-zoster virus. Ann Neurol 1994;34:569–672.
59. Luber AD, Flaherty JF. Famciclovir for treatment of herpesvirus infections. Ann Pharmacother 1996;30:978–985.
60. Stein GE. Pharmacology of new antiherpes agents: famciclovir and valacyclovir. J Amer Pharmaceut Assoc 1997;NS37:157–163.
61. Gheeraert P. Efficacy and safety of famciclovir in the treatment of uncomplicated herpes virus. In Program and Abstracts, 32nd ICAAC. Washington: American Society for Microbiology, 1992.
62. Navia BA, Jordan BD, Price RW. The AIDS dementia complex: I. Clinical features. Ann Neurol 1986;19:517–524.
63. Melton ST, Kirkwood CK, Ghaemi SN. Pharmacotherapy of HIV-dementia. Ann Pharmacother 1997;31:457–473.
64. American Academy of Neurology AIDS Task Force. Nomenclature and research case definitions for neurologic manifestations of human immunodeficiency virus type-1 (HIV-1) infection. Neurology 1991;41:778–785.
65. Bacellar H, Muñoz A, Miller EH, et al. Temporal trends in the incidence of HIV-1-related neurologic diseases. Neurology 1994;44:1892–1900.
66. McArthur JC, Hoover DR, Bacellar H, et al. Dementia in AIDS patients: incidence and risk factors. Neurology 1993;43:2245–2252.
67. Navia BA, Cho E-S, Petito CK, Price RW. The AIDS dementia complex: II. Neuropathology. Ann Neurol 1986;19:525–535.
68. Brew BJ, Rosenblum M, Cronin K, Price RW. AIDS dementia complex and HIV-1 brain infection: clinical-virological correlations. Ann Neurol 1995;38:563–570.
69. Sidtis JJ, Gatsonis C, Price RW, et al. Zidovudine treatment of the AIDS dementia complex: results of a placebo-controlled trial. Ann Neurol 1993;33:343–349.
70. Schmitt FA, Bigley JW, McKinnis R, et al. Neurophysiological outcome of zidovudine (AZT) treatment of patients with AIDS and AIDS-related complex. N Engl J Med 1988;319:1573–1578.
71. Portegies P, de Gans J, Lange MA, et al. Declining incidence of AIDS dementia complex after introduction of zidovudine treatment. Br Med J 1989;299:819–821.
72. Tozzi V, Narciso P, Galgani S, et al. Effects of zidovudine in 30 patients with mild to end-stage AIDS dementia complex. AIDS 1993;7:683–692.
73. Baldeweg T, Catalan J, Gazzard BG. Risk of HIV dementia and opportunistic brain disease in AIDS and zidovudine therapy. J Neurol Neurosurg Psychiatry 1998;65:34–41.
74. Butler KM, Husson RN, Balis FM, et al. Dideoxyinosine in children with symptomatic human immunodeficiency virus infection. N Engl J Med 1991;324:137–144.
75. Potegies P, Enting RH, de Jong MD, et al. AIDS dementia complex and didanosine. Lancet 1994;344:759.
76. Gulick RM, Mellors JW, Havir D, et al. Treatment with indinavir, zidovudine, and lamivudine in adults with human immunodeficiency virus infection and prior antiretroviral therapy. N Engl J Med 1997;337:734–739.

## 258 *Clinical Trials in Neurologic Practice*

77. Hammer SM, Squires KE, Hughes MD, et al. A controlled trial of two nucleoside analogues plus indinavir in persons with human immunodeficiency virus infection and CD4 cell counts of 200 per cubic millimeter or less. N Engl J Med 1997;337:725–733.
78. Brew BJ, Bhalla RB, Paul M, et al. Cerebrospinal fluid neopterin in human immunodeficiency virus type 1 infection. Ann Neurol 1990;28:556–560.
79. Heyes MP, Brew B, Martin A, et al. Cerebrospinal fluid quinolinic acid concentrations are increased in acquired immune deficiency syndrome. Adv Exp Med Biol 1991;294:687–690.
80. Brew BJ, Bhalla RB, Paul M, et al. Cerebrospinal fluid ß$_2$-microglobulin in patients with AIDS dementia complex: an expanded series including response to zidovudine treatment. AIDS 1992;6:461–465.
81. Brew BJ, Paul MO, Nakajima G, et al. Cerebrospinal fluid HIV-1 p24 antigen and culture: sensitivity and specificity for AIDS-dementia complex. J Neurol Neurosurg Psychiatry 1994;57:784–789.
82. Berger JR, Kaszovitz B, Post MJD, Dickinson G. Progressive multifocal leukoencephalopathy associated with human immunodeficiency virus infection. Ann Intern Med 1987;107:78–87.
83. Marriott PJ, O'Brien MD, MacKinzie ICK, Janota I. Progressive multifocal leukoencephalopathy: remission with cytarabine. J Neurol Neurosurg Psychiatry 1975;38:205–209.
84. O'Riordan T, Daly PA, Hutchinson M, et al. Progressive multifocal leukoencephalopathy—remission with cytarabine. J Infect 1980;20:51–54.
85. Conway B, Halliday WC, Brunham RC. Human immunodeficiency virus-associated progressive multifocal leukoencephalopathy: apparent response to 3'-azido-3'-deoxythymidine. Rev Infect Dis 1990;12:479–482.
86. Hall CD, Dafni U, Simpson D, et al. Failure of cytarabine in progressive multifocal leukoencephalopathy associated with human immunodeficiency virus infection. N Engl J Med 1998;338:1345–1351.
87. Cinque P, Casari S, Bertelli D. Progressive multifocal leukoencephalopathy, HIV and highly active antiretroviral therapy. N Engl J Med 1998;339:848–849.
88. Teófilo E, Gouveia J, Brotas V, da Costa P. Progressive multifocal leukoencephalopathy regression with highly active antiretroviral therapy. AIDS 1998;12:449.
89. Sadler M, Chinn R, Healy J, et al. New treatments for progressive multifocal leukoencephalopathy in HIV-infected patients. AIDS 1998;12:533–535.
90. Weber T, Turner RW, Frye S, et al. Specific diagnosis of progressive multifocal leukoencephalopathy by polymerase chain reaction. J Infect Dis 1994;169:1138–1141.
91. Powderly WG. Cryptococcal meningitis and AIDS. Clin Infect Dis 1993;17:837–842.
92. Saag MS, Powderly WG, Cloud GA, et al. Comparison of amphotericin B with fluconazole in the treatment of acute AIDS-associated cryptococcal meningitis. N Engl J Med 1992;326:83–89.
93. van der Horst CM, Saag MS, Cloud GA, et al. Treatment of cryptococcal meningitis associated with the acquired immunodeficiency syndrome. N Engl J Med 1997;377:15–21.
94. Bozzette SA, Larsen RA, Chiu J, et al. A placebo-controlled trial of maintenance therapy with fluconazole after treatment of cryptococcal meningitis in the acquired immunodeficiency syndrome. N Engl J Med 1991;324:580–584.
95. Bennett JE, Dismukes WE, Duma RJ, et al. A comparison of amphotericin B alone and combined with flucytosine in the treatment of cryptococcal meningitis. N Engl J Med 1979;301:126–131.
96. de Lalla F, Pellizzer G, Vaglia A, et al. Amphotericin B as primary therapy for cryptococcosis in patients with AIDS: reliability of relatively high doses administered over a relatively short period. Clin Infect Dis 1994;20:263–266.
97. Larsen RA, Bozzette SA, Jones BE, et al. Fluconazole combined with flucytosine for treatment of cryptococcal meningitis in patients with AIDS. Clin Infect Dis 1994;19:741–745.
98. Dismukes WE, Cloud G, Gallis HA, et al. Treatment of cryptococcal meningitis with combination amphotericin B and flucytosine for four as compared with six weeks. N Engl J Med 1987;317:334–341.
99. McCutchan JA. Cytomegalovirus infections of the nervous system in patients with AIDS. Clin Infect Dis 1995;20:747–754.
100. Cinque P, Vago L, Brytting M, et al. Cytomegalovirus infection of the central nervous system in patients with AIDS: diagnosis by DNA amplification from cerebrospinal fluid. J Infect Dis 1992;166:1408–1411.
101. Wolf DG, Spector SA. Diagnosis of human cytomegalovirus central nervous system disease in AIDS patients by DNA amplification form cerebrospinal fluid. J Infect Dis 1992;166:1412–1415.
102. Jacobson MA. Treatment of cytomegalovirus retinitis in patients with the acquired immunodeficiency syndrome. N Engl J Med 1997;337:105–114.
103. Wood AJJ. Antiviral drugs. N Engl J Med 1999;340:1255–1268.

## Clinical Trials in Central Nervous System Infections 259

104. Luft BJ, Remington JS. Toxoplasmic encephalitis in AIDS. Clin Infect Dis 1992;15:211–222.
105. DeMario MD, Liebowitz DN. Lymphomas in the immunocompromised patient. Sem Oncol 1998;25:492–502.
106. Ciricillo SF, Rosenbaum ML. Use of CT and MR imaging to distinguish intracranial lesions and to define the need for biopsy in AIDS patients. J Neurosurg 1990;73:720–724.
107. Ruiz A, Ganz WI, Post JD, et al. Use of thallium-201 brain SPECT to differentiate cerebral lymphoma from toxoplasma encephalitis in AIDS patients. Amer Soc Neuroradiol 1994;15:1885–1894.
108. Pierce MA, Johnson MD, Maciunas RJ, et al. Evaluating contrast-enhancing brain lesions in patients with AIDS by using positron emission tomography. Ann Inter Med 1995;123:594–598.
109. Cingolani A, De Luca A, Ammassari A, et al. PCR detection of *Toxoplasma gondii* DNA in CSF for the differential diagnosis of AIDS-related focal brain lesions. J Med Microbiol 1996;45:472–476.
110. DeAngelis LM, Wong E, Rosenblum M, Furneaux H. Epstein-Barr virus in acquired immune deficiency syndrome (AIDS) and non-AIDS primary central nervous system lymphoma. Cancer 1992;70:1607–1611.
111. Cinque P, Brytting M, Vago L, et al. Epstein-Barr virus DNA in cerebrospinal fluid from patients with AIDS-related primary lymphoma of the central nervous system. Lancet 1993;342:398–401.
112. Antinori A, Ammassari A, De Luca A, et al. Diagnosis of AIDS-related focal brain lesions. Neurology 1997;48:687–694.
113. Raffi F, Aboulker J-P, Michelet C, et al. A prospective study of criteria for the diagnosis of toxoplasmic encephalitis in 186 AIDS patients. AIDS 1997;11:177–184.
114. Roberts TC, Storch GA. Multiplex PCR for diagnosis of AIDS-related central nervous system lymphoma and toxoplasmosis. J Clin Microbiol 1997;35:268–269.
115. Leport C, Raffi F, Matheron S, et al. Treatment of central nervous system toxoplasmosis with pyrimethamine/sulfadiazine combination in 35 patients with the acquired immunodeficiency syndrome. Am J Med 1988;84:94–100.
116. Haverkos HW, The TE Study Group. Assessment of therapy for toxoplasma encephalitis. Am J Med 1987;82:907–914.
117. Dannemann B, McCutchan JA, Israelski D, et al. Treatment of toxoplasmic encephalitis in patients with AIDS. Ann Inter Med 1992;116:33–43.
118. Katlama C, De Wit S, O'Doherty E, et al. Pyrimethamine-clindamycin vs. pyrimethamine-sulfadiazine as acute and long-term treatment for toxoplasmic encephalitis in patients with AIDS. Clin Infect Dis 1996;22:268–275.
119. Kovacs JA, NIAID-Clinical Center Intramural AIDS Program. Efficacy of atovaquone in treatment of toxoplasmosis in patients with AIDS. Lancet 1992;340:637–638.
120. Katlama C, Mouthon B, Gourdon D, et al. Atovaquone as long-term suppressive therapy for toxoplasmic encephalitis in patients with AIDS and multiple drug intolerance. AIDS 1996;10:1107–1112.
121. Torres RA, Weinberg W, Stansall J, et al. Atovaquone for salvage treatment and suppression of toxoplasmic encephalitis in patients with AIDS. Clin Infect Dis 1997;24:422–429.
122. Formenti SC, Gill PS, Lean E, et al. Primary central nervous system lymphoma in AIDS: results of radiation therapy. Cancer 1989;63:1101–1107.
123. Baumgartner JE, Rachlin JR, Beckstead JH, et al. Primary central nervous system lymphomas: natural history and response to radiation therapy in 55 patients with acquired immunodeficiency syndrome. J Neurosurg 1990;73:206–211.
124. Kaufmann T, Nisce LZ, Coleman M. A comparison of survival of patients treated for AIDS-related central nervous system lymphoma with and without tissue diagnosis. Int J Radiat Oncol Biol Phys 1996;36:429–432.
125. Ling SM, Roach M, Larson DA, Ward WM. Radiotherapy of primary central nervous system lymphoma in patients with and without human immunodeficiency virus. Cancer 1994;73:2570–2582.
126. DeAngelis LM, Yahalom J, Thaler HT, Kher U. Combined modality therapy for primary CNS lymphoma. J Clin Oncol 1992;10:635–643.
127. Chamberlain MC. Long survival in patients with acquired immune deficiency syndrome-related primary central nervous system lymphoma. Cancer 1994;73:1728–1730.
128. Forsyth PA, Yahalom J, DeAngelis LM. Combined-modality therapy in the treatment of primary central nervous system lymphoma in AIDS. Neurology 1994;44:1473–1479.

# 13
## Peripheral Neuropathy Treatment Trials
Christopher Klein, Michael Polydefkis, and Vinay Chaudhry

In peripheral neuropathy, establishing a patient's diagnosis is the first step to successful treatment. A thorough clinical history and examination, coupled with electrophysiologic and laboratory testing, are essential to characterize the pathophysiology and etiology of peripheral neuropathy to guide specific treatments and predict prognoses. Guillain-Barré syndrome (GBS),[1-8] chronic inflammatory demyelinating polyneuropathy (CIDP),[9-14] and diabetic neuropathies (DNs)[15-23] have been identified with distinct subgroups as having varied treatment response and pathogeneses. Randomized and open trials have established the benefits of immune-regulating therapies in a number of peripheral neuropathies, such as GBS,[1,4,6] CIDP,[12,24,25] and multifocal motor neuropathy (MMN).[26-31] On the other hand, apart from good glycemic control, interventional treatment in diabetic peripheral neuropathy (DPN) has not met with similar benefit. Several immuno-modulating agents are available, including intravenous immunoglobulin (IVIG), plasma exchange (PE), corticosteroids, azathioprine, cyclosporine, and cyclophosphamide. In addition, a number of new immune modulating agents, including tumor necrosis factor-α antagonists (etanercept, infliximab, leflunomide) and the interferons, are available. Other drugs previously reserved for transplantation and chemotherapy are also being considered in peripheral neuropathy trials.

The choice of a specific therapy, dose, and length of treatment is complex and driven by an understanding of the realistic benefits and potential complications of each agent. Such an assessment should be based on frequent review of the literature and critical analyses of outcome measures used in each drug trial. Outcome measures can be classified into measures of impairment, disability, and handicap; these are essential in establishing the biologic effect of treatment. Studies that investigate whether patients benefit from treatment in terms of improvement of functional health require disability or handicap measures. Unlike stroke or multiple sclerosis, disability or handicap measures assessing quality-of-life have been infrequently used in patients with DN or CIDP.[32]

The most widely used clinical rating scales for monitoring peripheral nerve function have been the Neurologic Symptom Score (NSS),[33,34] Neurologic Symptom Profile (NSP),[35] and Neurologic Impairment Score (NIS).[34] NSS and NSP assess the

## 262 Clinical Trials in Neurologic Practice

presence or absence of bulbar and limb weakness, negative and positive sensory disturbances, and autonomic symptoms. NIS concentrates on grading the absence or presence of sensory or motor loss and reflex changes. Abnormalities in two or more of NSS, NIS, nerve conduction, and quantitative sensory testing (QST) are required for defining the presence or absence of neuropathy. This system, primarily designed to increase the sensitivity of detecting and grading DN, has been validated by the use of simultaneous sural nerve biopsies.[36] The Michigan Diabetic Neuropathy Score is another scoring system based on quantitative neurologic examination coupled with nerve conduction studies.[37,38] We have used the Total Neuropathy Score (TNS) (Table 13.1). TNS is a validated measure that can be used for monitoring peripheral

*Table 13.1*  Total neuropathy score (TNS)

| TNS | 0 | 1 | 2 | 3 | 4 |
|---|---|---|---|---|---|
| Sensory symptoms | None | Symptoms limited to fingers or toes | Symptoms extend to ankle or wrist | Symptoms extend to knee or elbow | Symptoms above knees or elbows or functionally disabling |
| Motor symptoms | None | Slight difficulty | Moderate difficulty | Require help/assistance | Paralysis |
| Autonomic symptoms* | None | 1 yes | 2 yes | 3 yes | 4 or 5 yes |
| Pin sensibility | Normal | Reduced in fingers/toes | Reduced up to wrist/ankle | Reduced up to elbow/knee | Reduced to above elbow/knee |
| Vibration sensibility | Normal | Reduced in fingers/toes | Reduced up to wrist/ankle | Reduced up to elbow/knee | Reduced to above elbow/knee |
| Strength | Normal | Mild weakness (MRC 4) | Moderate weakness (MRC 3) | Severe weakness (MRC 2) | Paralysis (MRC 0 or 1) |
| Tendon reflexes | Normal | Ankle reflex reduced | Ankle reflex absent | Ankle reflex absent/others reduced | All reflexes absent |
| Vibration sensation (QST using vibration) | Normal to 125% of ULN | 126–150% of ULN | 151–200% of ULN | 201–300% of ULN | >301% of ULN |
| Sural amplitude score | Normal/reduced <5% | 76–95% of LLN | 51–75% of LLN | 26–50% of LLN | 0–25% of LLN |
| Peroneal amplitude score | Normal/reduced <10% | 76–95% of LLN | 51–75% of LLN | 26–50% of LLN | 0–25% of LLN |

LLN = lower limits of normal; MRC = Medical Research Council; QST = quantitative sensory testing; ULN = upper limits of normal.

*Number of autonomic symptoms: postural fainting, impotence in men, loss of urinary control, night diarrhea, and gastroparesis.

*Peripheral Neuropathy Treatment Trials*   263

*Table 13.2*   Hughes' disability scale for Guillain-Barré syndrome

| | |
|---|---|
| 0 | Healthy |
| 1 | Minor symptoms or signs |
| 2 | Able to walk 15 feet (5 meters) without support but incapable of manual work |
| 3 | Able to walk 15 feet (5 meters) only with cane, appliance, or support |
| 4 | Bed- or chair-bound |
| 5 | Requires assisted ventilation |
| 6 | Dead |

neuropathy in clinical trials.[39–41] The TNS combines information obtained from grading of symptoms, signs, nerve conduction studies, and QST and provides a comprehensive and easily obtained measure for serial neurologic evaluation. Intra- and inter-rater reliability of TNS is excellent. The TNS arose from studies of chemotherapy-induced neuropathy in oncology patients,[40,41] in whom it was shown that TNS can be used to longitudinally assess the progression of neuropathy.

Most available measures including TNS, NSS, NSP, NIS, and the Michigan Diabetic Neuropathy Score, are designed for distal length–dependent axonal neuropathies. It has been shown that distal sensation (strength and reflexes) is the most reproducible component of the NDS and Michigan Diabetic Neuropathy Scale and is predictive of DN.[18,38] In addition, Dyck et al.[36] showed that sural and peroneal amplitudes had highly significant correlation with NSS, NIS, and neuropathology.

For peripheral neuropathies affecting proximal muscle function, neuropathic deficits have been graded using simple ordinal scales of disability. For GBS, the Hughes' six-grade disability scale is often used to measure outcome (Table 13.2). The scale is simple, reproducible, and clinically relevant.[42] A score that sums the strength of six or more muscle groups on each side, measured by Medical Research Council grading or by hand-held dynamometers, has also been used.[43] A clinical sensory scale was suggested by Merkies et al.[44] to evaluate sensory deficit in immune-mediated neuropathies (GBS, CIDP, and paraproteinemic neuropathies). This scale ranges from 0 (normal sensation) to 20 (maximum sensory deficit) and includes vibration sense, pinprick sense, and a two-point discrimination value.

QST with the CASE IV has been used in phase II DN trials and has demonstrated a positive effect of recombinant human nerve growth factor 9 (rhNGF) on heat threshold.[45] Punch skin biopsy is becoming a new tool for assessment of small-fiber sensory neuropathy. Intraepidermal fiber density measurement is a quantifiable and reproducible technique that can been used for longitudinal studies, as was shown in a phase II trial of nerve growth factor for sensory neuropathy associated with human immune deficiency virus infection.[46]

## IMMUNE-MEDIATED NEUROPATHIES

### Guillain-Barré Syndrome

GBS is an acquired disease of the peripheral nerves that is characterized clinically by rapidly progressing paralysis, areflexia, and albuminocytologic dissociation

264    *Clinical Trials in Neurologic Practice*

*Table 13.3*    Plasma exchange in Guillain-Barré syndrome

|  | North American (1985)[47,*] | | French (1987)[49,*] | |
|---|---|---|---|---|
|  | Plasma exchange (n = 122) | Control (n =23) | Plasma exchange (n = 109) | Control (n = 111) |
| Walking without assistance (days) | 53 | 85 | 70 | 111 |
| Time to wean from ventilator (days) | 9 | 23 | 18 | 31 |
| Time to improve one grade (days) | 19 | 40 | — | — |
| Ambulation in ventilator patients (days) | 97 | 169 | — | — |
| Percent improved 1 grade by 1 mo | 59 | 39 | — | — |
| Percent improved at 6 mos | 97 | 87 | — | — |
| Time in hospital (days) | — | — | 28 | 45 |
| Percentage requiring ventilator after entry | — | — | 21 | 42 |
| Percent long-term outcome (1 yr) | — | — | 71 | 55 |
| Percentage with residual weakness (1 yr) | — | — | 11 | 11 |

*All results were statistically significant.

and in the postpolio era, is the most common cause of an acute generalized paralysis. Advances have been made in understanding the clinical and electrodiagnostic features, immunopathogenesis, and management of the different variants of GBS, such as acute inflammatory demyelinating polyneuropathy, acute motor axonal neuropathy, acute motor sensory axonal neuropathy, and Fisher syndrome.

The mainstay of treatment of GBS is supportive care and prevention of complications. Respiratory failure and autonomic dysfunction are the common causes of death from GBS. Ten percent to 20% of patients with GBS need ventilatory assistance. Careful nursing is needed for prevention of pressure sores, and precautions for prevention of deep venous thrombosis should be instituted. Nasogastric or parenteral feeding is often needed if ileus or gastroparesis is present or if the patient is on a ventilator. Instituting means to communicate is important to reduce anxiety. Physical and occupational therapy need to be started soon after hospitalization to prevent contractures and maintain range of motion in joints.

Multiple well-controlled clinical trials have shown that plasma exchange (PE) and high-dose IVIG improve the rate of functional recovery by 50% (Table 13.3).[4,47–51] The first reported case of beneficial response to PE was published in 1978, and it was followed by many case reports. Four controlled trials in the 1980s showed that treated patients have a rapid recovery compared to their controls. In a large North American GBS trial, 245 patients were randomized to PE and control groups.[47] The patients treated with PE reached the point of ambulation 32 days

*Peripheral Neuropathy Treatment Trials* 265

*Table 13.4* Intravenous immunoglobulin versus plasma exchange in Guillain-Barré syndrome

| | Dutch (1992)[50] | | Bril et al. (1996)[51] | |
|---|---|---|---|---|
| | Plasma exchange (n = 73) | IV immuno-globulin (n = 74) | Plasma exchange (n = 24) | IV immuno-globulin (n = 26) |
| Percent improved 1 grade (4 wks) | 34* | 53 | 61 | 69 |
| Days to improve 1 grade (median) | 41 | 27 | 16.5 | 14 |
| Numbers of complications | 68 | 35 | 19 | 5 |
| Percent ventilator-dependent by 2 wks | 42 | 27 | — | — |

*No difference from control group in North American treatment trial 1985 (see Table 13.3).

before the control group. The mortality rates, however, were similar. This trial demonstrated the efficacy of PE in hastening the recovery process. Exploratory analyses showed that PE was more likely to be effective if given during the first week and if a continuous, rather than an intermittent, flow machine was used.[48] These results were corroborated by a French multicenter trial of similar size and design.[49] The French group also demonstrated that albumin should be used as the exchange fluid as fresh-frozen plasma is no more efficacious and may cause allergic reactions (see Table 13.3). In general, PE of 200–250 cc of plasma is divided over four to five exchanges. Complications from central line placement such as sepsis, thrombosis, bleeding, and injury to the lungs or thoracic duct, can occur.

IVIG prepared from large pools of plasma has also been shown to shorten the duration of the disease and has become the treatment of choice for GBS (Tables 13.4 and 13.5). The efficacy of IVIG in GBS was demonstrated in three clinical trials.[4,50,51] The multicenter Dutch study showed that the IVIG

*Table 13.5* Plasma exchange, intravenous immunoglobulin, or both in Guillain-Barré syndrome in Plasma Exchange/Sandoglobulin Trial Group (1997)[4]

| | IV immuno-globulin (n = 130) | Plasma exchange (n = 121) | Plasma exchange + IV immunoglobulin* (n = 128) |
|---|---|---|---|
| Mean change in disability grade (after 4 wks) | 0.8 | 0.9 | 1.1 |
| Number ventilated after randomization | 29 | 28 | 21 |
| Median time on ventilator (days) | 26 | 29 | 18 |
| Median days to walk unaided | 51 | 49 | 40 |
| Percent unable to walk unaided (after 40 wks) | 16.5 | 16.7 | 13.7 |
| Deaths (%) | 4.6 | 4.1 | 6.3 |

*Combination therapy was not statistically better.

266    *Clinical Trials in Neurologic Practice*

treatment at a total of 2,000 mg/kg was effective, and its effectiveness was comparable to PE in adults. Van der Meche et al.[50] studied 147 patients with GBS in a randomized, open, controlled clinical trial comparing IVIG (0.25–0.40 g/kg × 4 days) to PE. Clinical response was seen in 53% of patients treated with IVIG and 34% of patients treated with PE. Bril et al. studied 50 patients in a randomized open study of IVIG (0.5 g/kg daily for 4 days) versus PE.[51] At 1 month, clinical response was seen in 69% of patients treated with IVIG as compared to 61% of patients with PE. More complications were seen in the PE group. The PE Sandoglobulin GBS trial studied 359 patients randomized into three arms of IVIG, PE, and PE followed by IVIG (see Table 13.5).[4] There was no difference in the change in disability grade after 4 weeks, number of days on ventilation, number requiring ventilation, median days to walk unaided, and percent unable to walk unaided after 40 weeks. A trial assessing the efficacy of a second dose of IVIG should the patient fail to improve by one grade within the first 4 weeks is in progress (David Cornblath, personal communication).

IVIG is now considered equivalent to PE in the treatment of GBS and is more frequently used because of convenience and safety, particularly in children or patients with autonomic instability. Vascular complications, such as ischemic cardiovascular, cerebrovascular, and renovascular complications seen in older adults do not occur in children. Headache, fever, nausea, serum sickness, and, rarely, anaphylactic reaction can occur. All patients receiving IVIG should be screened for isolated immunoglobulin A (IgA) deficiency, as it increases the risk for severe anaphylactic reaction.

The results of most trials with corticosteroids have been negative.[42,52] In a multicenter, randomized trial, 21 patients were treated with prednisolone (60 mg daily for 1 week, 40 mg daily for 4 days, and then 30 mg daily for 3 days), and 19 did not have steroid treatment (Table 13.6). Reassessment at 1, 3, and 12 months consistently showed greater improvement in the control than the prednisolone group, but the only statistically significant result was in the improvement at 3 months among patients entering the trial within a week of onset of

*Table 13.6*    Corticosteroids in Guillain-Barré syndrome

| Hughes (1978)[42,a] | Prednisolone (n = 21) | Control (n = 19) |
|---|---|---|
| Median time to onset improvement (days) | 8 | 10 |
| Number of patients grade 2 or worse, 1 yr | 7 | 1 |
| Number of patients with relapses, 1 yr | 3 | 0 |
| GBS Steroid Trial Group (1993)[52,b] | IV methylprednisolone (n = 124) | Placebo (n = 118) |
| Median time to walk unassisted (days) | 38 | 50 |
| Time patients ventilated (days) | 39 | 44 |

[a]Overall, there was no significant benefit in oral prednisolone–treated patients. Prednisolone-treated patients randomized during the first week of illness fared worse than did the non–prednisolone-treated controls.

[b]No outcome measure was statistically better in the intravenous methylprednisolone group.

*Peripheral Neuropathy Treatment Trials* 267

illness. The results of this study indicated that steroid treatment is not beneficial and can be detrimental in GBS.[42] Another double-blind trial of intravenous methylprednisolone, 500 mg daily for 5 days, failed to show significant benefit in 124 patients treated with steroids compared to controls.[52]

## Chronic Inflammatory Demyelinating Neuropathy

CIDP is an acquired sensorimotor demyelinating polyneuropathy that is characterized clinically by progressive weakness of greater than 2 months' duration and areflexia; electrophysiologically by features of demyelination, including prolonged distal and F-wave latencies, reduced conduction velocity, and conduction block/temporal dispersion; laboratory features of albuminocytologic dissociation in the cerebrospinal fluid; and pathology of inflammation and demyelination/remyelination on nerve biopsy.[13,14,53–56] CIDP represents approximately 20% of all initially undiagnosed neuropathies and accounts for approximately 10% of all patients referred to tertiary neuromuscular clinics.[56] Two-thirds of cases are progressive, and the remainder show a relapsing course, although relapses are often closely linked to withdrawal of therapy.[13,57] The overall prognosis is favorable, and with treatment more than two-thirds of patients remain independent and able to work. Five percent to 10% of patients die of their illness or from complications of treatment.

Conventional therapy for CIDP has included corticosteroids, PE, and IVIG; 60–80% of patients improve with one of these treatments.[10–12,56–61] Each of these three modalities of treatment has been demonstrated to be superior to placebo in randomized, double-blind, controlled studies.[10,12,59,60] Numerous anecdotal reports demonstrate the efficacy of prednisone in CIDP with response rates between 40% and 95%.[14,58,62] Dyck and coworkers demonstrate that steroids were more effective than placebo in a 3-month, randomized, placebo-controlled trial of alternate-day, high-dose prednisone (120 mg) in 28 patients.[60] Of the 28 patients who completed the trial, 14 prednisone-treated patients improved by a median of 10 points on NDS, and the control patients deteriorated by a median of 1.5 points. The effect was similar between patients with a progressive and relapsing course. Barohn and colleagues[14] reported that the average time to induce a response with prednisone (60 mg/day) was approximately 2 months, and maximal improvement was not observed until after 6 months (Table 13.7). A minority remained in remission after tapering steroids, but most (up to 70%) relapsed after discontinuing treatment and required repeated courses of prednisone or alternative immunotherapy.[58] In some patients, the addition of azathioprine or other immunosuppressive agents may sustain a remission and reduce the requirement for high-dose corticosteroids,[13,14,56,63] but this benefit has not been confirmed in a randomized controlled trial.[64] Young age at onset, duration of symptoms of less than six months, slight neurologic impairment, and mild slowing of nerve conduction velocities have been associated with a favorable response to corticosteroids. A treatment period of less than 6 months and rapid tapering of prednisone may increase the risk of relapse.[13,14]

Two randomized, placebo-controlled trials have demonstrated that PE is superior to placebo with response rates between 33% and 80% (Table 13.8).[10,12] Improvement was observed in the mean Neurologic Disability, grip strength, and clinical disability grade. Mean compound motor action potential amplitudes and motor

268    *Clinical Trials in Neurologic Practice*

*Table 13.7*    Steroids in chronic inflammatory demyelinating polyneuropathy (CIDP)

**Prospective randomized controlled trial**

| | Dyck (1982)[60] | | |
| | (120 mg tapered over 13 weeks) | | |
| | Prednisone | Control | p value |
| | (n = 14) | (n = 14) | |
| Median NDS improvement | +10 | −1.5 | .016 |
| Other indices of improvement* | — | — | — |

**Case series**

| | |
|---|---|
| | McCombe (1987)[13] |
| | (prednisone; n = 92) |
| Total percent responding (%) | 65 |
| | Wertman (1988)[62] |
| | (prednisone alone; n = 16) |
| Improvement in FDS | 1.43 ± 1.12 (p <.001) |
| | Barohn (1989)[14] |
| | (prednisone, azathioprine, and/or plasma exchange; n = 60) |
| Total percent responding (%) | 94.9 (percent on steroid alone not reported) |
| | Gorson (1997)[58] |
| | (prednisone, plasma exchange, or IV immunoglobulin; n = 67) |
| First-line steroid response | Three of 11 patients |

FDS = functional disability score; NDS = neurologic disability score.

*Not shown: minor significant change in conduction velocity, hand grip, touch pressure hand; the *p* values were .029, .046, and .017, respectively.

nerve conduction velocities increased after PE in comparison to sham exchange. Patients improved within 4 weeks after initiating therapy, and those with a chronic progressive course apparently responded as well as patients with relapsing disease. Although the short-term efficacy of PE has been demonstrated, 50–67% of patients deteriorate weeks to months after treatment and require repeated exchanges or an alternative therapy to maintain improvement.[12,58,65] In these patients, combining prednisone or other immunosuppressive agents with PE may induce a prolonged remission.[12] Those with a short duration of disease and electromyographic or pathologic features of a primary demyelinating neuropathy without axonal loss are more likely to respond to PE.[12,66]

IVIG has been introduced as a therapy for CIDP. Although early studies showed variable results,[61] two well-controlled studies have demonstrated that 60–70% of patients respond to IVIG (Table 13.9).[11,59] Dyck et al.[11] studied 20 patients in a double-blind, randomized crossover study, comparing PE to IVIG, 0.4 g/kg once a week for 3 weeks, and then 0.2 g/kg once a week for another 3 weeks. All patients in both groups showed clinical improvement. Hahn et al.[59] studied 30 patients in a double-blind, randomized, placebo-controlled, crossover trial using IVIG at a dose of 0.4 g/kg daily for 5 days. Sixty-three percent of patients in the IVIG-treated group improved within 4 weeks, whereas 17% of the patients in the placebo group showed a nonsustained response. IVIG is the preferred treatment

*Table 13.8* Plasma exchange (PE) in chronic inflammatory demyelinating polyneuropathy (CIDP)

**Prospective randomized blinded placebo-controlled trials**

| | **Dyck (1986)[10]** | | |
| | (Six exchanges, ≈ 47 ml/kg plasma/treatment) | | |
| | **PE** | **Sham exchange** | **Open trial PE[a]** |
| | (n = 15) | (n = 14) | (n = 11) |
| NDS improvement over sham | 5 patients ( $p$ = .025) | — | — |
| Other indices of improvement[b–d] | — | — | — |

| | **Hahn (1996)[12]** | |
| | (10 exchanges, 40–50 ml/kg plasma/treatment) | |
| | **PE** | **Sham exchange** |
| | (n = 15) | (n = 15) |
| NDS improvement | 38 patients ($p$ < .001) | — |
| Improved functional clinical grade | 1.6 points | — |
| Grip strength | +13 kg ($p$ <.003) | — |
| Other indicis of improvement[e] | | |

NDS = neurologic disability score.

[a]Sham exchanged patients who had PE after the blinded trial.

[b]Total nerve conduction indicies improved status post-PE ( $p$ = .018).

[c]Similar NDS improvement was seen in the sham exchange patients who had PE after completion of the trial.

[d]All plasma exchange patients were crossed over to sham exchange after 5 weeks' washout.

[e]Statistical improvement in electrophysiologic measures Σ proximal compound motor action potential, ( $p$<.01); Σ motor conduction velocities, ( $p$ <.006); Σ distal motor latencies, ( $p$<.01).

for children, patients with poor venous access needed for PE, or those susceptible to the complications of long-term corticosteroid therapy. Improvement occurs within a few weeks, and recovery is rarely dramatic, appearing 1 or 2 days after treatment. Frequently, the benefit is transient (1–6 weeks), and 50% of patients relapse within weeks to months and require regular infusions to maintain maximum improvement.[58,65] Patients with a progressive course or predominantly sensory deficits with tremor may be less likely to improve.[59] IVIG can be considered the initial treatment of choice for patients with CIDP who do not have any complicating medical illness; its efficacy is similar to other first-line therapies. It has a low frequency of adverse effects, and it is easy to administer. As with PE, combining IVIG with prednisone or other immunosuppressive medications may increase the duration of remission and reduce the frequency of IVIG infusions.[59]

There have been no prospective, controlled trials comparing steroids, PE, and IVIG; however, retrospective studies suggest that the rate of response is similar among these therapies.[65] A small, randomized crossover trial demonstrated that IVIG and PE induce a comparable degree of improvement in patients with CIDP and are probably equivalent in terms of efficacy and cost.[11] Uncontrolled studies indicate that most patients who fail to improve with initial therapy will respond to an alternative treatment modality.[11,58,65]

Alternative immunosuppressive regimens have been used in patients who fail to respond to prednisone, PE, or IVIG, experience frequent relapses, or encounter

270    *Clinical Trials in Neurologic Practice*

*Table 13.9*    Intravenous immunoglobulin (IVIG) treatment in chronic inflammatory demyelinating polyneuropathy (CIDP)

**Prospective randomized blinded crossover controlled trials**

|  | Dyck (1994)[11,a] | |
| --- | --- | --- |
|  | **IVIG**[b] | **Plasma exchange**[c] |
|  | (n = 15) | (n = 17) |
| Mean NDS improvement | 36.1 ±32.0, $p$ <.006 | 38.3 ± 34.6, $p$ <.001 |
| Mean weakness subset improvement | 31.4 ± 31.5, $p$ <.003 | 33.4 ± 29.5, $p$ <.001 |
| Summated CMAP potentials | 3.3 ± 2.8 mV, $p$ <.001 | 3.7 ± 3.5 mV, $p$ >.001 |
|  | Hahn (1996)[59,d] | |
|  | **IVIG**[e] | **Sham** |
|  | (n = 25) | (n = 25) |
| Mean NDS improvement | 24.4 ± 5.4, $p$ <.002 | No improvement |
| Mean clinical grade improvement | 1 ± .03, $p$ <.001 | No improvement |
| Mean grip strength | +6.3 ± 1.7 kg, $p$ <.005 | No improvement |

CMAP = compound motor action potential; NDS = neurologic disability score.

[a]No statistical difference was found between IVIG and plasma exchange. The amount of strength improvement is significant and translatable to 50% weakness at bilateral limb or pelvic weakness improved to normal strength.

[b]IVIG dose equals 0.4 gm/kg once a wk × 3 wks, then 0.2 gm/kg once a wk × 3 wks.

[c]Plasma exchange dose twice a wk × 3 wks, then once a wk × 3 wks. Patients crossed over to the other treatment after a 6-week washout. Four patients did not worsen significantly to enter the other treatment, and 3 of 20 left the study.

[d]Additional support for IVIG is found in improved summated motor conduction velocities, CMAP potentials, and secondary subset analysis of the first trial period before crossover.

[e]IVIG dose, 0.4 g/kg × 5 consecutive days. The same 25 patients underwent both therapies with variable crossover times depending on response to treatment.

intolerable adverse effects. Anecdotal reports have indicated that azathioprine is an effective therapy for CIDP,[13,14,63] although one unblinded, randomized study of only 3 months' duration showed that the degree of improvement with azathioprine combined with prednisone was similar to prednisone alone (Table 13.10).[64] Oral cyclophosphamide has also been reported to be beneficial when administered for several months as monotherapy or in combination with prednisone.[13] Uncontrolled case series suggest that monthly, pulse intravenous cyclophosphamide is effective when combined with prednisone or administered after cycles of PE.[67] Cyclosporine A,[68–70] interferon-alpha (IFN-α) 2a,[71] interferon-beta (IFN-β),[72] total lymphoid irradiation,[73] and pulsed high-dose dexamethasone[74] may all be effective in patients who are refractory to other therapies. None of these has been studied systematically.

## Multifocal Motor Neuropathy

MMN is an acquired immune-mediated demyelinating neuropathy with distinctive clinical and electrophysiologic manifestations and a distinctive response to

*Peripheral Neuropathy Treatment Trials* 271

*Table 13.10*    Azathioprine in compound motor action potential (CIDP)

**Randomized unblinded**

| | Dyck (1985)[64] | |
| --- | --- | --- |
| | **Prednisone** | **Prednisone/Azathioprine**[a] |
| | (n = 10) | (n = 13) |
| Median NDS improvement at 9 mos[b, c] | −30 points | −29 points |
| **Case series** | | |
| **Dalakas (1981)**[63] | Three of four patients improved with azathioprine. | |
| **McCombe (1987)**[13] | Four of seven improved with azathioprine. | |
| **Barohn (1989)**[14] | Number not reported. | |

[a]Prednisone 120 mg every other day decreased over 9 mos with Azathioprine at 2 mg/kg/day.

[b]Indices improved, but not significantly. (Hand grip, pincher grip, and electrophysiology).

[c]Combining both groups, NDS improvement was statistically significant ($p < .03$).

treatment.[26–31] Patients present with progressive, asymmetric, predominantly distal weakness in named distribution of peripheral nerves without sensory symptoms or signs. The classic finding in MMN is well-localized, persistent, segmental, partial motor conduction block, along with other electrophysiologic features of demyelination. High titers of immunoglobulin M (IgM) antibody directed against ganglioside GM1 and other gangliosides are reported in 22–84% of patients.[27] Several immunomodulatory therapies have been tried, including prednisone, azathioprine, chlorambucil, cyclophosphamide, PE, and IVIG.

The efficacy of IVIG in MMN has been demonstrated in several open-label and small controlled clinical trials. Azulay et al.[75] studied five patients in a double-blind, placebo-controlled crossover trial using IVIG, 0.4 g/kg daily for 5 days. All five patients experienced a beneficial response to IVIG. Van den Berg et al.[31] studied six patients in a randomized, double-blind, placebo-controlled crossover trial. Five of the six patients treated with IVIG improved. Other case series with five or more patients are outlined in Table 13.11.[28] IVIG is the therapy of choice, alone or in combination with chemotherapy, for MMN. Beneficial effects from IVIG begin within days and sometimes hours after the infusion and peak at an average of 2 weeks; the effect lasts from weeks to months. Most patients require periodic maintenance doses of IVIG. The dose and frequency of IVIG administration need to be individualized depending on the length of benefit received; this appears to vary between patients but is relatively constant in individual patients. In Azulay's group,[26] follow-up extended from 9 to 48 months, and many patients needed repeat dosing to prevent relapse. Computerized isometric testing revealed 32–97% improved strength, which translated into functional improvement.

Prednisone and PE, two therapies used in the standard treatment of chronic inflammatory demyelinating polyneuropathy, have rarely been effective in the treatment of MMN.[2,4,11,25–29,76–80] It is important to note that some patients with MMN may worsen in strength after initiation of corticosteroids treatment or after PE.[78,80,81]

Among the immunosuppressive agents available, cyclophosphamide is perhaps the only one shown to have consistent efficacy in the treatment of

272    *Clinical Trials in Neurologic Practice*

*Table 13.11*    Intravenous immunoglobulin (IVIG) treatment in multifocal motor neuropathy

**Controlled Trials**

|  | Van den Berg (1995)[31,a] | |
|---|---|---|
|  | **IVIG** | **Plasma** |
|  | (n = 6) | (n = 6) |
| Improvement in muscle strength (50% or more in at least two muscles) | Five of six | One of six |
| Improvement in condition block | One of six | None of six |
| Change in antiGM$_1$ antibody | 0 | — |

|  | Azulay (1994)[75,b] | |
|---|---|---|
|  | **IVIG** | **Saline** |
|  | (n = 5) | (n = 5) |
| Improvement in muscle strength (%) (day 5) | $18 \pm 34$ | $9 \pm 19$ |
| Improvement in muscle strength (%) (day 28) | $103 \pm 19$ | $30 \pm -2, p < .05$ |
| Improvement in muscle strength (%) (day 56) | $61 \pm 21$ | $22 \pm 24$ |

**Case series**

| | |
|---|---|
| **Chaudhry (1993)[28]** | IVIG, nine of nine; steroids, none of six; plasma exchange, none of three; CTX, three of three improved. |
| **Nobile-Orazio (1993)[29]** | Five of seven improved with IVIG. |
| **Leger (1994)[167]** | Five of six improved with IVIG. |
| **Comi (1994)[168]** | Five of five improved with IVIG. |
| **Bouche (1995)[169]** | Seventeen of 19 improved. |
| **Jaspert (1996)[170]** | Eight of eight improved with IVIG, CB improved in five. |
| **Azulay (1997)[26]** | Twelve of 18 improved with IVIG. |
| **Meucci (1997)[83]** | IVIG and CTX; able to stop IVIG in three patients. |

CB = chlorambucil; CTX = cyclophosphamide.

[a]0.4 g/kg for 5 consecutive days versus pasteurized plasma solution for 5 days in randomized order.

[b]No change in GM$_1$ antibody titers or electrophysiology.

MMN.[26,28,76,78–80,82–84] The largest group reported in an open trial was of 13 patients who had failed oral prednisone, four of whom had failed PE.[79] Nine showed clinical improvement, and in three patients clinical relapse resulted in discontinuation. Patients were treated with high-dose cyclophosphamide (3 g/m$^2$ of body surface given in five divided doses over 8 days), followed by oral maintenance therapy at 2 mg/kg per day. Meaningful improvement was seen in 3–6 months.

## Antimyelin-Associated Glycoprotein Neuropathy

The antimyelin-associated glycoprotein (antiMAG) syndrome is a clinically distinct demyelinating neuropathy associated with an IgM monoclonal gammopathy. The M protein binds to myelin and is directed against an oligosaccharide moiety that is shared by MAG and the glycolipids sulphoglucuronyl paragloboside and sulphoglucuronyl lactosaminyl paragloboside.[85–90] Clinically, the patients present with a long history of sensory ataxia and postural tremor. Nerve conduction studies show demyelinating features most accentuated at the distal end of nerve fibers. The pathologic hallmarks include the presence of mono-clonal IgM and complement bound to myelin and widening of the myelin lamel-lae at the minor dense line.

There is only one randomized trial assessing the treatment of neuropathy asso-ciated specifically with the antiMAG antibody (Table 13.12). Mariette et al.[91] per-formed a 12-month multicenter, prospective, randomized open-label crossover trial comparing IVIG and recombinant human IFN-α. Ten patients were enrolled in each arm. All patients had evidence of neuropathy for at least 3 months, positive antiMAG titers, and a clinical neuropathy disability score (CNDS) greater than 10. Enrolled patients who demonstrated evidence of worsening of neuropathy (more than 20% of the CNDS) before 6 months or absence of improvement at 6 months were switched to the other treatment arm. After 6 months, one of the 10 patients in the IVIG group had a clinical improvement of more than 20%, whereas eight of 10 in the IFN-α arm had such an improvement. The mean CNDS decreased (improved) by 7.5 units (31%) in the IFN-α group, whereas it increased (wors-ened) by 2.3 units in the IVIG group. The improvement seen in the IFN-α arm was due primarily to improvements in the sensory score and in patients' subjective assessments of their status. Neither group had any improvement in motor or reflex scores. Among the nine patients unsuccessfully treated in the IVIG group, five switched to IFN-α. Of these, one had an improvement in CNDS of greater than 20%. The two patients in the IFN-α group who switched to IVIG saw no improve-

*Table 13.12*    Antimyelin-associated glycoprotein neuropathy

**Randomized blinded placebo-controlled trial**

| | Mariette (1997)[91] | |
| | IV immunoglobulin[a] | Interferon-alpha[b,c] |
| --- | --- | --- |
| | (n = 10) | (n = 10) |
| CNDS change (>20%) | 1 | 8 (*p* = .005) |
| Mean improvement CNDS | –2.3 (SD, 7.6) 8% | 7.5 (SD, 11.1) (31%) (*p* = .02) |

**Case series**

**Blume (1995)[92]**
Plasma exchange (×2) followed by cyclophosphamide (1 g/m$^2$): Five of five patients improved.
**Nobile-Orazio (1988)[93]**
Chlorambucil 10 mg/day for 1–2 months: Two of five patients improved.
**Wilson (1999)[94]**
IV fludarabine: All four patients improved.
**Levine (1999)[95]**
Rituximab: Improvement in all five patients.

CNDS = clinical neuropathy disability score.
[a]IV immunoglobulin; 2 g/kg and then 1 g/kg every 3 weeks.
[b]Recombinant interferon-alpha; 3 MU/m$^2$ subcutaneously 3 times weekly.
[c]The main end point was a CNDS.

274    *Clinical Trials in Neurologic Practice*

ment in their CNDS. More importantly, the differences between the two treatment groups persisted after 12 months. The one responder in the IVIG group subsequently returned to his or her baseline CNDS at 12 months. Among the eight patients responding to IFN-α at 6 months, one returned to his or her baseline score, one remained stable at 75% of his or her initial CNDS, and the remaining six patients experienced continued improvement. Five of the six attained CNDS smaller than 50% of their entry scores. The differences between the two groups were statistically significant, although the instrument used to measure improvement was not validated. Electrophysiologically, there was a trend for patients in the IVIG group to have further prolongation of their ulnar distal latencies, whereas the trend for those in the IFN-α treatment group was a regaining of median sensory nerve action potentials that had initially been absent. Of note, two of the responding patients in the IFN-α group had a greater than 50% decrease in their antiMAG IgM titer. The dose of IFN-α used was 3 MU/m$^2$ twice a week. This regimen was decreased in three patients to 2 MU/m$^2$ twice a week due to systemic adverse affects, which were mainly flulike symptoms. No local adverse effects were noted, and none of the patients in the IFN-α group dropped out.

Blume et al.[92] treated four patients with antiMAG activity with a combination regimen of PE on 2 consecutive days followed by cyclophosphamide (1 g/m$^2$) monthly for 5–7 months. Effects of treatment were quantitatively measured with hand-held dynamometry. All four patients showed improvement in strength and sensation in the 5–24 months after treatment.

A nonrandomized trial of chlorambucil was performed in five patients with antiMAG IgM-associated neuropathy.[93] Two patients were diagnosed with Waldenström's macroglobulinemia on the basis of bone marrow plasma cell infiltrates. All patients were treated with chlorambucil 10 mg per day for 1–2 months. Subsequent therapy varied in each patient according to response and tolerance to treatment and included prednisone, cyclophosphamide, or both. Two of the five patients experienced significant improvement, walking normally after 9 months of treatment. Both patients' improvements coincided with a decline in the anti-MAG IgM titer, whereas none of the nonresponders had a decrease in their titer. Furthermore, temporary cessation of treatment was associated with neurologic deterioration in one patient that remitted after chlorambucil was reinstated.

A recent study by Wilson et al. reported four patients with IgM paraproteinemic neuropathy and treated them with intravenous pulses of fludarabine.[94] Two of the four patients had antibodies to MAG and characteristic widely spaced myelin on nerve biopsy, and a third had characteristic widely spaced myelin only. The fourth had an endoneurial lymphocytic infiltrate on nerve biopsy and a diagnosis of Waldenström's macroglobulinemia. Subjective and objective clinical improvement was associated with a significant fall in the IgM paraprotein concentration in three cases. Neurophysiologic parameters improved in the three patients examined. All patients developed mild, reversible lymphopenia, and 50% developed mild, generalized myelosuppression.[94]

Last, Levine et al.[95] in a five-patient pilot trial of rituximab, a human monoclonal protein directed against B-cell surface membrane marker CD20, showed that all five patients with neuropathy and IgM antibodies to GM1 ganglioside or MAG experienced improvement within 3–6 months. Along with improvement in function with increased quantitative strength, there was reduction in titers of serum autoantibodies.

*Peripheral Neuropathy Treatment Trials* 275

### Neuropathies with Monoclonal Gammopathy of Uncertain Significance

Many neuropathies occur in the setting of nonmalignant monoclonal gammopathies.[96–102] These conditions are referred to as monoclonal gammopathies of unclear significance or monoclonal gammopathy of uncertain significance. They are heterogeneous both in the immunoglobulin subtype involved and in the clinical course of the neurologic disease. One percent of the population older than 65 years will have a paraprotein, but approximately 10% of patients with neuropathy have a paraprotein.[103] The most common paraprotein is immunoglobulin G, whereas the most common with neuropathy is IgM. IgA monoclonal proteins are uncommon, and their presence should lead to the search for solitary osteosclerotic myeloma.[104]

Dyck et al.[105] performed a randomized double-blind trial assessing the efficacy of PE in patients with monoclonal gammopathy–associated neuropathy (Table 13.13). Of the 39 patients treated, 21 had IgM gammopathies and 18 had IgG or IgA gammopathies. The prevalence of antiMAG activity in the IgM group was not reported. Patients receiving PE experienced near–statistically significant improvement as measured by a validated neurologic disability score (NDS). When patients were segregated into IgA and IgG versus IgM gammopathies, improvement was greater in the IgA and IgG group. Among patients with IgM gammopathies who underwent sham exchange followed by PE, there were no statistically significant differences between the treatments. Although this trial did not specifically address antiMAG-associated neuropathy, the lack of improvement in the IgM group argues that PE is not effective in this population.

A prospective randomized open trial of 44 patients with IgM gammopathy–associated neuropathy was performed by Oksenhendler et al.[106] AntiMAG activity was not identified. Patients were randomly assigned to treatment with chloram-

*Table 13.13*  Monoclonal gammopathy and plasma exchange

**Randomized blinded-placebo controlled trial**

| | Dyck (1991)[105] | |
| --- | --- | --- |
| | **Plasma exchange**[a] <br> (n = 11 IgM and 8 IgA or IgG) | **Sham exchange** <br> (n = 10 IgM and 10 IgA or IgG) |
| NDS improvement IgG and IgA | 20 ± 24 (*p* = .08) | 2 ± 18 |
| NDS improvement in IgM | No statistically significant change | |
| | Oksenhandler (1995)[106] | |
| | **Cholarambucil + plasma exchange*** <br> (n = 22) | **Chlorambucil** <br> (n = 22) |
| Clinical neuropathy disability score improvement | 1.8 points | 2.1 points |

IgA = immunoglobulin A; IgG = immunoglobulin G; IgM = immunoglobulin M; NDS = neurologic disability score.

*Plasma exchange consisted of six treatments in 3 weeks with follow up NDS and electrophysiologic testing.

276  *Clinical Trials in Neurologic Practice*

bucil plus PE or chlorambucil alone. Outcome was measured by a validated neurologic disability score (CNDS) and nerve conduction studies. After 12 months, both groups experienced modest improvements in their CNDS scores. This improvement was small and limited to sensory symptoms. There was no significant change in the motor component of the CNDS, nor was there a significant difference between the two treatment groups.

## DIABETIC NEUROPATHY

DN is an umbrella term that encompasses many heterogeneous disorders with different etiologies, natural histories, and treatment approaches.[107-114] The heterogeneity in clinical presentation speaks to the complex pathogenesis. In general two types of neuropathy exist: focal and diffuse. The focal neuropathies are further divided into those with acute onset and those with gradual onset. DNs of abrupt onset include disorders such as diabetic lumbosacral radiculoplexus neuropathy (DLSRPN) and oculomotor neuropathy. These conditions are generally believed to be attributable to vascular mechanisms, such as infarction, and are typically monophasic. Those of more gradual onset are typically attributed to entrapment or compression and include median neuropathy at the wrist, ulnar neuropathy at the elbow, tarsal tunnel syndrome, and meralgia paresthetica. Why focal entrapment and compressive mononeuropathies are more common in diabetic patients than in the general population is not known.

Most clinical trials in DN have focused on diffuse length-dependent DPN. This form has the highest prevalence and long-term impact on morbidity and mortality. DPN has an insidious, progressive course involving sensory and autonomic function typically long before motor nerves. Abnormal nerve function is believed to be due to both metabolic and structural factors. These alterations lead to the clinical signs and symptoms that predispose the patient to painful or insensitive extremities, foot ulcers, and amputation. Experimental and clinical studies have demonstrated hyperglycemia as the trigger for DPN.

The pathogenesis of DPN is complex and multifactorial; vascular, metabolic, autoimmune, and genetic factors are implicated as contributory.[107,109,111,113] The alteration of normal metabolic pathways in diabetes has provided the rationale for the most extensive treatment trials. In brief, hyperglycemia leads excess glucose to be converted to sorbitol (aldose reductase enzyme), which is converted to fructose (sorbitol dehydrogenase enzyme). Conversion of glucose to sorbitol results in decreased nicotinamide adenine dinucleotide phosphate:oxidized form of nicotinamide adenine dinucleotide phosphate ratio, and reduction of sorbitol to fructose also causes a decrease of the nicotinamide adenine dinucleotide:oxidized form of nicotinamide adenine dinucleotide ratio. This depletion is theorized to result in an overall oxidative stress with mitochondrial dysfunction, nerve ischemia, and damage. Increased flux through the sorbitol pathway has been shown to result in reduction of nerve conduction velocity. Increased sorbitol also results in a decrease of nerve myoinositol, which has been shown to cause structural damage to the nerves. Clinical experience, complemented by the understanding of hyperglycemia's role as the primary trigger in pathogenesis, has, arguably, led to the greatest benefit by simple sugar control.

## Glycemic Control

The importance of early intervention with tight glycemic control has been the focus of many trials (Table 13.14). The most successful study was carried out by the Diabetes Control and Complications Trial Research Group.[115,116] A large group of 1,441 insulin-dependent diabetes mellitus (IDDM) patients were enrolled and randomized to conventional insulin therapy (once- or twice-daily insulin) or tight glucose control (three or more daily insulin injections or insulin delivered by insulin pump) (see Table 13.14). Patients randomized to the tight-control group averaged 2 points lower on routine glycosylated hemoglobin testing and were followed for a mean of 6.5 years with testing focused on nephropathy, retinopathy, and neuropathy. There were many strengths in the study: 99% of patients completed the 10-year study, and of patients in the conventional and tight-control groups, 98% and 97%, respectively, were able to abide by the study treatment requirements. The tight-control group reduced its risk for neuropathy as well as nephropathy and retinopathy. In particular, 10% of patients having conventional therapy developed neuropathy, compared to 3% in the tightly controlled group, for a 60% reduction (95% CI, 38–74%) (see Table 13.14). All measures of neuropathy, including clinical examination, autonomic testing, and nerve conductions, had significant improvement compared to traditional therapy. The adverse events included a

Table 13.14   Glucemic control in diabetic neuropathy

**Randomized tight glucose control**

| | The Diabetic Research Group (1993)[115] (n = 1,441 IDDM)[a] | | |
|---|---|---|---|
| | Tight glucose control[b] | Conventional therapy | p value |
| Percent at 5 years developing neuropathy[c] | 3 | 10 | .0006 |
| Abnormal neurologic examination (%) | ≈ 9 | ≈ 19 | <.001 |
| Abnormal autonomic testing (%) | ≈ 5 | ≈ 7 | <.04 |
| Abnormal nerve-conduction study (%) | ≈ 18 | ≈ 35 | <.001 |

| | The Stockholm Trial (1993)[118] (n = 102 IDDM)[a] | |
|---|---|---|
| | Tight glucose control (n = 48) | Conventional therapy (n = 54) |
| Neuropathy at baseline | 5 (12%) | 8 (17%) |
| Neuropathy at 7.4 yrs | 6 (14%) | 13 (28%) |
| Nerve conduction velocity | — | Decreased by 4.1 m/sec |
| Foot ulcers | 0% | 3 (5%) |

IDDM = insulin-dependent diabetes mellitus.

[a]Patients were stratified by having mild retinopathy at onset or no retinopathy.

[b]Defined by either 3-times-a-day insulin injection or pump. Average glycosylated hemoglobin was approximately 2 percentage points lower than conventional insulin therapy.

[c]Defined by clinical examination consistent with peripheral neuropathy plus two abnormal nerve conductions in two nerves or unequivocally abnormal autonomic testing. Patients were without neuropathy at onset.

278    *Clinical Trials in Neurologic Practice*

threefold increase in the incidence of severe hypoglycemia and a mean weight gain of 4.6 kg compared to the traditional therapy. Most patients were not type I diabetics, and many already had DPN.

Supportive data of the importance of tight control in type II diabetics comes from Japan, where 110 type II diabetics also were randomized to conventional insulin treatment or multiple insulin injections. End points included nephropathy, retinopathy, and neuropathy. The tightly controlled group had average glycosylated hemoglobin of less than 6.5% over 6 years. Nerve conductions, vibratory threshold, electrocardiogram R-R ratio, and postural hypotension improved in the tightly controlled group compared to the traditional group, in which indices worsened.[117]

In the Stockholm trial, 102 patients with IDDM were randomized to intensified insulin treatment (48 patients) or standard insulin treatment (54 patients). Mean ($\pm$ standard deviation) glycosylated hemoglobin values were reduced from $9.5 \pm 1.3\%$ to $7.1 \pm 0.7\%$ in the group receiving intensified treatment and from $9.4 \pm 1.4\%$ to $8.5 \pm 0.7\%$ in the group receiving standard treatment ($p = .001$). The conduction velocities of the ulnar, tibial, peroneal, and sural nerves decreased significantly more in the standard-treatment group than in the intensified-treatment group.[118]

In another study from Scandinavia, 45 IDDM patients without clinical signs of neuropathy were randomly assigned to treatment with continuous insulin infusion, multiple injections (4–6 times daily), or conventional treatment (twice daily) for 4 years and then followed prospectively for 8 years. Motor and sensory nerve conduction velocities were measured at the start of the study and after 8 years. Autonomic nerve function tests were performed only once, after 8 years. A significant reduction of nerve conduction velocity was observed during 8 years in patients with mean HbA1 (major component of adult hemoglobin) greater than 10% (n = 12, group mean 10.9%, 10.1–13.2%) compared to patients with HbA1 less than 10% (n = 33, group mean 9.0%, 7.5–9.9%). Multiple regression analysis showed that a change in HbA1 of 1% resulted in a 1.3 ms change in nerve conduction velocity during 8 years.[119]

Pancreatic transplantation provides further evidence for the value of tight glucose control in DPN in which euglycemia is the end result and many patients have neuropathy before transplantation. Several factors, however, complicate investigation; these include concomitant uremia, immunosuppressants, and a bias toward non–insulin-dependent diabetes mellitus, in which most transplants are performed. The studies of Kennedy,[120] Solders,[121] and Navarro[122] have attempted to exclude bias through careful randomization and identification of uremia (Table 13.15). Long-term follow-up, more than 10 years, demonstrates the statistically significant benefit in which neuropathy status is halted or improved after pancreas transplantation.[122] Of additional note is the observation that in control groups having a kidney transplant alone for uremia, neuropathy progressed at approximately the same rate as non-transplanted diabetics.[123,124] This argues that the benefit of transplantation is largely due to sugar control and not immunosuppression; it has been suggested that autoimmune mechanisms play a possible role in DN. Clinical and autonomic improvement, however, was only slightly improved compared to motor and sensory conductions.[121,123] These findings argue that even with the best glycemic control additional therapies are still needed.

*Table 13.15*  Pancreatic Transplantation in Diabetic Neuropathy

| | Kennedy (1990)[120] | |
| --- | --- | --- |
| | IDDM with transplant[a] | IDDM with conventional therapy[b] |
| | (n = 61) | (n = 48) |
| Neurologic clinic examination (12, 24, 42 mos) | No significant change | Worse clinically |
| Electrophysiology (12 mos) | Significant motor, sensory improvement, $p < .001$ | No significant worsening |
| | **Solders (1992)[121]** | |
| | IDDM with kidney/pancreas | IDDM with kidney transplant |
| | (n = 18) | (n = 18) |
| Autonomic improvement (48 mos) | Slight | Slight |
| Electrophysiology (1 yr) | Slightly improved | Slightly improved |
| Electrophysiology (2 and 4 yrs) | Continued improvement | Stable to worse |
| | **Navarro (1997)[122]** | |
| | IDDM with pancreas transplant | IDDM treated with insulin[c] |
| | (n = 115) | (n = 92) |
| **10-year follow-up** | | |
| Functional examination | Slight but significant improvement | Progressive worsening |
| Electrophysiology | Significant improvement | Progressive worsening |
| **Large case series** | | |
| **Nusse (1991)[124,d]** | 26 IDDM patients with simultaneous pancreas kidney transplant (suggests euglycemia halts autonomic neuropathy) | |

IDDM = insulin-dependent diabetes mellitus.

[a]Patients were euglycemic after transplant, requiring no insulin with $A_{1c}$ 7.2 ± 0.2% (12 mos) compared to 9.6 ± 0.4 % before transplantation. Twenty-six also were with renal allograft. No patients were uremic.

[b]Patients had no worse neuropathy compared to their transplanted counterparts, and 21 had previous renal allograft. None had uremia.

[c]Thirty control patients had previous kidney transplant with uremia. Subset analysis in this group showed their neuropathy progressed despite immunosuppression.[22] Previous work in diabetic neuropathy had shown that after kidney transplant for uremia, neuropathy progresses.

[d]Large case series.

## Aldose Reductase Inhibitors

Aldose reductase inhibitors (ARIs) have been a focus for more than 25 years and have had more than 30 human trials directed at the treatment and prevention of diabetic complications through the use of ARIs. ARIs offer an attractive theoretical treatment in diabetes.[125–127] Both human and animal studies have demonstrated that nerve sorbitol concentrations are reduced with treatment using ARIs and sorbitol plays a role in pathogenesis.[107] Trials involving ARIs can be divided into those aimed at functional changes, symptomatic improvement, or structural changes. One of the first trials used sorbinil, a potent inhibitor of the key polyol pathway enzyme aldose reductase, and measured nerve conduction velocity in 39 diabetics in a ran-

280    *Clinical Trials in Neurologic Practice*

domized, double-blind, crossover trial. During 9 weeks of treatment with sorbinil (250 mg per day), nerve conduction velocity was greater than during a 9-week placebo period for all three nerves tested. Conduction velocity for all three nerves declined significantly within 3 weeks of cessation of the drug.[128] Sima et al.[129] showed regeneration and repair of myelinated fibers in sural nerves of 10 sorbinil-treated patients (Table 13.16). In the Sorbinil Retinopathy Trial, 497 IDDM patients were randomized to treatment with sorbinil or placebo. Nearly 30% of patients showed worsening of clinical measures of distal symmetric polyneuropathy at maximum follow-up, with very little difference in rates between the two groups. Nerve conduction velocity in the peroneal nerve, at the 30-month and maximum follow-up visits, showed an overall improvement in the sorbinil group and a decline in the placebo group; nerve conductions in the other groups remained normal.[130]

On the other hand, no beneficial effect was demonstrated on the clinical manifestation or on the neurophysiologic measurements made in DN patients over 12 months of treatment in a double-blind, placebo-controlled trial of sorbinil (250 mg daily).[131]

The effects of tolrestat, an ARI, on chronic symptomatic diabetic sensorimotor neuropathy were studied during a placebo-controlled, randomized, 52-week mul-

*Table 13.16*    Aldose reductase inhibitor trials

| | Sima (1998)[129] | | |
|---|---|---|---|
| | **Sorbinil** | **Placebo** | ***p* Value** |
| | (n = 10) | (n = 6) | |
| Clinical improvement[a] | 8.1 ± 0.6 | 3.3 ± 2.0 | *p* <.01 |
| Sural nerve sorbitol levels | −41.8 ± 8.0% | 9.0 ± 15.3 | *p* <.01 |
| Myelinated fiber density | 33% | −68 ± 385 | *p* <.013 |
| Fiber regeneration | 4 fold | 0 fold | *p* = .0009 |

| | Greene(1999)[134] | | | | |
|---|---|---|---|---|---|
| | **Zenerastat** | | | **Placebo** | ***p* Value** |
| | (150 mg bid) | (300 mg bid) | (600 mg bid) | | |
| | (n = 33) | (n = 44) | (n = 54) | (n = 33) | |
| Peroneal motor nerve conduction velocity[b] | ≈ 0.75 | ≈ 1.25 | ≈ 1.90 | ≈ −0.25 m/s | — |
| Myelinated nerve fiber density[c] (<5 μm) | ≈ −50 | ≈ 120 | ≈ 250 | ≈ −200 fibers/ mm$^2$ | *p* = .014 |
| Nerve sorbitol | −70% | −80% | −80% | — | — |

[a]Neurologic clinical testing consisted of a patient questionnaire and a ranking via the physician, automated tactile and thermal testing, and standard electrophysiology.

[b]*p* values in the 300-mg and 600-mg dosings were statistically significant at .007 and .008, respectively. Composite rank score for all nerve conduction velocity (peroneal motor, sural sensory, median sensory) improved 1.0–1.5 m/sec in the 600-mg group, compared to a more than 0.25-m/sec decline in the placebo. Composite amplitudes in similar nerves showed a similar trend, but the *p* value was less impressive at .13.

[c]Sural nerves were compared at initiation and completion of the study at 52 weeks. The numbers shown are myelinated fibers smaller than 5 μm, in which statistically significant improvement was seen at 300 mg bid and 600 mg bid. Neurologic disability score is not reported.

ticenter trial of 550 DN patients.[132] Of the four tolrestat doses investigated, only the highest-dose group, 200 mg once daily, showed subjective and objective benefit over baseline and placebo. Improvement in paresthetic symptoms was seen at one year ($p = .04$), although painful symptoms improved on placebo and active therapies. Significant improvements in tibial and peroneal motor nerve conduction velocities were seen at 52 weeks. In meta-analysis to review the evidence on the effectiveness of tolrestat in the treatment of DPN patient data on 738 subjects from the three randomized clinical trials published showed a significant treatment effect on nerve conduction velocities after treatment duration between 24 and 52 weeks.[133] Treatment-related differences were associated with pathologic changes in the tolrestat group; sural nerve biopsies revealed reduced evidence of axonal degeneration, myelin abnormalities, and increased signs of nerve regeneration. Tolrestat was approved for use in Europe and South America, but was taken off the market in 1996 after being associated with increase in liver function enzymes.

Greene et al.[134] used the ARI zenerastast and demonstrated statistically significant improvement in a number of parameters, including nerve sorbitol content, small diameter myelinated nerve fiber density, and nerve conduction indices.

It is worth mentioning that a series of studies involving ponalrestat, a potent ARI failed to demonstrate any significant effect.[135] Similarly, a number of DN patients treated with epalrestat, another ARI available in Japan, showed improvement in subjective symptoms (e.g., spontaneous pain, numbness, coldness, hypoesthesia) with 75% (slightly improved or better) and mild improvement in nerve function tests (e.g., motor nerve conduction velocity, sensory nerve-conduction velocity, vibration threshold).[136]

As a group, the ARIs hold promise in slowing the progression of DN, although it appears unlikely that they will reverse the process. No single agent appears to be safe and efficacious, but ARI trials are ongoing. Despite several intense trials, no ARI has been considered sufficiently beneficial to gain acceptance by the regulatory commissions in the United States.

## Myoinositol

Myoinositol depletion in peripheral nerves has been shown to cause a reduction in nerve conduction velocity and structural changes in experimental diabetes[137] and can be reproduced in normal rats by providing diets enriched in L-fucose, a competitive inhibitor of sodium-dependent myoinositol transport.[138] Dietary myoinositol supplementation prevented these changes and increased nodal remyelination, supporting a role of myoinositol depletion in the genesis of early DN.[139] In a double-blind study of 59 diabetic patients, dietary myoinositol (3 g/day) was not able to change motor conduction velocity or vibratory perception threshold over 24 weeks.[140] Two other studies using different dosages of myoinositol did not show an improvement in nerve conduction parameters.[141,142]

## Trophic Factors

Initial treatment with nerve growth factors was supported by the observation that nerve regeneration is reduced in diabetics while others noted deficiency

## 282  Clinical Trials in Neurologic Practice

of neurotrophic factors.[143–146] In a large double-blind controlled study, 250 patients with symptomatic DPN randomly received placebo or one of two doses of rhNGF for 6 months. Patients were assessed for symptoms and signs of polyneuropathy before and after treatment. Compared with placebo, rhNGF led to significant improvement after 6 months of treatment, as measured by the sensory component of the neurologic examination, two quantitative sensory tests, and the impression of most subjects that their neuropathy had improved. RhNGF was well tolerated, with injection site discomfort reported as the most frequent adverse event (Table 13.17).[45] The study, however, was complicated by the fact that 81% of those receiving rhNGF knew they were not receiving placebo secondary to local reaction. Others left the study because of hyperalgesia at the injection site or myalgia. This was consistent with the earlier observations by Dyck.[147] During the subsequent large phase III investigation, Genentech discontinued the trial with efficacy as a major concern. Others have met with similar disappointment, including insulin-like growth factor-1 secondary to the observation in phase III trials of increased rate of diabetic retinopathy, secondary to insulin-like growth factor-1's known role in neovascularization.[148] Others are under investigation, including neurotrophin-3, brain-derived neurotrophic factor, acetyl-L-carnitine, and cil-

*Table 13.17*   Nerve growth factors in diabetic neuropathy

**rhNGF (Genentech, San Francisco, CA)**

### Dyck (1997)[147]

(Healthy volunteers; n = 15)
Increased allodynia and lowered heat-pain threshold were felt related to injection reaction versus neurotropism.

### Apfel (1998)[45]

|  | (n = 84: 0.1 µg/kg rhNGF) | (n = 84: 0.3 µg/kg rhNGF) | (n = 84: placebo) | *p* value |
|---|---|---|---|---|
| Δ NIS (6 mos)[a,b] | −1.05 | −1.41 | −0.64 | .170 |
| Δ Cooling threshold | −0.16 | −0.08 | −0.01 | .049 |
| Δ Heat-perceived pain | −0.045 | −0.38 | −0.02 | .150 |

(This phase II trial showed minimal benefit and phase III trials were aborted with multiple factors suspected.)

**Insulin-like growth factor-1 (Genentech)**

Discontinued at phase III secondary to possible role in speeding diabetic retinopathy.

**Neurotrophin-3, brain-derived NF, acetyl-L-carnitine, ciliary NF**

Currently under investigation in diabetic neuropathies and others.

NF = neurotrophic factor; rhNGF = recombinant human nerve growth factor.
[a]Patients with symptomatic diabetic neuropathy and randomization resulted in equivalent demographics between groups. Patients and observers were blinded; however, 81% correctly predicted they were on NGF because of local reaction, compared to 57% on placebo. Sixteen patients treated with rhNGF left the study early because of adverse events.
[b]Δ NIS = change in neuropathy impairment score. Patients were also asked if they subjectively improved, and the rhNGF group reported a global improvement above placebo with chi square of 0.001.

iary neurotrophic factor (NF).[144] Further growth factors will be discovered. No trophic factor has been identified for the C-fiber group, in which many of the painful and painless symptoms of DN originate. It is unclear what ultimate role these agents will play, as they have not been demonstrated to alter the well-established aldose and sorbitol pathways.

## Investigational

Multiple other agents have been attempted in DPN with failure. Still others are unproved with inconsistent or incomplete controlled trials. In a small double-blinded study, gangliosides showed no statistical significance on disease.[149] A review of the literature has failed to show reproduction of the report by Keen et al.[150] with γ-linolenic acid. Supplementation with γ-linolenic acid is predicted to be helpful, as diabetics have deficient synthesis of n-6 essential fatty acids. Keen et al. treated 111 patients with mild DN using 480 mg per day of γ-linolenic acid versus placebo for 1 year. Thirteen of 16 parameters were improved, including conductions and clinical deficit scores.[150]

Other treatments have included α-lipoic acid, which is a powerful antioxidant that presumably provides protection from free-radical injury related to hyperglycemia.[151–154] Two double-blind placebo trials, ALADIN II and III (ALADIN: alpha-lipoic acid in DN), showed mixed results. In ALADIN II, oral agents were given after a 5-day intravenous therapy. Patients were followed up with serial nerve conductions and believed to have statistically significant improvement compared to controls, but no improvement was noted after 24 months. Interpatient test variability impaired the number of patients who could be included at the end of the trial.[153] In the ALADIN III group, nerve conductions were not reported; rather, a total symptom score was obtained between treatment groups and placebo. No statistically significant improvement was noted after 7 months.[154] Two agents have been attempted in diabetes for their potential roles in improving vascularization (cilostazol and prostaglandin $E_1$). The cilostazol was used on 30 diabetic patients with non–insulin-dependent diabetes mellitus and demonstrated increased blood flow to the dorsalis pedis artery.[155,156] Its role in DPN is unclear. Prostaglandin $E_1$, however, was shown in a randomized placebo study of 38 diabetic patients to statistically increase vibratory threshold and improve symptoms.[157] Further work on cilostazol, prostaglandin $E_1$, and others is needed to show consistent robust effect. Sixty-two patients were randomized in a double-blind, placebo-controlled trial to evaluate the effect of ORG 2766, a five-peptide fragment of adrenocorticotropic hormone, in IDDM patients with peripheral neuropathy. After 1 year of treatment, there was a significant improvement in vibration threshold.[158] A controlled double-blind neurophysiologic study (uridine versus placebo) in 40 diabetic patients with peripheral neuropathy showed improvement of neurophysiologic parameters compared with baseline.[159]

## Diabetic Lumbosacral Radiculoplexus Neuropathy

Of the abrupt onset DNs, DLSRPN has been shown to be most amenable to interventional therapy with immunosuppression.[160–162] These diabetic patients are typ-

284    *Clinical Trials in Neurologic Practice*

*Table 13.18*    Diabetic lumbosacral radiculoplexus neuropathy (DLSRN) treatment trials

| |
|---|
| **Bradley (1984)**[160] |
| (n = 6; all with elevated ESR 56-123; three with diabetes) |
| Five of six patients improved. All three diabetics improved when treated with high-dose prednisone.[a] |
| **Krendel (1995)**[161] |
| (n = 21; all diabetics; 15 consistent with DLSRN) |
| Fifteen of 15 improved when treated with prednisone/IVIG/azathioprine, cyclophosphomide, or a combination. |
| **Younger (1996)**[162] |
| (n = 5; with "proximal diabetic neuropathy" pathology microvasculitis) |
| Five of 5 improved with IVIG 2 g/kg over 5 days.[b] |

IVIG = intravenous immunoglobulin.

[a]All three patients had worsening of diabetes on steroids. These patients are unusual for diabetic lumbosacral radiculoplexus due to increased erythrocyte sedimentation rate, and the authors did not believe that despite the sural biopsy findings of epineurial lymphocytic perivasculitis, this inflammation was related to diabetes.

[b]Two patients went from walker to independent ambulation. One progressed from wheelchair to walker. One improved ambulation. Clinical follow-up was 1 year. No control comparisons.

ically older, with mild type II diabetes, and they may or may not have good sugar control. Typically, patients have severe debilitating unilateral focal leg, buttock, or thigh involvement with spread to the other side with similar involvement. Atrophy with weight loss is often a component. The entity has many descriptors, the most famous of which is *diabetic amyotrophy*.[163] Previous studies have suggested multiple pathogenesis including ischemia, metabolic derangement, inflammation, vasculitis, or inflammatory demyelination.[162,164] Bradley,[160] Krendel,[161] and Younger[162] have noted a subset of patients that has an ischemic inflammatory process. In Bradley's group, an elevation of erythrocyte sedimentation rate (ESR) and other features left doubt about the diagnosis of DLSRPN. Treatment with immunosuppression aided most (Table 13.18). Others have proposed a more diverse pathology and have not attempted immunosuppression when no clear evidence for inflammation was documented. Recent prospective pathologic work by Dyck and Norell[165] noted in 33 such patients that all had evidence of a primary microscopic vasculitis (i.e., epineurial perivascular mononuclear inflammation [all patients], vessel wall inflammation [half of patients], previous bleeding [more than half of patients]). This work supports the earlier observations of Said, and has provided the emphasis for further consideration of aggressive immunotherapy in this group.[166]

## SUMMARY

Immune-mediated and DPNs hold unique sets of problems in establishing useful treatment trials. Perhaps the greatest impediment is the insidious course, making the choice of a good study design with specific outcome measures essential. Of the outcome measures of impairment, disability, and handicap, most trials have concentrated on impairment. Demonstrating biologic effects on nerve conduction parameters or biopsy is often inadequate; functional improvement should be the ultimate outcome measure. Future drug trials will require additional validated measures of functional health with disability or handicap measures. Clear end points will need to be established based on normative progression data or, better still, demographically matched placebo groups. This is especially important in insidious illnesses such as diabetes, in which placebo effect often exceeds intervention outcome in the short run.

# REFERENCES

1. Hahn AF. Guillain-Barré syndrome. Lancet 1998;352:635–641.
2. Hartung H-P, Pollard JD, Harvey GK, Toyka KV. Immunopathogenesis and treatment of the Guillain-Barré syndrome--Part I. Muscle Nerve 1995;18:137–153.
3. Hartung H-P, Pollard JD, Harvey GK, Toyka KV. Immunopathogenesis and treatment of the Guillain-Barré syndrome--Part II. Muscle Nerve 1995;18:154–164.
4. Plasma Exchange/Sandoglobulin Guillain-Barré Syndrome Trial Group. Randomised trial of plasma exchange, intravenous immunoglobulin, and combined treatments in Guillain-Barré syndrome. Lancet 1997;349:225–230.
5. Sheikh KA, Ho TW, Nachamkin I, et al. Molecular mimicry in Guillain-Barré syndrome. Ann N Y Acad Sci 1998;845:307–321.
6. Toyka KV. Eighty three years of the Guillain-Barré syndrome: clinical and immunopathologic aspects, current and future treatments. Rev Neurol (Paris) 1999;155:849–856.
7. Visser LH, Schmitz PI, Meulstee J, et al. Prognostic factors of Guillain-Barré syndrome after intravenous immunoglobulin or plasma exchange. Dutch Guillain-Barré Study Group. Neurology 1999;598–604.
8. Hadden RD, Cornblath DR, Hughes RA, et al. Electrophysiological classification of Guillain-Barré syndrome: clinical associations and outcome. Plasma Exchange/Sandoglobulin Guillain-Barré Syndrome Trial Group. Ann Neurol 1998;780–788.
9. Ad Hoc Subcommittee of the American Academy of Neurology AIDS Task Force. Research criteria for diagnosis of chronic inflammatory demyelinating polyneuropathy (CIDP) [Review]. Neurology 1991;41:617–618.
10. Dyck PJ, Daube J, O'Brien P, et al. Plasma exchange in chronic inflammatory demyelinating polyradiculoneuropathy. N Engl J Med 1986;314:461–465.
11. Dyck PJ, Litchy WJ, Kratz KM, et al. A plasma exchange versus immune globulin infusion trial in chronic inflammatory demyelinating polyradiculoneuropathy. Ann Neurol 1994;36:838–845.
12. Hahn AF, Bolton CF, Pillay N, et al. Plasma-exchange therapy in chronic inflammatory demyelinating polyneuropathy (CIDP). A double-blind, sham-controlled, cross-over study. Brain 1996; 119:1055–1066.
13. McCombe PA, Pollard JD, McLeod JG. Chronic inflammatory demyelinating polyradiculoneuropathy. A clinical and electrophysiological study of 92 cases. Brain 1987;110:1617–1630.
14. Barohn RJ, Kissel JT, Warmolts JR, Mendell JR. Chronic inflammatory demyelinating polyneuropathy: Clinical characteristics, course, and recommendations for diagnostic criteria. Arch Neurol 1989;46:878–884.
15. Asbury AK. Understanding diabetic neuropathy. N Engl J Med 1988;319:577–578.
16. Boulton AJM, Levin S, Comstock J. A multicenter trial of the aldose-reductase inhibitor, Tolrestat, in patients with symptomatic diabetic neuropathy. Diabetologia 1990;33:431.
17. Capsaicin Study Group. Treatment of painful diabetic neuropathy with topical capsaicin: a multicenter, double-blind, vehicle-controlled study. Arch Intern Med 1991;151:2225–2229.
18. Dyck PJ, Kratz KM, Lehman KA, et al. The Rochester Diabetic Neuropathy Study: Design, criteria for types of neuropathy, selection bias, and reproducibility of neuropathic tests. Neurology 1991;41:799–807.
19. Dyck PJ, Karnes JL, O'Brien PC, et al. The Rochester Diabetic Neuropathy Study: Reassessment of tests and criteria for diagnosis and staged severity. Neurology 1992;42:1164–1170.
20. Dyck PK, Dratz KM, Karnes JL, et al. The prevalence by staged severity of various types of diabetic neuropathy, retinopathy, and nephropathy in a population-based cohort: the Rochester Dia-

## 286 *Clinical Trials in Neurologic Practice*

betic Neuropathy Study [published erratum in Neurology 1993;43:2345]. Neurology 1993;43:817–824.

21. Vinik A, Mitchell B. Clinical aspects of diabetic neuropathies. Diabetes Metab Rev 1988;4:223–253.

22. Wilbourn AJ. Diabetic Neuropathies. In WF Brown, CF Bolton (eds), Clinical Electromyography. London: Butterworth–Heinemann, 1993:477–515.

23. DCCT Research Group. Factors in development of diabetic neuropathy: Baseline analysis of neuropathy in feasibility phase of diabetes control and complications trial (DCCT). Diabetes 1988; 37:476–481.

24. Mahattanakul W, Crawford TO, Griffin JW, et al. Treatment of chronic inflammatory demyelinating polyneuropathy with cyclosporin-A. J Neurol Neurosurg Psychiatry 1996;60:185–187.

25. Ropper AH, Zuniga G, Wijdicks E. Comparison of treatments for chronic inflammatory demyelinating polyneuropathy. Ann Neurol 1990;28:238–239.

26. Azulay JP. Long term follow up of multifocal motor neuropathy with conduction block under treatment. J Neurol Neurosurg Psychiatry 1997;62:391–394.

27. Pestronk A. Multifocal motor neuropathy: diagnosis and treatment. Neurology 1998;51:S22–S24.

28. Chaudhry V, Corse AM, Cornblath DR, et al. Multifocal motor neuropathy: Response to human immune globulin. Ann Neurol 1993;33:237–242.

29. Nobile-Orazio E, Meucci N, Barbieri S, et al. High-dose intravenous immunoglobulin therapy in multifocal motor neuropathy. Neurology 1993;43:537–544.

30. Biessels GJ. Multifocal motor neuropathy. J Neurol 1997;244:143–152.

31. Van den Berg LH, Kerkhoff H, Oey PL, et al. Treatment of multifocal motor neuropathy with high dose intravenous immunoglobulins: a double blind, placebo controlled study. J Neurol Neurosurg Psychiatry 1995;59:248–252.

32. Molenaar DSM, de Haan R, Vermeulen M. Impairment, disability or handicap in peripheral neuropathy. Analysis of the use of outcome measures in clinical trials in patients with peripheral neuropathy. J Neurol Neurosurg Psychiatry 1995;59:165–169.

33. Dyck PJ, Bushek W, Spring EM, et al. Vibratory and cooling detection thresholds compared with other tests in diagnosing and staging diabetic neuropathy. Diabetes Care 1987;10:432–440.

34. Dyck PJ, Sherman WR, Hallcher LM, et al. Human diabetic endoneurial sorbitol, fructose, and myo-inositol related to sural nerve morphometry. Ann Neurol 1980;8:590–596.

35. Dyck PJ, Karnes J, O'Brien PC, Swanson CJ. Neuropathy symptom profile in health, motor neuron disease, diabetic neuropathy, and amyloidosis. Neurology 1986;36:1300–1308.

36. Dyck PJ, Karnes JL, Daube J, et al. Clinical and neuropathological criteria for the diagnosis and staging of diabetic polyneuropathy. Brain 1985;108:861–880.

37. Feldman EL, Stevens MJ. Clinical testing in diabetic peripheral neuropathy. Can J Neurol Sci 1994;21(Suppl 4):S3–S7.

38. Feldman EL, Brown MB, Stevens MJ, et al. A practical two-step quantitative clinical and electrophysiological assessment for the diagnosis and staging of diabetic neuropathy. Diabetes Care 1994;17:1281–1289.

39. Cornblath DR, Chaudhry V, Carter K, et al. Total Neuropathy Score: Validation and reliability study. Neurology 1999;53:1660–1664.

40. Chaudhry V, Eisenberger MA, Sinibaldi VJ, et al. A prospective study of suramin-induced peripheral neuropathy. Brain 1996;119:101–114.

41. Chaudhry V, Rowinsky EK, Sartorius SE, et al. Peripheral neuropathy from taxol and cisplatin combination chemotherapy: Clinical and electrophysiological studies. Ann Neurol 1994;35:304–311.

42. Hughes RA, Newsom-Davis JM, Perkin GD, Pierce JM. Controlled trial of prednisolone in acute polyneuropathy. Lancet 1978;1902:750–753.

43. Kleyweg RP, van der Meche FG, Schmitz PI. Interobserver agreement in the assessment of muscle strength and functional abilities in Guillain-Barré syndrome. Muscle Nerve 1991;1103–1109.

44. Merkies IS, Schmitz PI, van der Meche FG, Van Doorn PA. Psychometric evaluation of a new sensory scale in immune-mediated polyneuropathies. Inflammatory Neuropathy Cause and Treatment (INCAT) Group. Neurology 2000;54:943–949.

45. Apfel SC, Kessler JA, Adornato BT, et al. Recombinant human nerve growth factor in the treatment of diabetic polyneuropathy. NGF Study Group [see comments]. Neurology 1998;695–702.

46. McArthur JC, Yiannoutsos C, Simpson DM, et al. A phase II trial of nerve growth factor for sensory neuropathy associated with HIV infection. AIDS Clinical Trials Group Team 291. Neurology 2000;54:1080–1088.

47. Guillain-Barré Study Group. Plasmapheresis and acute Guillain-Barré syndrome. Neurology 1985; 35:1096–1104.

*Peripheral Neuropathy Treatment Trials* 287

48. McKhann GM, Griffin JW, Cornblath DR, et al. Plasmapheresis and Guillain-Barré syndrome: Analysis of prognostic factors and the effect of plasmapheresis. Ann Neurol 1988;23:347–353.
49. French Cooperative Group. Cooperative randomized trial of plasma exchange (P.E.) in Guillain-Barré syndrome (GBS). Preliminary results. Ann Med Interne 1984;135:8.
50. van der Meché FGA, Schmitz PIM, Dutch Guillain-Barré Study Group. A randomized trial comparing intravenous immune globulin and plasma exchange in Guillain-Barré syndrome. N Engl J Med 1992;326:1123–1129.
51. Bril V, Ilse WK, Pearce R, et al. Pilot trial of immunoglobulin versus plasma exchange in patients with Guillain-Barré syndrome. Neurology 1996;100–103.
52. Anonymous. Double-blind trial of intravenous methylprednisolone in Guillain-Barré syndrome. Guillain-Barré Syndrome Steroid Trial Group. Lancet 1993;341:586–590.
53. Dyck PJ, Lais AC, Ohta M, et al. Chronic inflammatory polyradiculoneuropathy. Mayo Clin Proc 1975;50:621–637.
54. Cornblath DR, Asbury AK, Albers JW, et al. Research criteria for diagnosis of chronic inflammatory demyelinating polyneuropathy (CIDP). Neurology 1991;41:617–618.
55. Dyck PJ. Chronic Inflammatory Demyelinating Polyradiculopathy. In PJ Dyck, PK Thomas, EH Lambert, R Bunge (eds), Peripheral Neuropathy (Vol. II) Philadelphia: WB Saunders, 1984;2101–2114.
56. Barohn RJ, Saperstein DS. Guillain-Barré syndrome and chronic inflammatory demyelinating polyneuropathy. Semin Neurol 1998;18:49–61.
57. Briani C, Brannagan TH III, Trojaborg W, Latov N. Chronic inflammatory demyelinating polyneuropathy. Neuromuscul Disord 1996;311–325.
58. Gorson KC, Allam G, Ropper AH. Chronic inflammatory demyelinating polyneuropathy: clinical features and response to treatment in 67 consecutive patients with and without a monoclonal gammopathy. Neurology 1997;321–328.
59. Hahn AF, Bolton CF, Zochodne D, Feasby TE. Intravenous immunoglobulin treatment in chronic inflammatory demyelinating polyneuropathy: A double-blind, placebo-controlled, cross-over study. Brain 1996;119:1067–1077.
60. Dyck PJ, O'Brien PC, Oviatt KF, et al. Prednisone improves chronic inflammatory demyelinating polyradiculoneuropathy more than no treatment. Ann Neurol 1982;11:136–141.
61. Van Doorn PA, Vermeulen M, Brand A, et al. Intravenous immunoglobulin treatment in patients with chronic inflammatory demyelinating polyneuropathy. Arch Neurol 1991;48:217–220.
62. Wertman E, Argov Z, Abrmasky O. Chronic inflammatory demyelinating polyradiculoneuropathy: features and prognostic factors with corticosteroid therapy. Eur Neurol 1988;28:199–204.
63. Dalakas MC, Engel WK. Chronic relapsing (dysimmune) polyneuropathy and treatment. Ann Neurol 1981;9(Suppl):134–145.
64. Dyck PJ, O'Brien P, Swanson C, et al. Combined azathioprine and prednisone in chronic inflammatory demyelinating polyneuropathy. Neurology 1985;35:1173–1176.
65. Choudhary PP, Hughes RA. Long-term treatment of chronic inflammatory demyelinating polyradiculoneuropathy with plasma exchange or intravenous immunoglobulin. QJM 1995;493–502.
66. Pollard JD, McLeod JG, Gatenby P, Kronenberg H. Prediction of response to plasma exchange in chronic relapsing polyneuropathy. A clinico-pathological correlation. J Neurol Sci 1983;269–287.
67. Prineas JW, McLeod JG. Chronic relapsing polyneuritis. J Neurol Sci 1976;27:427–458.
68. Barnett MH, Pollard JD, Davies L, McLeod JG. Cyclosporine A in resistant chronic inflammatory demyelinating polyradiculoneuropathy. Muscle Nerve 1998;21:454–460.
69. Mahattanakul M, Crawford, TO, Griffin JW, et al. Cyclosporine-A therapy in chronic inflammatory demyelinating polyneuropathy. J Neurol Neurosurg Psychiatry 1996;60:185–187.
70. Hodgkinson SJ, Pollard JD, McLeod JG. Cyclosporine A in the treatment of chronic demyelinating polyradiculopathy. J Neurol Neurosurg Psychiatry 1990;53:327–330.
71. Gorson KC, Ropper AH, Clark BD, et al. Treatment of chronic inflammatory demyelinating polyneuropathy with interferon-alpha 2a. Neurology 1998;84–87.
72. Choudhary PP, Thompson N, Hughes RAC. Improvement following interferon beta in chronic inflammatory demyelinating polyradiculoneuropathy. J Neurol 1995;242:252–253.
73. Rosenberg NL, Lacy JR, Kennaugh RC, et al. Treatment of refractory chronic demyelinating polyneuropathy with lymphoid irradiation. Muscle Nerve 1985;8:223–232.
74. Molenaar DS, Van Doorn PA, Vermeulen M. Pulsed high dose dexamethasone treatment in chronic inflammatory demyelinating polyneuropathy: a pilot study. J Neurol Neurosurg Psychiatry 1997;388–390.
75. Azulay J-P, Blin O, Pouget J, et al. Intravenous immunoglobulin treatment in patients with motor neuron syndromes associated with anti-GM$_1$ antibodies: a double-blind, placebo-controlled study. Neurology 1994;44:429–432.

288  *Clinical Trials in Neurologic Practice*

76. Pestronk A, Cornblath DR, Ilyas AA, et al. A treatable multifocal motor neuropathy with antibodies to GM1 ganglioside. Ann Neurol 1988;24:73–78.
77. Krarup C, Stewart JD, Sumner AJ, et al. A syndrome of asymmetrical limb weakness and motor conduction block. Neurology 1990;40:118–127.
78. Pestronk A, Chaudhry V, Feldman EL, et al. Lower motor neuron syndromes defined by patterns of weakness, nerve conduction abnormalities, and high titers of antiglycolipid antibodies. Ann Neurol 1990;27:316–326.
79. Feldman EL, Bromberg MB, Albers JW, Pestronk A. Immunosuppressive treatment in multifocal motor neuropathy. Ann Neurol 1991;30:397–401.
80. Donaghy M, Mills KR, Boniface SJ, et al. Pure motor demyelinating neuropathy: deterioration after steroid treatment and improvement with intravenous immunoglobulin. J Neurol Neurosurg Psychiatry 1994;57:778–783.
81. Van den Berg LH, Lokhorst H, Wokke JH. Pulsed high-dose dexamethasone is not effective in patients with multifocal motor neuropathy. Neurology 1997;48:1135.
82. Tan E, Lynn DJ, Amato AA, et al. Immunosuppressive treatment of motor neuron syndromes. Attempts to distinguish a treatable disorder. Arch Neurol 1994;51:194–200.
83. Meucci N. Long term effect of intravenous immunoglobulins and oral cyclophosphamide in multifocal motor neuropathy. J Neurol Neurosurg Psychiatry 1997;63:765–769.
84. Katz JS. Electrophysiologic findings in multifocal motor neuropathy. Neurology 1997;48:700–707.
85. Chassande B, Leger JM, Younes-Chennoufi AB, et al. Peripheral neuropathy associated with IgM monoclonal gammopathy: correlations between M-protein antibody activity and clinical/electrophysiological features in 40 cases. Muscle Nerve 1998;55–62.
86. Dalakas MC, Quarles RH, Farrer RG, et al. A controlled study of intravenous immunoglobulin in demyelinating neuropathy with IgM gammopathy. Ann Neurol 1996;792–795.
87. Leger JM, Chassande B, Bouche P. (Peripheral neuropathies associated with IgM monoclonal gammopathy: clinical and electrophysiological aspects). Rev Neurol (Paris) 1996;152:394–399.
88. Van den Berg L, Hays AP, Nobile-Orazio E, et al. Anti-MAG and anti-SGPG antibodies in neuropathy. Muscle Nerve 1996;19:637–643.
89. Trojaborg W, Hays AP, Van den Berg L, et al. Motor conduction parameters in neuropathies associated with anti-MAG antibodies and other types of demyelinating and axonal neuropathies. Muscle Nerve 1995;730–735.
90. Latov N, Steck AJ. Neuropathies Associated with Anti-Glycoconjugate Antibodies and IgM Monoclonal Gammopathies. In AK Asbury, PK Thomas (eds), Peripheral Nerve Disorders II. Woburn, MA: Butterworth–Heinemann, 1995.
91. Mariette X, Chastang C, Clavelou P, et al. A randomised clinical trial comparing interferon-alpha and intravenous immunoglobulin in polyneuropathy associated with monoclonal IgM. The IgM-associated Polyneuropathy Study Group. J Neurol Neurosurg Psychiatry 1997;28–34.
92. Blume G, Pestronk A, Goodnough LT. Anti-MAG antibody-associated polyneuropathies: improvement following immunotherapy with monthly plasma exchange and IV cyclophosphamide. Neurology 1995;1577–1580.
93. Nobile-Orazio E, Baldini L, Barbieri S, Marmiroli P, et al. Treatment of patients with neuropathy and anti-MAG IgM M-proteins. Ann Neurol 1988;24:93–97.
94. Wilson HC, Lunn MP, Schey S, Hughes RA. Successful treatment of IgM paraproteinaemic neuropathy with fludarabine. J Neurol Neurosurg Psychiatry 1999;575–580.
95. Levine TD, Pestronk A. IgM antibody-related polyneuropathies: B-cell depletion chemotherapy using Rituximab. Neurology 1999;1701–1704.
96. Simmons Z. Paraproteinemia and neuropathy. Curr Opin Neurol 1999;589–595.
97. Gorson KC. Clinical features, evaluation, and treatment of patients with polyneuropathy associated with monoclonal gammopathy of undetermined significance (MGUS). J Clin Apheresis 1999; 14;149–153.
98. Ponsford S, Willison H, Veitch J, et al. Long-term clinical and neurophysiological follow-up of patients with peripheral, neuropathy associated with benign monoclonal gammopathy [see comments]. Muscle Nerve 2000;164–174.
99. Latov N. Prognosis of neuropathy with monoclonal gammopathy [editorial; comment]. Muscle Nerve 2000;150–152.
100. Notermans NC, Franssen H, Eurelings M, et al. Diagnostic criteria for demyelinating polyneuropathy associated with monoclonal gammopathy. Muscle Nerve 2000;73–79.

## Peripheral Neuropathy Treatment Trials   289

101. Di Troia A, Carpo M, Meucci N, et al. Clinical features and anti-neural reactivity in neuropathy associated with IgG monoclonal gammopathy of undetermined significance. J Neurol Sci 1999;164:64–71.

102. Simovic D, Gorson KC, Ropper AH. Comparison of IgM-MGUS and IgG-MGUS polyneuropathy. Acta Neurol Scand 1998;194–200.

103. Kelly JJ, Kyle RA, O'Brien PC, Dyck PJ. Prevalence of monoclonal protein in peripheral neuropathy. Neurology 1981;31:1480–1483.

104. Miralles GD, O'Fallon JR, Talley NJ. Plasma-cell dyscrasia with polyneuropathy. The spectrum of POEMS syndrome. N Engl J Med 1992;327:1919–1923.

105. Dyck PJ, Low PA, Windebank AJ, et al. Plasma exchange in polyneuropathy associated with monoclonal gammopathy of undetermined significance. N Engl J Med 1991;325:1482–1486.

106. Oksenhendler E, Chevret S, Leger JM, et al. Plasma exchange and chlorambucil in polyneuropathy associated with monoclonal IgM gammopathy. IgM-associated Polyneuropathy Study Group. J Neurol Neurosurg Psychiatry 1995;243–247.

107. Feldman EL, Russell JW, Sullivan KA, Golovoy D. New insights into the pathogenesis of diabetic neuropathy [editorial]. Curr Opin Neurol 1999;553–563.

108. Greene DA, Stevens MJ, Feldman EL. Diabetic neuropathy: scope of the syndrome. Am J Med 1999;107:2S–8S.

109. Feldman EL, Stevens MJ, Greene DA. Pathogenesis of diabetic neuropathy. Clin Neurosci 1997; 4:365–370.

110. Parry GJ. Management of diabetic neuropathy. Am J Med 1999;107:27S–33S.

111. Vinik AI. Diabetic neuropathy: pathogenesis and therapy. Am J Med 1999;107:17S–26S.

112. Arezzo JC. New developments in the diagnosis of diabetic neuropathy. Am J Med 1999;107:9S–16S.

113. Zochodne DW. Diabetic neuropathies: features and mechanisms. Brain Pathol 1999;369–391.

114. Illa I. Diagnosis and management of diabetic peripheral neuropathy. Eur Neurol 1999;1941:3–7.

115. The Diabetes Control and Complications Trial Research Group. The effect of intensive treatment of diabetes on the development and progression of long-term complications in insulin-dependent diabetes mellitus. N Engl J Med 1993;329:977–986.

116. The Diabetes Control and Complications Trial Research Group. The effect of intensive diabetes treatment on the development and progression of neuropathy. Ann Intern Med 1995;122:561–568.

117. Ohkubo Y, Kishikawa H, Araki E, et al. Intensive insulin therapy prevents the progression of diabetic microvascular complications in Japanese patients with non-insulin-dependent diabetes mellitus: a randomized prospective 6-year study [see comments]. Diabetes Res Clin Pract 1995;103–117.

118. Reichard P, Nilsson BY, Rosenqvist U. The effect of long-term intensified insulin treatment on the development of microvascular complications of diabetes mellitus [see comments]. N Engl J Med 1993;329:304–309.

119. Amthor KF, Dahl-Jorgensen K, Berg TJ, et al. The effect of 8 years of strict glycaemic control on peripheral nerve function in IDDM patients: the Oslo Study. Diabetologia 1994;579–584.

120. Kennedy WR, Navarro X, Goetz FC, et al. Effects of pancreatic transplantation on diabetic neuropathy [see comments]. N Engl J Med 1990;322:1031–1037.

121. Solders G, Wilczek H, Gunnarsson R, et al. Effects of combined pancreatic and renal transplantation on diabetic neuropathy: a two-year follow-up study. Lancet 1987;(2):1232–1235.

122. Navarro X, Sutherland DE, Kennedy WR. Long-term effects of pancreatic transplantation on diabetic neuropathy [see comments]. Ann Neurol 1997;727–736.

123. Muller-Felber W, Landgraf R, Scheuer R, et al. Diabetic neuropathy 3 years after successful pancreas and kidney transplantation. Diabetes 1993;1482–1486.

124. Nusser J, Scheuer R, Abendroth D, et al. Effect of pancreatic and/or renal transplantation on diabetic autonomic neuropathy. Diabetologia 1991;S118–S120

125. Gabbay KH, Merola LO, Field RA. Sorbitol pathway: Presence in nerve and cord with substrate accumulation in diabetes. Science 1966;151:209–210.

126. Judzewitsch RG, Jaspan JB, Polonsky KS, et al. Aldose reductase inhibition improves nerve conduction velocity in diabetic patients. N Engl J Med 1983;308:119–125.

127. Dyck PJ, Zimmerman BR, Vilen TH, et al. Nerve glucose, fructose, sorbitol, myo-inositol, and fiber degeneration and regeneration in diabetic neuropathy. N Engl J Med 1988;319:542–548.

128. Judzewitsch RG, Jaspan JB, Polonsky KS, et al. Aldose reductase inhibition improves nerve conduction velocity in diabetic patients. N Engl J Med 1983;308:119–125.

## 290 Clinical Trials in Neurologic Practice

129. Sima AAF, Bril V, Nathaniel V, et al. Regeneration and repair of myelinated fibers in sural nerve biopsy specimens from patients with diabetic neuropathy treated with sorbinil. N Engl J Med 1988; 319:548–555.
130. Anonymous. The sorbinil retinopathy trial: neuropathy results. Sorbinil Retinopathy Trial Research Group. Neurology 1993;1141–1149.
131. O'Hare JP, Morgan MH, Alden P, et al. Aldose reductase inhibition in diabetic neuropathy: clinical and neurophysiological studies of one year's treatment with sorbinil. Diabetic Med 1988;537–542.
132. Boulton AJ, Levin S, Comstock J. A multicentre trial of the aldose-reductase inhibitor, tolrestat, in patients with symptomatic diabetic neuropathy. Diabetologia 1990;431–437.
133. Nicolucci A, Carinci F, Graepel JG, et al. The efficacy of tolrestat in the treatment of diabetic peripheral neuropathy. A meta-analysis of individual patient data. Diabetes Care 1996;1091–1096.
134. Greene DA, Arezzo JC, Brown MB. Effect of aldose reductase inhibition on nerve conduction and morphometry in diabetic neuropathy. Zenarestat Study Group. Neurology 1999;580–591.
135. Faes TJ, Yff GA, DeWeerdt O, et al. Treatment of diabetic autonomic neuropathy with an aldose reductase inhibitor. J Neurol 1993;240:156–160.
136. Hotta N, Sakamoto N, Shigeta Y, et al. Clinical investigation of epalrestat, an aldose reductase inhibitor, on diabetic neuropathy in Japan: multicenter study. Diabetic Neuropathy Study Group in Japan. J Diabetic Complications 1996;168–172.
137. Greene DA. Sorbitol, myo-inositol and sodium-potassium ATPase in diabetic peripheral nerve. Drugs 1986;32;6–14.
138. Greene DA, DeJesus PV, Winegrad AI. Effects of insulin and dietary myoinositol on impaired peripheral motor nerve conduction velocity in acute streptozotocin diabetes. J Clin Invest. 1975; 55:1326–1336.
139. Sima AA, Dunlap JA, Davidson EP, et al. Supplemental myo-inositol prevents L-fucose-induced diabetic neuropathy. Diabetes 1997;301–306.
140. Gregersen G, Borsting H, Theil P, Servo C. Myoinositol and function of peripheral nerves in human diabetics. A controlled clinical trial. Acta Neurol Scand 1978;58:241–248.
141. Salway JG, Whitehead L, Finnegan JA, et al. Effect of myo-inositol on peripheral-nerve function in diabetes. Lancet 1978;2:1282–1284.
142. Gregersen G, Bertelsen B, Harbo H, et al. Oral supplementation of myoinositol: effects on peripheral nerve function in human diabetics and on the concentration in plasma, erythrocytes, urine and muscle tissue in human diabetics and normals. Acta Neurol Scand 1983;67:164–172.
143. Apfel SC. Neurotrophic factors in the therapy of diabetic neuropathy. Am J Med 1999;107:34S–42S.
144. Apfel SC. Neurotrophic factors in peripheral neuropathies: therapeutic implications. Brain Pathol 1999;9:393–413.
145. Apfel SC. Neurotrophic factors and diabetic peripheral neuropathy. Eur Neurol 1999;41:27–34.
146. Apfel SC, Kessler JA. Neurotrophic factors in the therapy of peripheral neuropathy. Baillieres Clin Neurol 1995;593–606.
147. Dyck PJ, Peroutka S, Rask C, et al. Intradermal recombinant human nerve growth factor induces pressure allodynia and lowered heat-pain threshold in humans. Neurology 1997;501–505.
148. Smith LE, Shen W, Perruzzi C, et al. Regulation of vascular endothelial growth factor-dependent retinal neovascularization by insulin-like growth factor-1 receptor. Nat Med 1999;1390–1395.
149. Horowitz SH. Ganglioside therapy in diabetic neuropathy. Muscle Nerve 1986;531–536.
150. Keen H, Payan J, Allawi J, et al. Treatment of diabetic neuropathy with gamma-linolenic acid. The gamma-Linolenic Acid Multicenter Trial Group [see comments]. Diabetes Care 1993;8–15.
151. Ruhnau KJ, Meissner HP, Finn JR, et al. Effects of 3-week oral treatment with the antioxidant thioctic acid (alpha-lipoic acid) in symptomatic diabetic polyneuropathy. Diabetic Med 1999;1040–1043.
152. Ziegler D, Reljanovic M, Mehnert H, Gries FA. Alpha-lipoic acid in the treatment of diabetic polyneuropathy in Germany: current evidence from clinical trials. Exp Clin Endocrinol Diabetes 1999; 107:421–430.
153. Reljanovic M, Reichel G, Rett K, et al. Treatment of diabetic polyneuropathy with the antioxidant thioctic acid (alpha-lipoic acid): a two year multicenter randomized double-blind placebo-controlled trial (ALADIN II). Alpha Lipoic Acid in Diabetic Neuropathy. Free Radic Res 1999;171–179.
154. Ziegler D, Hanefeld M, Ruhnau KJ, et al. Treatment of symptomatic diabetic polyneuropathy with the antioxidant alpha-lipoic acid: a 7-month multicenter randomized controlled trial (ALADIN III Study). ALADIN III Study Group. Alpha-Lipoic Acid in Diabetic Neuropathy. Diabetes Care 1999;1296–1301.
155. Yamamoto Y, Yasuda Y, Kimura Y, Komiya Y. Effects of cilostazol, an antiplatelet agent, on axonal regeneration following nerve injury in diabetic rats. Eur J Pharmacol 1998;352:171–178.

## Peripheral Neuropathy Treatment Trials    291

156. Okuda Y, Mizutani M, Ikegami T, et al. Hemodynamic effects of cilostazol on peripheral artery in patients with diabetic neuropathy. Arzneimittelforschung 1992;540–542.
157. Shindo H, Tawata M, Inoue M, et al. The effect of prostaglandin E1.alpha CD on vibratory threshold determined with the SMV-5 vibrometer in patients with diabetic neuropathy. Diabetes Res Clin Pract 1994;173–180.
158. Bravenboer B, Hendrikse PH, Oey PL, et al. Randomized double-blind placebo-controlled trial to evaluate the effect of the ACTH4-9 analogue ORG 2766 in IDDM patients with neuropathy. Diabetologia 1994;408–413.
159. Gallai V, Mazzotta G, Montesi S, Sarchielli P, Del Gatto F. Effects of uridine in the treatment of diabetic neuropathy: an electrophysiological study [see comments]. Acta Neurol Scand 1992;3–7.
160. Bradley WG, Chad D, Verghese JP, et al. Painful lumbosacral plexopathy with elevated erythrocyte sedimentation rate: a treatable inflammatory syndrome. Ann Neurol 1984;457–464.
161. Krendel DA, Costigan DA, Hopkins LC. Successful treatment of neuropathies in patients with diabetes mellitus [see comments]. Arch Neurol 1995;1053–1061.
162. Younger DS, Rosoklija G, Hays AP, et al. Diabetic peripheral neuropathy: A clinicopathologic and immunohistochemical analysis of sural nerve biopsies [see comments]. Muscle Nerve 1996;722–727.
163. Chokroverty S, Sander HW. AAEM case report #13: Diabetic amyotrophy [published erratum appears in Muscle Nerve 1996 Dec;19(12):1655]. Muscle Nerve 1996;939–945.
164. Younger DS, Rosoklija G, Hays AP. Diabetic peripheral neuropathy. Semin Neurol 1998;18:95–104.
165. Dyck PJ, Norell JE. Microvasculitis and ischemia in diabetic lumbosacral radiculoplexus neuropathy. Neurology 1999;2113–2121.
166. Said G, Goulon-Goeau C, Lacroix C, Moulonguet A. Nerve biopsy findings in different patterns of proximal diabetic neuropathy. Ann Neurol 1994;35:559–569.
167. Leger JM, Ben Younes-Chennoufi A, Chassande B, et al. Human immunoglobulin treatment of multifocal motor neuropathy and polyneuropathy associated with monoclonal gammopathy. J Neurol Neurosurg Psychiatry 1994;57(Suppl):46–49.
168. Comi G, Amadio S, Galardi G, et al. Clinical and neurophysiological assessment of immunoglobulin therapy in five patients with multifocal motor neuropathy. J Neurol Neurosurg Psychiatry 1994; 57(Suppl):35–37.
169. Bouche P, Moulonguet A, Ben Younes-Chennoufi A, et al. Multifocal motor neuropathy with conduction block: a study of 24 patients. J Neurol Neurosurg Psychiatry 1995;59:38–44.
170. Jaspert A, Claus D, Grehl H, Neundörfer B. Multifocal motor neuropathy: clinical and electrophysiological findings. J Neurol 1996;243:684–69.

# 14
## Myasthenia Gravis: A Clinical Trials Perspective

Robert M. Pascuzzi

Myasthenia gravis (MG) is an autoimmune disorder of neuromuscular transmission involving the production of autoantibodies directed against the nicotinic acetylcholine receptor. The acetylcholine receptor antibodies are detectable in the serum of 80–90% of patients with autoimmune MG.[1] The prevalence of MG is estimated at approximately one in ten to twenty thousand. Women are affected twice as often as men. Symptoms can begin at virtually any age, with a peak in women in the second and third decades, whereas the peak in men occurs in the fifth and sixth decades. Associated autoimmune diseases, such as rheumatoid arthritis, systemic lupus erythematous, and pernicious anemia, are present in approximately 5% of patients. Thyroid disease occurs in approximately 10% of patients with MG, often in association with antithyroid antibodies. Abnormalities of the thymus gland have been noted in MG since Weigert's initial observation of thymoma in 1901.[2] Ten percent to 15% of patients have thymoma, which is typically a benign tumor; lymphoid hyperplasia with proliferation of germinal centers has been observed in 50–70% of patients with MG.

## CLINICAL MANIFESTATIONS

The hallmark of MG is fluctuating or fatigable weakness. Ocular symptoms are common. In Grob's retrospective review of 1,487 patients with MG, 25% presented with diplopia, 25% with ptosis, and by 1 month into the course of illness, 80% of patients had some degree of ocular involvement.[3] Presenting symptoms in his series were bulbar (dysarthria and dysphagia) in 10% of patients, whereas 10% presented with lower extremity weakness and nearly 10% presented with generalized weakness. Isolated respiratory failure as the presenting symptom occurred in 1% of patients.[3]

293

294   *Clinical Trials in Neurologic Practice*

Overall, patients typically complain of symptoms from focal muscle dysfunction, such as diplopia, ptosis, dysarthria, dysphagia, inability to work with the arms raised over the head, or disturbance of gait. In contrast, patients with MG tend not to complain of generalized weakness, generalized fatigue, sleepiness, or muscle pain.

In the classic MG patient, weakness tends to fluctuate; it is worse with exercise and better with rest. Symptoms tend to progress as the day goes on. Many different factors can precipitate or aggravate weakness, including fever, physical or emotional stress, infection or exposure to medications that interfere with neuromuscular transmission (e.g., neuromuscular blocking drugs, aminoglycoside antibiotics, quinidine, quinine).

## NATURAL COURSE

A clear understanding of the natural course of MG would seem essential to the optimal design of therapeutic trials. The natural course of autoimmune MG is inadequately known. Reports from the first half of the twentieth century noted a high mortality of 30–70%. With the advent of intensive technology, mechanical ventilation, the introduction of cholinesterase inhibitors, and immunosuppressive therapy, mortality has dramatically declined, such that myasthenic death is relatively rare. In 1934, Dr. Mary Walker, a house officer at St. Alfege's Hospital in London, observed her patient improved with the cholinesterase inhibitor physostigmine.[4,5] Blalock reported a favorable response after removing a thymic tumor from a patient in 1939, leading to widespread interest in thymectomy in the treatment of MG.[6] The subsequent use of corticosteroids, other immunosuppressive drugs, plasmapheresis, and intravenous immunoglobulin (IVIG) has hampered efforts to observe and define the untreated natural course of the disease. Because nearly all patients in the modern era are treated with one or more therapeutic modalities, it is unlikely that we will ever completely understand the "natural course" of MG.

In 1937, Kennedy and Moersch reported on the course of MG in 87 untreated patients seen at the Mayo Clinic between 1915 and 1932.[7] Remission occurred in 31% of patients and lasted from 1 month to 15 years (mean, 2.2 years). Partial remission occurred in an additional 13 of 87 patients. Therefore, 46 of the untreated patients spontaneously improved, whereas 28% died from MG. Kennedy and Moersch concluded, "Needless to say, it is this tendency to remissions in this disease that makes the benefits of any form of treatment so difficult to evaluate."[7]

In Grob's series, symptoms remained purely ocular in 14% of patients.[3] Of those patients who presented with ocular symptoms and later developed generalized weakness, 87% did so within 1 year. Maximal weakness occurred within the first 3 years in 70% of patients. Spontaneous, long-lasting remission occurred in approximately 10% of his patients. After the initial 3-year observation period, most patients achieved a steady state of clinical symptoms or actually improved.[3]

Oosterhuis reported on the natural course of MG in 73 patients from Amsterdam who presented before 1965 and were treated with cholinesterase inhibitors alone.[8] Follow-up through 1985 showed that 29% died (eight with thymoma), 22% were in complete clinical remission, and 18% were in a state of marked improvement. Bever et al. studied the course of 269 patients seen between 1957 and 1967.[9] Ocular symptoms were initially noted in 84%, of which 53% were purely ocular. Of 108

*Myasthenia Gravis: A Clinical Trials Perspective* 295

patients who presented with isolated ocular disease treated only with cholinesterase inhibitors and followed for 1–39 years (mean, 14 years), subsequent generalized weakness occurred in 49%, and progression occurred within the first 2 years in 85% of cases. Those who eventually had a myasthenic respiratory crisis or died did so within the first 2 years of illness in 17 of 20 cases. One or more episodes of remission lasting from 1 month to 20 years (mean, 4.8 years) occurred in 17%. These "spontaneous" remissions occurred within 1 year in 30% and as late as 13 years into the clinical course. Complete long-lasting remission occurred in 11%.[9]

Simpson, who originally developed the autoimmune hypothesis for MG, described an initial "active stage" or progressive weakness with a labile course, generally lasting 5–10 years, which was followed by a second "inactive stage" with less fluctuation and less lability.[10] Finally, patients entered a "burned-out stage" 14–20 years after the onset of symptoms, with minimal fluctuation and relatively stable weakness.

These observations illustrate the variability of the natural course of MG. Many, and perhaps most, MG patients develop progression of clinical symptoms during the initial 2–3 years, with a tendency for stabilization or improvement after that point. However, the progression of weakness is not uniform, as illustrated by the tendency for ocular weakness to remain isolated in 14–40% of cases and the observation that approximately 10% of patients experience a spontaneous long-lasting complete clinical remission.

The short-term course of MG is equally variable. Howard and colleagues reported on a small prospective double-blind controlled study of alternate-day prednisone.[11] Patients received prednisone 100 mg alternate day or placebo and were followed for 6 months. Three of the six patients on prednisone improved. More interesting is that, of the seven patients on placebo, "three were improved and had minimal disability, while controlled by small amounts of cholinesterase inhibitors." Howard concluded that "any evaluation of treatment of MG must take into consideration the potential for spontaneous improvement. . . ."[11]

Patten, in a discussion of the use of plasmapheresis, stated the following:

> We did imaginary exchanges in six very severe generalized myasthenics. The referring physicians and residents felt that these patients had reached a point in their therapy program at which time they needed exchange. I informed the patients that we would exchange, but this was carried out only in our imagination. We watched the patients over three weeks. All improved. All left the hospital. The imaginary exchanges had no side effects. The cost was less. MG is a very complex disease, and the patients themselves are very complex. If you look at them the wrong way they get weak. If you look at them the right way they get better. Proper medication and rest in the hospital may be just as effective as some of the things we are talking about now.[12]

## TREATMENT OPTIONS

### Thymectomy

Blalock reported the first improvement in MG after removal of the thymus gland in his seminal article in 1941.[6] He operated on a woman with moderately severe

296    *Clinical Trials in Neurologic Practice*

generalized MG who had a mediastinal mass detected by radiographic studies. The mediastinal mass was treated with radiation therapy but continued to expand; therefore, he took the patient to surgery, removing a cystic lesion. The patient's MG improved after surgery. Thereafter, Blalock performed thymectomy on a series of patients with MG and subsequently documented clinical improvement.[13] Since then, thymectomy has been commonplace in the treatment of autoimmune MG, particularly for younger patients, and in all of those suspected of having thymoma. Prospective controlled trials of thymectomy for MG have not been performed. Retrospective data from Perlo et al. illustrate the traditionally held view of effectiveness of thymectomy.[14] Of 267 patients having a thymectomy in Perlo's series, most with severe MG, 76% improved, with 35% in total remission. Remission developed 1–10 years after surgery, with approximately half occurring within 3 years. The remission rate was better than in a medically treated group (17%). The surgical mortality was said to be 2.8% in this series, which was reported in 1971.[14] Buckingham and colleagues from the Mayo Clinic performed a retrospective comparison of results of thymectomy versus medical therapy in 80 patients who were matched (retrospectively) for age, gender, and severity and duration of disease.[15] In this retrospective comparative study, the patients who had a thymectomy fared significantly better with regard to remission, rate, improvement, and mortality, including death from MG.[15] Not all experts have been impressed with the benefits of thymectomy. In 1950, Eaton and Clagett reported little benefit in 87 thymectomy patients compared with 225 controls.[16]

Whereas most centers use a maximal type of thymectomy with a trans-sternal approach, the goal being complete removal of the thymus gland, some surgeons prefer a more limited surgical approach, although a more limited transcervical approach has been largely abandoned because of the likelihood of incomplete removal.[17,18] The embryologic development of the thymus gland from multiple brachial arches and complex migration to form the mature thymus provide anatomic support for the trans-sternal approach. Masoaki et al. found ectopic thymic rests in 72% of patients.[19] Re-exploration with removal of residual thymic tissue has been associated in some patients with significant clinical improvement in MG patients who had previously received surgical thymectomy.[20] Jaretzki and colleagues advocated "maximal thymectomy" to ensure complete removal of the gland.[17] This procedure involves a combined trans-sternal and transcervical exposure with the in-block removal of the thymus. In Jaretski's retrospective series, morbidity was exceedingly low, and the majority of patients substantially improved 1–4 years after surgery.[17]

The role of thymectomy in isolated ocular myasthenia is less clear. However, Schumm et al. performed thymectomy on 18 patients having purely ocular symptoms with suspected thymoma, resistance to cholinesterase inhibitors, or relapse of their MG after immunosuppression.[21] In these patients, thymic abnormalities were noted in all; clinical improvement of MG occurred in 80% after thymectomy, with remission in 17%. None of Schumm's patients was noted to progress to generalized myasthenic weakness, although the duration of follow-up was limited to 3 years.[21]

Thymectomy is often avoided in children because of the theoretical concerns of adverse effects on the developing immune system; however, reports in the literature of thymectomy in children as young as 2–3 years have shown favorable results without adverse immunologic effects.

Thymectomy has generally been discouraged in those patients older than 55 years because of several factors. An increased morbidity with increasing age, the delay in clinical benefit, and the frequent observation of an atrophic involuted gland contributed to the general view not to perform thymectomy in an older patient unless there is suspicion for thymoma. However, Olanow et al. found that 11 of 12 patients older than 55 years became free of symptoms, with nine requiring no subsequent long-term medication after thymectomy.[22] The presence of an atrophic involuted thymus gland may not preclude immunologic activity.

Major complications from thymectomy are uncommon in the recent literature, but this author has observed postoperative hemothorax in one patient (with recurrent pleural fluid accumulation and pulmonary fibrosis) and death from postoperative pulmonary embolus in another patient. Both patients were men in their twenties with stable early MG. Common, although less serious, aspects of thymectomy include postoperative chest pain that may last for several weeks and a 4- to 6-week convalescence, as well as the possibility of incisional scarring. There have been more than 100 reports in the literature of thymectomy for the treatment of MG, with nearly all of them emphasizing the benefits of the treatment. Nonetheless, the absence of a controlled prospective trial, the lack of standardized or well-defined measurements, the variable natural course of the disease, and the use of a multitude of other concomitant therapies have made it difficult to know the exact role of thymectomy in improving patient symptoms. In addition, the shortcomings of clinical trials of thymectomy are emphasized in a recent "Practice parameter: Thymectomy for autoimmune myasthenia gravis (an evidence-based review)," in which the authors conclude, "for patients with nonthymomatous autoimmune MG, thymectomy is recognized as an option to increase the probability of remission or improvement."[23] Alfred Jaretzki, a pioneer in the treatment of MG with thymectomy, has headed a task force for the Myasthenia Gravis Foundation of America to define a uniform classification system for severity of symptoms, to define such terms as *remission* or *improvement*, and to develop a standardized approach to evaluating and monitoring patients long term, including those who undergo thymectomy (see the section Future of Clinical Trials in Myasthenia Gravis).[24]

## Medical Therapy

Clinical Trials

### Cholinesterase Inhibitors

There have been no prospective placebo-controlled trials of cholinesterase inhibitors in MG. Due to the safety profile of cholinesterase inhibitors, such drugs remain the first-line therapy for all patients with mild to moderate MG.

### Corticosteroids

Kupersmith et al. reported on the beneficial effects of corticosteroids in ocular MG.[25] The authors studied 32 patients with ocular MG and their response to pred-

298     *Clinical Trials in Neurologic Practice*

nisone; patients were observed for at least 2 years. Patients were treated with initial high-dose daily prednisone, 40–80% per os daily and withdrawn over 4–6 weeks. In six patients, low-dose prednisone, 2.5–20.0 mg per os alternate day was used on a long-term basis. The outcome measures included diplopia in the primary position or downgaze diplopia and generalized MG after 2 years of follow-up. The authors found that in patients treated as described, diplopia was present in the primary position in 29 patients initially, in the downgaze position in 26 patients, and resolved in 21 patients at 2 years. Generalized MG occurred in three patients at 2 years. Abnormal levels of acetylcholine receptor antibodies and abnormal electromyographic findings did not predict the eventual worsening or generalization. The authors concluded that moderate-dose daily prednisone for 4–6 weeks, followed by low-dose alternate-day therapy, can control double vision in patients with ocular myasthenia. The majority of patients was treated with limited courses of prednisone for 4–6 weeks as opposed to long-term maintenance therapy; however, the majority of patients improved on a long-term basis.[25]

In a letter published by Kupersmith, McQuillen commented on the study and emphasized that Kupersmith and colleagues "neglected to mention the only controlled clinical trial of anything in myasthenia—namely of corticotropin" and cited the article by Mount.[26,27]

However, there have been other controlled clinical trials of medical therapy in MG, including corticosteroid therapy. In 1976, Howard et al. from the Mayo Clinic reported that prednisone, 100 mg alternate day, was given to patients with moderately severe MG. Thirteen patients were observed for up to 6 months.[11] Six of the patients received prednisone, three of whom improved. Seven patients received placebo, of whom "three were improved and had minimal disability well controlled by small amounts of anticholinesterase medication."[11] Howard concluded, "Finally, any evaluation of treatment of myasthenia gravis must take into consideration the potential for spontaneous improvement as demonstrated by 3 (of 7) of the patients treated with placebo." In a personal communication from Dr. Howard (May 14, 1998), the following comments are made regarding the Mayo Clinic prospective controlled double-blind trial:

> The study on the use of prednisone in M.G. was, of course, limited by being a small number of patients. We were surprised by the three patients on the placebo that improved. The study was not extended for two reasons; 1) lack of funding and 2) because one of the placebo patients died and I felt that she would have survived if she had been on prednisone. Prior to the study I was convinced of the benefits of prednisone and I just didn't have the scientific zeal to continue to withhold the use of a life saving drug for the sake of accumulating more data.[28]

Although no optimal placebo-controlled clinical trials of corticosteroid therapy in MG have been performed, decades of extensive clinical experience support the general conclusion that such therapy is an effective and appropriate option for patients with severe MG.

### Azathioprine

Azathioprine has been used for the treatment of MG since the 1960s, initially receiving widespread use in Europe.[29,30] Azathioprine is often given along with corticosteroids for chronic immunosuppressive therapy. Some authorities choose to use the drug as a sole immunosuppressive drug. Large uncontrolled studies have consistently suggested substantial benefit with a conservative estimate of 50% of patients showing some improvement, with onset of improvement approximately 6 months after beginning therapy and maximal improvement 1–2 years after beginning therapy. Patients withdrawn from azathioprine have been observed to develop recurrence of clinical symptoms of MG, typically within 6 months of stopping the drug.[31,32] The use of azathioprine may allow for lower prednisone doses in patients requiring long-term immunosuppressive therapy.[33] An unblinded prospective comparative trial that compared patients on prednisone with those being treated with azathioprine after 4 months suggested more treatment failures in the prednisone group.[34,35]

## Comparison of Corticosteroids and Azathioprine for Long-Term Treatment of Myasthenia Gravis

Palace et al., with the MG Study Group, performed a prospective comparative trial in the treatment of MG.[34–36] One group of patients received prednisolone and azathioprine, whereas the second group received prednisolone alone. Thirty-four patients were randomized and followed in a double-blind study for a 3-year period. The group receiving prednisolone and azathioprine received alternate-day prednisolone plus azathioprine, 2.5 mg/kg. The group receiving prednisolone alone also received a placebo to control for the effects of azathioprine. The initial prednisolone dose was 1.5 mg/kg on alternate days and was gradually reduced when patients were clinically stable to allow for the minimal dose necessary to keep the patient in clinical remission. The prednisolone dosage was similar in the two groups at 1 year (37.5 mg alternate-day prednisolone plus azathioprine compared with 45 mg alternate-day prednisolone plus placebo). However, at 2 and 3 years, the prednisolone plus azathioprine group had a statistically significantly lower dose of prednisolone than the prednisolone plus placebo group (median value at 3 years: prednisolone plus azathioprine, 0 mg prednisolone on alternate day, compared with prednisolone plus placebo, 40 mg on alternate day; $p = .02$). Clinical exacerbation or relapse and failure to reach remission during a 3-year follow-up period were more frequent in the prednisolone plus placebo group. In addition, there was a rise in the acetylcholine receptor antibody titers in the prednisolone plus placebo group at 2 years. Overall side effects were somewhat less prominent in the prednisolone plus azathioprine group.[36]

The authors concluded that azathioprine is a meaningful adjunctive treatment to alternate-day prednisolone in the treatment of autoimmune MG, in that it reduces the long-term maintenance dose of prednisolone, is associated with fewer treatment failures, is associated with longer clinical remissions, and has fewer side effects.[36]

## Cyclosporine

Cyclosporine A has been the subject of a prospective controlled double-blind trial for the treatment of MG. Tindall et al. studied the effect of cyclospo-

300    *Clinical Trials in Neurologic Practice*

rine in MG in a prospective double-blind randomized placebo-controlled trial, in which 20 patients with generalized progressive MG of recent onset who were inadequately controlled by cholinesterase inhibitors were randomized to 6 mg/kg per day cyclosporine or placebo and followed for the next 12 months.[37,38] At 6 months, the cyclosporine group demonstrated significantly better muscle strength and had an associated reduction in acetylcholine receptor antibody titer that continued to be apparent at the 12-month follow-up point. Renal toxicity occurred in three patients but seemed to be dose dependent and reversible. Nausea occurred in three patients, thus limiting the use of medication. The onset of improvement appeared to occur several months after initiating cyclosporine.[37,38]

Goulon et al. performed an open trial of cyclosporine A in 10 patients with severe generalized myasthenia who were poorly controlled with other therapies.[39] They used a dose of 2 mg/kg two or three times daily, progressively increased, aiming for a peak serum level below 200 ng/ml. The mean dosage during the course of the study was 5.5 mg/kg per day. At 12 months, two patients were unimproved, four moderately improved, and four markedly improved. The response was gradual, occurring 3–9 months after starting medication. In most patients, the acetylcholine receptor antibody titers declined over 12 months. Reversible renal toxicity and hypertension were noted, and additional side effects included hypertrichosis, increased libido, gum sensitivity, and muscle cramps.[39]

Cyclosporine appears to inhibit the production of interleukin 2 by helper T cells. The onset of improvement is typically in 1 or 2 months, with maximum improvement in 6 months. Most of the patients on cyclosporine seem to require some dose of corticosteroid if they have severe disease, but the steroid-sparing effect can be substantial.[37,38]


## INTRAVENOUS IMMUNOGLOBULIN AND PLASMA EXCHANGE, SEVERE MYASTHENIA, AND MYASTHENIC CRISIS

Regarding treatment with high-dose IVIG as compared with plasma exchange (PE), Ronager et al. reported a clinical effect of high-dose IVIG compared to PE in patients with moderate to severe MG, comparing the two treatments in patients with moderate to severe MG.[40] The study used a randomized crossover design. Twelve patients with generalized, moderately severe MG were on immunosuppressive therapy for at least 3 months; azathioprine, prednisone, or both, with stable dose for 1 month before randomization. One group of patients received IVIG 400 mg/kg per day for 5 consecutive days and were observed for 16 weeks. After 16 weeks, the patients were treated with PE every other day for five exchanges and then observed for the subsequent 16 weeks. The second group of patients was treated initially with PE and later with IVIG. The patients were evaluated using a quantified MG clinical score (QMGS) and were evaluated at 1, 4, 8, and 16 weeks after the end of each treatment. Additional measures included immunoglobulin concentrations, titers of acetylcholine receptor antibodies, and repetitive stimulation studies at baseline and 1 week after each treatment.[40]

The results of this study showed that 1 week after treatment, those who received PE had significantly improved QMGS, whereas such improvement could not be shown 1 week after IVIG treatment. Four weeks after treatment, there was significant improvement in QMGS in both the PE and IVIG groups; 1 week and 4 weeks after treatment, no significant difference between the two treatments was found. A higher number of adverse events was noted during and after IVIG treatment, but the adverse events were relatively minor and transient. On the other hand, with PE, there were less adverse events, but those that occurred included some that were judged to be more serious, including one patient with septicemia and another patient with arterial bleeding. There were no significant changes in the electromyographic studies (repetitive stimulation).[40]

The authors conclude that both treatments have clinically significant benefits in patients with chronic stable MG. In these limited studies, the authors believed that improvement was more rapid after PE compared with IVIG, but that the side effects observed with IVIG were more benign than those seen with PE.[40]

Gajdos and colleagues reported on the clinical trial of PE and high-dose IVIG in MG.[41] Eighty-seven patients with exacerbation of MG were randomized to one of two treatment groups. Group one received PE (n = 41), three exchanges total. The second group received IVIG (n = 46), 0.4 gm/kg per day for 3 days (n = 23) or 5 days (n = 23). The primary end point was the myasthenic muscular score with the change in score from time of randomization to day 15. The results showed that the myasthenic muscular score variation was similar in both the PE and IVIG patient groups, with improved score of 18 points in the PE group and of 15.5 in the IVIG group ($p = .65$). The two different schedules of IVIG administration provided similar degree of improvement, but there was a trend toward reduced improvement in the 5-day group compared with the 3-day group.[41]

Regarding side effects, the PE group had eight patients with side effects, and only one patient in the IVIG group had side effects. The authors concluded that although there was no difference in the efficacy of both treatments, the less frequent side effects in the IVIG group suggest that this is an important alternative therapy for treatment of myasthenic crisis.[41]

Qureshi et al. reported a retrospective multicenter chart review comparing tolerance and efficacy of PE and IVIG in 54 episodes of myasthenic crisis.[42] The decision to treat with PE or IVIG was at the physician's discretion. In this retrospective review, the authors found that PE was somewhat more effective than IVIG with regard to the ability to extubate the patient at 2 weeks and the 1 month functional outcome. However, patients in the PE group had more adverse complications than those receiving IVIG. The complications tended to be hemodynamic in the PE group. The authors concluded that IVIG provided a good alternative treatment, particularly in patients at risk for hemodynamic complications or in those who did not adequately respond to PE, and suggested a formal prospective randomized trial.[42]

Thomas et al. retrospectively reviewed the records of 53 patients having 73 myasthenic crises at Columbia Presbyterian Medical Center from 1983 to 1994.[43] Age at time of crisis was 20–82 years, with a median age of 55 years. Women were more often affected than men at a ratio of 2:1, and the average interval from initial myasthenic symptoms to initial episode of crisis was 8

302   *Clinical Trials in Neurologic Practice*

months. Precipitating factors were headed by infection, typically pneumonia or an upper respiratory infection, which occurred in 38%, whereas in 30% of patients there was no clear-cut precipitating event. In 10% of patients, aspiration seemed to precipitate the myasthenic crisis. Twenty-five percent of patients were extubated by 7 days, 50% by 13 days, and 75% by 1 month; the longest duration of intubation was more than 5 months. There were three independent predictors of prolonged intubation, including a preintubation serum bicarbonate level of 30 mg/dl or less, a peak vital capacity on day 1–6 of postintubation of less than 25 ml/kg, and age older than 50 years. Of the patients intubated longer than 2 weeks, 0% had none of the three risk factors, 21% had one risk factor, 46% had two risk factors, and 88% had three risk factors. Complications in this series of prolonged intubation were atelectasis, anemia, *Clostridia difficile* gastrointestinal infection, and congestive heart failure. Three episodes were fatal leading to an overall mortality rate of 4% (three deaths in 73 crises). Four other patients died after extubation. All deaths were apparently related to multiple medical complications. Of those who survived, half were functionally dependent at home or in a facility at the time of discharge.[43]

The authors emphasize that not only are immunotherapies important in addressing myasthenic crisis, but also that the prevention and management of multiple medical complications is central to optimal outcome for myasthenic crisis. These authors defined *crisis* as respiratory failure requiring mechanical ventilation.[43]

Berrouschot et al. reviewed therapy of myasthenic crisis, reviewing their experience with causes, course, and outcome of 63 myasthenic crises treated by their group over a 26-year period (1970–1995), with an interest in the effect of the following therapeutic modalities: pyridostigmine intravenous, pyridostigmine plus prednisolone, and PE.[44] Of 235 patients with MG treated at the University of Leipzig, 44 experienced myasthenic crises, for a total of 63 presentations. The average annual incidence of myasthenic crisis during this time period in these patients was 2.5%, a figure that was fairly consistent through the 26-year monitoring period. The 44 patients with crisis included 26 women and 18 men with mean age of 43 years. Twenty-five patients had a single crisis, 14 patients had two episodes, four patients had three episodes, and one patient had four episodes. The precipitating factors included myasthenic weakness alone in 32%, respiratory infection in 27%, post-thymectomy in 17%, start of corticosteroid therapy in 5%, overdose of cholinergic drugs in 3%, underdose of cholinergic drugs in 2%, emotional stress in 2%, and no specific cause in 12%. The average time from onset of MG to the occurrence of crisis was a mean of 37 months with a broad range. Fourteen (22%) crises preceded thymectomy, whereas 46% followed thymectomy and 20 occurred in patients who never had thymectomy. Precrisis treatment included pyridostigmine in 33%; pyridostigmine plus azathioprine in 25%; pyridostigmine, azathioprine, and prednisolone in 16%; pyridostigmine and prednisolone in 11%; and neostigmine in 2%. In eight patients (13%), crisis was the first manifestation of MG. The evolution of crisis was 1–3 days from onset of deterioration to requiring mechanical ventilation in 68%, 4–7 days in 22%, and 14–21 days in 10%. Precrisis treatment included increasing medication dosage in 40%, PE in one patient, and an

*Myasthenia Gravis: A Clinical Trials Perspective* 303

unchanged regimen in 58% of patients. The mean duration of mechanical ventilation was 9 days, with an overall range of 2–51 days.[44]

With regard to treatment of crisis, 24 patients received pyridostigmine from 1 to 2 mg per hour, as a continuous intravenous infusion. Eighteen patients received pyridostigmine at 1–2 mg per hour continuous intravenous infusion, along with 100 mg of prednisolone over 5 days, with a subsequent decrease in dosage. Two patients were given azathioprine and one received IVIG. Twenty-one patients received PE every 2 days. A variety of other immunosuppressive drugs was administered in some of these patients as well.[44]

Overall, the three treatment groups showed no significant overall differences in the interval between start of crisis and ventilation, and the outcome in the three groups was similar. After 3 months, all but two patients reached their precrisis status. Eight patients (13%) died during crisis, with the causes being cardiac arrhythmia in six patients, cardiac arrest in five, defibrillation in one, and infection with pneumonia and sepsis after long-term ventilation in two patients. Autopsy was performed on seven of the eight patients, and four were found to have malignant thymoma. One patient had evidence of a viral myocarditis; otherwise, the heart autopsy was normal. The authors emphasized the importance of general support for the patient in crisis with early ventilation, mechanical ventilation, and treatment of infection when present.[44]

## FUTURE OF CLINICAL TRIALS IN MYASTHENIA GRAVIS

The task force for the development of evaluation standards of the Myasthenia Gravis Foundation of America (MGFA), led by Alfred Jaretzki, addressed a long-standing need in the arena of clinical trials in MG.[24] There has been a clear need for universally accepted classifications, grading systems, and methods of analysis for patients undergoing therapy for MG. The task force was formed in 1996 by the Medical Advisory Board of the MGFA with an initial view toward standardizing classification and outcomes for evaluation of thymectomy. The task force recognized that prospective randomized clinical trials, although preferred, may be difficult to perform—particularly with regard to such treatments as thymectomy. Nonetheless, the task force believed that prospective risk-adjusted outcome analysis with a central data bank may be helpful in resolving questions regarding optimal therapy. To do so, a uniform classification system defining the disease with appropriate grading systems and methods of analysis has been developed by the task force. The consensus guidelines are as follows[24]:

- *MGFA clinical classification of MG.* The purpose of the classification is to identify subgroups of patients with clinical features that may be important in defining the illness or appropriate therapy. A quantitative assessment of muscle strength is determined using the quantitative MG score for disease severity and response to therapy is assessed using the MGFA postintervention status along with the quantitative MG score. In addition,

304    *Clinical Trials in Neurologic Practice*

*Table 14.1*    Myasthenia Gravis Foundation of America clinical classification of myasthenia gravis

| | |
|---|---|
| Class I | Any ocular muscle weakness |
| | May have weakness of eye closure |
| | No limb, trunk, oropharyngeal, or respiratory muscle weakness |
| Class II | Mild weakness affecting more than just ocular weakness (may also have ocular muscle weakness of any severity) |
| Class IIa | Predominantly affecting limb and/or axial muscles (may also have lesser involvement of oropharyngeal muscles) |
| Class IIb | Predominantly affecting oropharyngeal and/or respiratory muscles (may also have lesser or equal involvement of limb and/or axial muscles) |
| Class III | Moderate weakness affecting more than just ocular muscles (may also have ocular muscle weakness of any severity) |
| Class IIIa | Predominantly affecting limb and/or axial muscles (may also have lesser involvement of oropharyngeal muscles) |
| Class IIIb | Predominantly affecting oropharyngeal and/or respiratory muscles (may also have lesser or equal involvement of limb and/or axial muscles) |
| Class IV | Severe weakness affecting more than just ocular muscles (may also have ocular muscle weakness of any severity) |
| Class IVa | Predominantly affecting limb and/or axial muscles |
| Class IVb | Predominantly affecting oropharyngeal and/or respiratory muscles (may also have lesser or equal involvement of limb and/or axial muscles) |
| Class V | Defined by intubation with or without mechanical ventilation, except when used in routine postoperative management |

Source: Adapted from A Jaretzki, RJ Barohn, RM Ernstoff, et al. Myasthenia gravis. Recommendations for clinical research standards. Neurology 2000;55:16–23.

the status of treatment or medication is assessed with the therapy status classification.

The task force recommended that the most severely affected muscles be used to define the patient's class and that the most severe pretreatment measurement of the classification be used as the reference point and termed the *maximum severity* to which future clinical status be compared, including the postintervention status. The clinical classification is outlined in Table 14.1.[24]

- *Quantitative MG score for disease severity.* Because a quantitative system is necessary to properly evaluate results of treatment in MG, the task force endorsed the use of the quantitative MG score, as modified by Barohn et al., to be used in all prospective studies of therapy in MG.[45,46] The scoring system tests sentinel muscle groups, noting the time of the examination in relationship to therapy. The quantitative MG score has been assessed with regard to interexaminer reliability, and a formal manual and videotape demonstrating the appropriate use of the test is available.[45,46] The score is not intended to replace the clinical evaluation of the patient in the office setting or to compare severity between patients. The quantitative MG scale is shown in Table 14.2.

*Myasthenia Gravis: A Clinical Trials Perspective* **305**

*Table 14.2*   Quantitative myasthenia gravis (MG) score for disease severity

| Test items weakness | None | Mild | Moderate | Severe |
|---|---|---|---|---|
| Grade | 0 | 1 | 2 | 3 |
| Double vision on lateral gaze, right or left (circle one) (secs) | 61 | 11–60 | 1–10 | Spontaneous |
| Ptosis (upward gaze) (secs) | 61 | 11–60 | 1–10 | Spontaneous |
| Facial muscles | Normal lid closure | Complete, weak, some resistance | Complete, without resistance | Incomplete |
| Swallowing 4 ounces of water ($\frac{1}{2}$ cup) | Normal | Minimal coughing or throat clearing | Severe coughing/ choking or nasal regurgitation | Cannot swallow (test not attempted) |
| Speech after counting aloud from 1 to 50 (onset of dysarthria) | None at 50 | Dysarthria at 30–49 | Dysarthria at 10–29 | Dysarthria at 9 |
| Right arm outstretched (90 degrees sitting) (secs) | 240 | 90–239 | 10–89 | 0–9 |
| Left arm outstretched (90 degrees sitting) (secs) | 240 | 90–239 | 10–89 | 0–9 |
| Vital capacity (% predicted) | ≥ 80 | 65–79 | 50–64 | Less than 50 |
| Right hand grip (kgW): men | ≥ 45 | 15–44 | 5–14 | 0–4 |
| Right hand grip (kgW): women | ≥ 30 | 10–29 | 5–9 | 0–4 |
| Left hand grip (kgW): men | ≥ 35 | 15–34 | 5–14 | 0–4 |
| Left hand grip (kgW): women | ≥ 25 | 10–24 | 5–9 | 0–4 |
| Head, lifted (45 degrees supine) (secs) | 120 | 30–119 | 1–29 | 0 |
| Right leg outstretched (45 degrees supine) (secs) | 100 | 31–99 | 1–30 | 0 |
| Left leg outstretched (45 degrees supine) (secs) | 100 | 31–99 | 1–30 | 0 |
| **Total quantitative MG score (range, 0–39)** | | | | |

kgW = kilogram watt.

Source: Adapted from A Jaretzki, RJ Barohn, RM Ernstoff, et al. Myasthenia gravis. Recommendations for clinical research standards. Neurology 2000;55:16–23.

- *MGFA MG therapy status.* The therapy status for long-term follow-up of MG patients is defined in Table 14.3.
- *MGFA postintervention status.* To clarify clinical status after a specific form of therapy, the MGFA postintervention status has been developed. Postintervention status is as listed in Table 14.4.
- *Grouping by age.* The task force suggested that patients be grouped by decade (e.g., up to 10 years, 11–20 years, 21–30 years).

## 306    Clinical Trials in Neurologic Practice

*Table 14.3*    Myasthenia Gravis Foundation of America therapy status

| NT | No therapy |
|---|---|
| SPT | Status post-thymectomy (record type of resection) |
| CH | Cholinesterase inhibitors |
| PR | Prednisone |
| IM | Immunosuppression therapy other than prednisone (define) |
| PE(a) | Plasma exchange therapy, acute (for exacerbations or preoperative) |
| PE(c) | Plasma exchange therapy, chronic (used on regular basis) |
| IG(a) | IVIG therapy, acute (for exacerbations or preoperative) |
| IG(c) | IVIG therapy, chronic (used on a regular basis) |
| OT | Other forms of therapy (define) |

Source: Adapted from A Jaretzki, RJ Barohn, RM Ernstoff, et al. Myasthenia gravis. Recommendations for clinical research standards. Neurology 2000;55:16–23.

- *Thymic pathology.* The task force recommended that a pathology task force be appointed to address issues of classification of malignant and nonmalignant thymic tissues.
- *Thymectomy classification.* The task force recommended that the goal of thymectomy always be "total thymectomy," as there is a variety of surgical techniques for performance of thymectomy and extent of thymus removal, and overall benefit (as well as complications) may vary. The task force's designation of various thymectomy types for data collection is shown in Table 14.5.
- *Outcomes analysis.*
- *Survival instruments, levels of clinical improvement, quality-of-life instruments, and the need for future development and design of outcome studies.* Quality-of-life instruments, quality-adjusted survival, and cost effectiveness have been emphasized by the task force.[24,47] Details of the outcome analysis may be found in the formal task force report.
- *Data bank.* In addition to the recommendation of performing prospective controlled randomized trials to evaluate therapeutic options, the use of prospective risk-adjusted outcome analysis, in which the clinical information is stored centrally and monitored long term, is recognized by the task force as a method of acquiring important data on clinical course, response to therapy, and outcomes.

The members of the task force for the Development and Evaluation Standards of the Myasthenia Gravis Foundation of America, Incorporated included Alfred Jaretzki, III, MD, Chairman; Richard J. Barohn, MD; Raina M. Ernstoff; Henry J. Kaminski; John C. Keesey; Audrey S. Penn; and Donald B. Sanders, MD.[24]

MG, characterized by a plethora of clinical manifestations and presentations, variable natural course, and a multitude of therapeutic options, will be

*Myasthenia Gravis: A Clinical Trials Perspective* 307

*Table 14.4* Myasthenia Gravis Foundation of America postintervention status

| Status | Definition |
| --- | --- |
| Complete stable remission (CSR) | Patient has had no symptoms or signs of MG for at least 1 year and received no therapy for MG during that time. There is no weakness of any muscle on careful examination by someone skilled in the evaluation of neuromuscular disease. Isolated weakness of eyelid closure is accepted. |
| Pharmacologic remission (PR) | The same criteria as for CSR, except that patient continues to take some form of therapy for MG. Patients receiving cholinesterase inhibitors are excluded. |
| Minimal manifestations (MM) | Patient has no symptoms or functional limitations from MG, but has weakness on examination of some muscles. This class recognizes that some patients who otherwise meet the definition of CSR or PR have weakness that is only detectable by careful examination. |
| MM-0 | Patient has received no MG treatment for at least 1 year. |
| MM-1 | Patient continues to receive some MG treatment but no cholinesterase inhibitors. |
| MM-2 | Patient has received only low-dose cholinesterase inhibitors for at least 1 year. |
| MM-3 | Patient has received cholinesterase inhibitors and some other MG treatment during the past year. |
| Improved (I) | A substantial decrease in pretreatment clinical manifestations or a sustained substantial reduction in MG medications, as defined in the protocol. In prospective studies, this should be defined as a specific decrease in QMG score. |
| Unchanged (U) | No substantial change in pretreatment clinical manifestations or reduction in MG medications as defined in the protocol. In prospective studies, this should be defined in terms of a maximum change in QMG score. |
| Worse (W) | A substantial increase in pretreatment clinical manifestations or a substantial increase in MG medications as defined in the protocol. In prospective studies, this should be defined as a specific increase in QMG score. |
| Exacerbation (E) | Patients who fulfilled criteria of CSR, PR, or MM but subsequently developed clinical findings greater than permitted by these criteria. |
| Died of MG (D of MG) | Patients who died of MG, of complications of MG therapy, or within 30 days after thymectomy. |

MG = myasthenia gravis; QMG = quantitative myasthenia gravis.

Note: The postintervention status definitions are designed to assess the status of MG patients at any time after beginning treatment for MG. Use of this classification requires that specific forms of therapy be recorded separately. When comparing the results of the various thymectomy techniques, the CSR status is recommended as the most definitive measure.

This classification requires a careful neurologic examination by someone skilled in the evaluation of neuromuscular disease. Criteria of change in the status of the patient should be defined in the protocol by quantitative assessment of strength in pertinent or sentinel muscles. A sustained substantial change in medication should also be specifically defined in the protocol. The bundling of postintervention categories is discouraged. If the patient has attained the CSR, PR, or MM status, one of the other five responses should be indicated as well.

Source: Adapted from A Jaretzki, RJ Barohn, RM Ernstoff, et al. Myasthenia gravis. Recommendations for clinical research standards. Neurology 2000;55:16–23.

308   *Clinical Trials in Neurologic Practice*

*Table 14.5*   Thymectomy classification

| Classification | Definition |
| --- | --- |
| T-1 transcervical thymectomy | (a) Basic: This resection uses an intracapsular extraction of the mediastinal thymus via a cervical incision and is limited to the removal of the central cervical-mediastinal lobes (A and B). No other tissue is removed in the neck or mediastinum. |
| T-1 transcervical thymectomy | (b) Extended: The original extended procedure uses a special manubrial retractor for improved exposure of the mediastinum. The mediastinal dissection is extracapsular and includes resection of the visible mediastinal thymus and fat. The neck dissection is limited to removal of the cervical-mediastinal extensions. Variations include the addition of a partial median sternotomy and the associated use of mediastinoscopy. |
| T-2 videoscopic thymectomy | (a) "Classic": This procedure uses unilateral videoscopic exposure of the mediastinum with removal of variable amounts of anterior mediastinal fat. The cervical extensions of the thymus are usually removed from below. |
| T-2 videoscopic thymectomy | (b) "Vatet": This technique uses bilateral thoracoscopic exposure of the mediastinum for improved visualization of both sides of the mediastinum. Extensive removal of the mediastinal thymus and perithymic fat is obtained, the thymus and fat being removed separately. A cervical incision is performed with removal of the cervical thymic lobes and pretracheal fat. |
| T-3 trans-sternal thymectomy | (a) Standard: This technique was originally designed to remove the well-defined central cervical-mediastinal lobes. Although a complete or partial sternotomy may be performed, the resection is more extensive than originally described with removal of all visible mediastinal thymus. The cervical extensions of the thymus are removed from below. A variation of this technique adds a transverse cervical incision with a formal exploration of the neck. |
| T-3 trans-sternal thymectomy | (b) Extended: This procedure is also known as *aggressive trans-sternal thymectomy* and *trans-sternal radical thymectomy*. These resections remove the entire mediastinal thymus and most of the mediastinal perithymic fat. They vary somewhat in extent in the mediastinum and may or may not include all tissue removed by the T-4 techniques. The superior poles of the central lobes of the thymus are removed from below without a formal neck dissection. |
| T-4 transcervical and trans-sternal maximal thymectomy | This procedure is also known as *extended cervicomediastinal thymectomy*. These resections use generous exposure in the neck and a complete median-sternotomy with en bloc removal of all tissue in the neck and mediastinum that anatomically may contain gross and/or microscopic thymus. The resections include removal of both sheets of mediastinal pleura and sharp dissection of the pericardium. |

Source: Adapted from A Jaretzki, RJ Barohn, RM Ernstoff, et al. Myasthenia gravis. Recommendations for clinical research standards. Neurology 2000;55:16–23.

*Myasthenia Gravis: A Clinical Trials Perspective* 309

the target of clinical trials during the twenty-first century, using a standardized approach to classification, management, and outcomes. Those investigators who have tread before us should be congratulated for their efforts and induce the rest of us to use the great wealth of experience and data to enrich our understanding of this disorder.

# REFERENCES

1. Howard FM Jr, Lenin VA, Finley J, et al. Clinical correlations of antibodies that bind, block, or modulate human acetylcholine receptors in myasthenia gravis. Ann N Y Acad Sci 1987;505:526–538.
2. Lacquer L, Weigert C. Beitrage zur Lehre von der Erb'schen krankheit ueber die Erb-sche krankheit (myasthenia gravis). Neurol Zentralblatt 1901;20:594–601.
3. Grob D, Arsura EL, Brunner NG, Namba T. The course of myasthenia gravis and therapies affecting outcome. Ann N Y Acad Sci 1987;505:472–499.
4. Walker MB. Case showing the effect of prostigmin on myasthenia gravis. Proc R Soc Med 1935; 28:759–761.
5. Walker MB. Myasthenia gravis: a case in which fatigue of the forearm muscles could induce paralysis of the extraocular muscles. Proc R Soc Med 1937;31:722.
6. Blalock A, Mason MF, Morgan HJ, Riven SS. Myasthenia gravis in tumors of the thymic region. Report of a case in which tumor was removed. Ann Surg 1939;110:544–561.
7. Kennedy FS, Moersch FP. Myasthenia gravis: a clinical review of 87 cases observed between 1915 and the early part of 1932. Can Med Assoc J 1937;37:217.
8. Oosterhuis HJGH. The natural course of myasthenia gravis: a long term follow up study. J Neurol Neurosurg Psychiatry 1989;52:1121–1127.
9. Bever CT Jr, Aquino AV, Penn AS, et al. Prognosis of ocular myasthenia. Ann Neurol 1983; 14:516–519.
10. Simpson JA. Myasthenia gravis: a personal view of pathogenesis and mechanism, Part 1. Muscle Nerve 1978;1:45–46.
11. Howard FM, Duane DD, Lambert EH, Daube JR. Alternate-day prednisone: preliminary report of a double-blind controlled study. Ann N Y Acad Sci 1976;274:596–607.
12. Patten BM. (Referenced as an article discussant). Keesey J, Buffkin D, Kebo D, et al. Plasma Exchange Alone as Therapy for Myasthenia Gravis. In D Grob (ed), Myasthenia Gravis: Pathophysiology and Management. Ann N Y Acad Sci 1981;377:742.
13. Blalock A. Thymectomy in the treatment of myasthenia gravis. Report of 20 cases. J Thorac Surg 1944;13:316–339.
14. Perlo VP, Arnason B, Poskanzer D, et al. The role of thymectomy in the treatment of myasthenia gravis. Ann N Y Acad Sci 1971;183:308–315.
15. Buckingham JM, Howard FM, Bernatz PE, et al. The value of thymectomy in myasthenia gravis: computer assisted match study. Ann Surg 1976;184:453–458.
16. Eaton LM, Clagett OT. Thymectomy in the treatment of myasthenia gravis. Results in 72 cases compared with 142 cases. JAMA 1950;142:963–967.
17. Jaretzki A, Pen AS, Younger DS, et al. Maximal thymectomy for myasthenia gravis. J Thorac Cardiovasc Surg 1988;95:747–757.
18. Jaretzki A. Thymectomy for myasthenia gravis: analysis of the controversies regarding technique and results. Neurology 1997;48(4):52S–63S.
19. Masoaka A, Negaoka Y, Kotake Y. Distribution of thymic tissue in the anterior mediastinum: current procedures in thymectomy. J Thorac Cardiovasc Surg 1975;70:747–754.
20. Pirskanen R, Matell G, Henze A. Results of transsternal thymectomy after failed transcervical thymectomy. Ann N Y Acad Sci 1987;505:866–867.
21. Schumm JF, Wietholter H, Fateh-Moghadam A, Dichgans J. Thymectomy in myasthenia with pure ocular symptoms. J Neurology Neurosurg Psychiatry 1985;48:332–337.
22. Olanow CW, Lane RJM, Roses AD. Thymectomy in late onset myasthenia gravis. Arch Neurol 1982;39:82–83.

## 310    *Clinical Trials in Neurologic Practice*

23. Gronseth GS, Barohn RJ. Practice parameter: Thymectomy for autoimmune myasthenia gravis (an evidence-based review). Report of the Quality Standards Subcommittee of the American Academy of Neurology. Neurology 2000;55:7–15.
24. Jaretzki A, Barohn RJ, Ernstoff RM, et al. Myasthenia gravis. Recommendations for clinical research standards. Neurology 2000;55:16–23.
25. Kupersmith MJ, Moster M, Bhuiyan S, et al. Beneficial effects of corticosteroids on ocular myasthenia gravis. Arch Neurol 1996;53:802–804.
26. McQuillen MP. Ocular myasthenia gravis. Arch Neurol 1997;54:229.
27. Mount FW. Corticotropin in the treatment of ocular myasthenia. Arch Neurol 1964;11:114–124.
28. Howard FM. Personal communication. 1998.
29. Mertens HG, Balzereit F, Leipert M. The treatment of severe myasthenia gravis with immunosuppressive agents. Eur Neurol 1969;2:323–339.
30. Matell G, Bergstrom K, Franksson C, et al. Effects of some immunosuppressive procedures on myasthenia gravis. Ann N Y Acad Sci 1979;274:659–676.
31. Scherpbier HJ, Oosterhuis HJ. Factors influencing the relapse risk at steroid dose reduction to myasthenia gravis. Clin Neurol Neurosurg 1987;89:145–150.
32. Hohlfeld R, Toyka KV, Besinger UA, et al. Myasthenia gravis: reactivation of clinical disease and of autoimmune factors after discontinuation of long-term azathioprine. Ann Neurol 1985;17:238–242.
33. Miano MA, Bosley TM, Heiman-Patterson TD, et al. Factors influencing outcome of prednisone dose reduction in myasthenia gravis. Neurology 1991;41:919–921.
34. Myasthenia Gravis Clinical Study Group. A randomized clinical trial comparing prednisone and azathioprine in myasthenia gravis. Results of the second interim analysis. J Neurol Neurosurg Psychiatry 1993;56:1157–1163.
35. Palace J, Newsome-Davis J, Lecky B, the Myasthenia Study Group. A multicenter randomized double-blind trial of prednisolone plus azathioprine versus prednisolone plus placebo in myasthenia gravis. Neurology 1996;46:A332.
36. Palace J, Newsome-Davis J, Lecky B, the Myasthenia Gravis Study Group. A randomized double-blind trial of prednisolone alone or with azathioprine in myasthenia gravis. Neurology 1998;50(6):1778–1783.
37. Tindall RSA, Rollins JA, Phillips JT, et al. Preliminary results of a double-blind, randomized, placebo-controlled trial of cyclosporine in myasthenia gravis. N Engl J Med 1987;316:719–724.
38. Tindall RSA, Phillips JT, Rollins JA, et al. A clinical therapeutic trial of cyclosporin in myasthenia gravis. Ann N Y Acad Sci 1993;681:539 551.
39. Goulon M, Elkharrat D, Lokiec F, Gajdos P. Results of a One Year Open Trial of Cyclosporine in 10 Patients with Severe Myasthenia Gravis. In BD Kahan (ed), Cyclosporine Applications in Autoimmune Diseases. Philadelphia: Grune and Stratton, 1988;211–217.
40. Ronager J, Ravnborg M, Vorstrup S. Clinical effect of high-dose intravenous immunoglobulin compared to plasma exchange in patients with moderate to severe myasthenia gravis. American Academy of Neurology 51st Annual Meeting. Scientific Program: Scientific Sessions. 1999; 52(6)S:184–185.
41. Gajdos P, Chevret S, Clair B, et al. Clinical trial of plasma exchange and high-dose intravenous immunoglobulin in myasthenia gravis. Myasthenia Gravis Clinical Study Group. Ann Neurol 1997;41(6):789–796.
42. Qureshi AI, Choundry MA, Akbar MS, et al. Plasma exchange versus intravenous immunoglobulin treatment in myasthenic crisis. Neurology 1999;52:629–632.
43. Thomas CE, Mayer SA, Gungor Y, et al. Myasthenic crisis: clinical features, mortality, complications and risk factors for prolonged intubation. Neurology 1997;48(5)1253–1260.
44. Berrouschot J, Baumann I, Kalischewski P, et al. Therapy of myasthenic crisis. Crit Care Med 1997;25(7):1228–1235.
45. Barohn RJ, McIntire D, Herbelin L, et al. Reliability testing of the quantitative myasthenia score. Ann N Y Acad Sci 1998;841:769–772.
46. Barohn RJ. How to administer the quantitative myasthenia test. Manual and video available through the Myasthenia Gravis Foundation of America, 1996.
47. Wolfe GI, Herbelin JR, Nations SP, et al. Myasthenia gravis activities of daily living profile. Neurology 1999;52(7):1487–1489.

# 15
# Clinical Trials in Muscle Disorders

Renato Mantegazza, Carlo Antozzi, Ferdinando Cornelio, and Stefano Di Donato

Because of the relatively rare occurrence of muscle disorders, and the lack of specific markers to support their diagnosis, clinical trials have not been performed until recently. The application of molecular biology to the investigation of muscle diseases is reshaping the classification of hereditary myopathies; several new disorders, such as ion channel diseases, and mitochondrial and metabolic myopathies, have been identified or better characterized from clinical and pathogenetic standpoints. Moreover, the improvement of neuroimmunologic studies has greatly enhanced our knowledge of autoimmune disorders of the neuromuscular junction and inflammatory myopathies. The advancement promoted by molecular genetics, gene therapy techniques, and neuroimmunologic studies constantly provides new research tools that make clinical trials more feasible in this particular field of neurology.

The main goal of any clinical trial should be to demonstrate that a new therapeutic approach can modify the natural course of the disease or at least improve treatment protocols. To pursue a clinical trial in patients with muscle diseases, the following should be known:

1. The clinicopathologic features and the natural history of the disease
2. The quantitation of muscular deficits
3. The evaluation of functional impairments
4. The definition of primary (and secondary) end points to evaluate the effectiveness of treatments

The knowledge of a given disease's natural history is crucial for its evaluation in the perspective of new treatments. Longitudinal studies are essential for this aim, but most of our knowledge of the clinical course and natural history is derived from cross-sectional and retrospective studies. Because some of the genetically based muscle diseases have a very low prevalence, multicenter studies are needed to identify clinical features and describe the natural history of a disorder. Prospective and quantitative studies of the natural history of muscle diseases

312    *Clinical Trials in Neurologic Practice*

would also provide guidelines to determine sample size and duration of follow-up for clinical trials. Identification of standardized protocols enables us to evaluate patients homogeneously. These protocols should include (1) evaluation of muscle strength by manual muscle testing or maximum voluntary isometric contraction testing, (2) functional testing by ad hoc scales, and (3) laboratory data (e.g., serum or urine tests, muscle biopsy evaluation, lean body mass, muscle imaging). End points may vary considerably according to each muscle disease under investigation; for instance, in boys with Duchenne muscular dystrophy (DMD), the end-point is the time to become wheelchair bound, whereas in myotonic dystrophy two different end points can be considered: lack of myotonia or improvement of muscle weakness.

Because of their relatively low frequency and difficulties in classification, clinical trials have only recently been introduced in the field of muscle diseases when compared to other areas of neurology. However, open and controlled clinical trials have been reported, thereby improving quality in the care of patients with muscle disorders. This review focuses on the three main areas of muscle diseases in which clinical trials have been or are being performed: (1) autoimmune ion channel disorders, (2) inflammatory myopathies, and (3) primary hereditary myopathies.

## AUTOIMMUNE NEUROMUSCULAR ION CHANNEL DISORDERS

This group of autoimmune disorders shares a common pathogenesis, mediated by autoantibodies against different ion channels of motor nerve terminals. Myasthenia gravis (MG) and Lambert-Eaton myasthenic syndrome (LEMS) are due to antibodies to postsynaptic acetylcholine receptors (AChRs) and presynaptic voltage-gated calcium channels, respectively.[1,2] Antibodies against voltage-gated potassium channels have been reported in acquired neuromyotonia.[3,4]

MG is the most commonly observed disease in this group. Its natural course has been modified by the introduction of immunosuppressive drugs and thymectomy.[5-8] According to the features and severity of the disease, and due to ethical reasons, treatments available for MG have been rarely evaluated in a controlled fashion. The introduction of corticosteroids and the improvement of intensive care management have greatly reduced mortality due to respiratory insufficiency. Corticosteroids (e.g., prednisone, prednisolone, and methylprednisolone) are rapidly effective in most MG patients; their efficacy is usually evident within 2 months after the start of a full daily schedule of 1 mg/kg of body weight of prednisone, a dosage that must be slowly tapered to an alternate-day regimen and then slowly reduced to keep the disease under control and minimize side effects.[9] However, it must be emphasized that the required long-term treatment with corticosteroids is often associated with side effects, the severity of which must not be overlooked. Immunosuppressive drugs have been investigated in open and controlled studies with positive results. Among these, azathioprine is the most widely used, due to its low toxicity and good tolerability, although it takes at least 6 months to exert its positive effects.[10,11] The efficacy and steroid-sparing effects of azathioprine have been confirmed by a randomized double-blind placebo-controlled trial comparing prednisolone alone or combined with azathioprine. Patients treated with this combination showed a lower incidence of treatment failures, longer remissions, and fewer side effects.[12] A possible alternative in unresponsive patients is cyclophosphamide, which must be carefully monitored due to its possible side effects.[13] Cyclosporine A was evaluated in a 12-month double-blind randomized placebo-controlled trial that concluded that the drug can be effective in some patients with MG[14]; again, patients must be carefully monitored for signs of nephrotoxicity when doses higher than 6 mg/kg of body weight are used.

Thymectomy has been introduced as a therapeutic measure able to modify the natural history of the disease (i.e., to increase the percentage of remission).[8] The rationale for its use is based on the assumption that the initial sensitization to the AChR and its maintenance might occur in the thymus.[1] The usual approach is through the extended trans-sternal technique, which provides the widest approach to the mediastinum to remove the whole thymus as well as ectopic thymic islets frequently found in the fat tissue extending from the pericardium to the thyroid gland. Although no controlled studies are available, data from open series on several hundreds of patients support the conclusion that thymectomy can modify the natural course of the disease. Thymectomy is performed in the majority of MG patients, and the best response is observed in young patients who show thymic hyperplasia histologically and are operated on early in the course of the disease. We have introduced a new thoracoscopic approach (video-assisted thoracoscopic extended thymectomy) that avoids sternotomy and is more easily tolerated by patients.[15] This new approach allows a detailed, severalfold-magnified observation of the mediastinal space for maximal removal of the thymus and mediastinal fat as reported with the classical extended approach. Results obtained after 2 years of clinical follow-up are in line with, if not better than, findings reported with extended thymectomy.[15]

Plasma exchange has also considerably modified the natural course of MG since its first introduction in 1976.[16] No controlled studies have been reported on plasma exchange alone, but the time-related association between plasmapheresis and clinical improvement has always been considered proof of its efficacy.[16,17] Plasma exchange must be considered as a short-term treatment for severely compromised patients, to avoid worsening of a myasthenic crisis, or as a way to improve muscle strength before thymectomy. In selected patients, it can be taken into consideration as a chronic intermittent therapy in case of inadequate response to pharmacologic therapy. The clinical response to plasma exchange is usually rapid, and the recommended protocols require the removal of at least one plasma volume per session. Each course should consist of at least two exchanges. In our experience, 70% of patients respond to two exchanges (of one plasma volume each) performed every other day.[18] There is no evidence that prolonged, intensive plasma exchange protocols are needed if two courses of two sessions each do not exert any demonstrable effect. The use of plasma exchange in a chronic fashion has not been addressed in detail, and no definite protocols have been established. We have introduced a promising new approach in the apheretic treatment of MG, and that is the use of long-term immunoglobulin G (IgG) immunoadsorption with protein A. Staphylococcal protein A, a component of the bacterial cell wall, has unique properties: It has a very high affinity for human IgG without a significant interaction with other plasma proteins, it is resistant to wide variations in temperature and pH, and it can be easily regenerated. These features make staphylococcal protein A suitable for its extensive reuse as a chromatographic reagent for chronic removal of IgG from

314    *Clinical Trials in Neurologic Practice*

human plasma. We chose this approach to treat selected severely compromised MG patients who failed to respond to prolonged pharmacologic treatment or to plasma exchange or who required frequent exchanges to maintain a satisfactory level of improvement. However, due to the need for fluid replacement, it is difficult to perform intensive plasma exchange protocols for long periods of time. The advantage of staphylococcal protein A over conventional plasma exchange is that it can be continuously regenerated throughout the procedure; this allows the treatment of an unlimited amount of plasma during each session without the need for replacement fluid. Two to three plasma volumes can be exchanged during each session, an amount that cannot be achieved with plasma exchange unless fresh-frozen plasma is given to the patient. We observed a significant improvement in the patients we treated. Interestingly, immunoadsorption was also effective in patients who had not responded to traditional plasma exchange or to high-dose intravenous immunoglobulins (IVIG).[19,20]

IVIG represents an alternative to plasma exchange and shares the same indications. Several uncontrolled series appeared in the literature, and no definite protocols as far as dosage, duration, and definition of response have surfaced.[21] The most widely used protocol is similar to that used in patients with Guillain-Barré syndrome, consisting of five consecutive daily infusions of 400 mg of immunoglobulins per kg of body weight. The majority of patients seemed to improve after IVIG infusion, but the degree of improvement is variable and the onset of improvement is not as rapid as that reported for plasma exchange. Moreover, the association with corticosteroids and immunosuppressive drugs makes the evaluation even more difficult. Only one randomized trial has been reported so far; it compared the efficacy of IVIG to that of plasma exchange in MG patients with acute forms of the disease. The study concluded that IVIG (400 mg/kg per day for 3 or 5 days) was as effective as plasma exchange (three sessions of 1.5 plasma volumes).[22] A positive response to plasma exchange after failure with IVIG has also been reported, although in a small, uncontrolled group of patients.[23] However, IVIG can always be considered as a treatment option for severely compromised patients when plasma exchange is not readily available or feasible due to inadequate vascular access.

LEMS is an antibody-mediated neuromuscular junction disorder in which muscle weakness is caused by reduced calcium-dependent release of acetylcholine from motor nerve terminals due to antibodies to presynaptic voltage-gated P/Q calcium channels.[2] The association with small cell lung cancer has been reported in more than 50% of patients. Removal of the underlying malignancy is often followed by clinical improvement, suggesting a pathogenetic linkage between antigenic determinants on neoplastic tissues and the autoimmune response against calcium channels. A favorable response has also been reported with immunosuppression with corticosteroids and azathioprine and with plasma exchange.[24,25] However, when compared to MG, the response to plasma exchange and immunosuppression is considerably slower. A positive response has also been reported with IVIG. In this regard, a randomized, double-blind placebo-controlled crossover trial has been performed on nine LEMS patients during an 8-week period.[26] A significant improvement of indices of limb, respiratory, and bulbar muscle strength was observed and correlated with the decline of serum calcium channel antibody levels. The peak of clinical improvement was noted after 2–4 weeks and declined after 8 weeks. No controlled trials in large series on the use of plasma exchange in LEMS have been performed. Because LEMS shows a more chronic

*Clinical Trials in Muscle Disorders*   315

course, and response to pharmacologic treatment is not as rapid as observed in MG patients, we consider LEMS a good candidate for chronic IgG immunoadsorption with protein A. We adopted the same treatment protocol reported for MG patients and had promising results that deserve further investigation.[27]

Neuromyotonia is a heterogeneous disorder characterized by continuous muscle fiber activity. Apart from a genetic form,[28] acquired neuromyotonia[29] has been associated with antibodies to voltage-gated potassium channels.[3,4] Evidence for a pathogenic humoral factor has been suggested by the efficacy of plasmapheresis in reducing muscle discharges recorded by electromyography and by passive transfer studies.[3,4,29] These findings indicate that in some forms of neuromyotonia, besides antiepileptic drugs, treatment with plasma exchange and immunosuppressive drugs can be of value in some patients affected with this rare syndrome.[29]

The immunosuppressive approach to autoimmune ion channel disorders can be considered effective in a considerable proportion of patients. However, we must emphasize again that available treatments are sources of severe side effects in the long term, and we are striving for new, less toxic, and more specific therapies. Immunosuppressive drugs exert their effect nonspecifically on the immune system. The ideal approach should therefore inhibit only the pathogenic autoimmune response, leaving the overall function of the immune system unaltered.[6] Novel immunotherapies for autoimmune diseases are an area of active research; promising results have been reported in several models of autoimmune disorders. Different approaches have been investigated with the aim of inhibiting the autoimmune response selectively or specifically. Although the majority of experimental studies has been performed in T-cell–mediated disorders, such as experimental autoimmune encephalitis, adjuvant arthritis, and uveitis or the diabetic mouse,[30] interesting data have been reported in experimental autoimmune MG (EAMG) studies. The aim of these studies is to induce a state of tolerance to the AChR by the administration of the native antigen or its fragments. It has been demonstrated that EAMG can be prevented by the oral administration of AChR purified from Torpedo electroplax tissue, and also that the disease can be prevented or cured by the nasal administration of Torpedo Receptor (TAChR).[31–34] These results have prompted further studies using fragments of the receptor itself, chosen according to the major immunodominant epitopes of the AChR recognized by autoreactive antigen-specific T lymphocytes. These fragments, administered as synthetic peptides via the nasal, subcutaneous, and oral routes, have been effective in the mouse model of EAMG.[35–37] The availability of synthetic peptides and recombinant fragments of the AChR[38] opens new perspectives in the search for new forms of treatment of the experimental disease that will constitute the basis for clinical trials in human MG.

## INFLAMMATORY MYOPATHIES

Inflammatory myopathies (IM) encompass a heterogenous group of disorders in which clinical, histopathologic, and laboratory data define three major entities: polymyositis (PM), dermatomyositis (DM), and inclusion body myositis (IBM).[39] Although several clinical features are shared by the different forms,

316    *Clinical Trials in Neurologic Practice*

pathogenetic mechanisms differ considerably among PM, DM, and IBM. The hallmark of IM is the presence of mononuclear cell infiltrates in muscle tissue. Inflammation involves effector cells (e.g., T or B lymphocytes, macrophages, natural killer cells) and muscle tissue as targets of the immune response. However, the antigen against which the immune response is mounted has not been identified, and the causative agents involved in each form are unknown. Studies based on immunocytochemical analysis of infiltrating mononuclear cells, as well as on molecular biology, have increased our knowledge of the immuno-pathogenetic mechanism underlying IM. Considerable evidence exists on the pivotal role of cytotoxic T lymphocytes in surrounding, invading, and hence, destroying muscle fibers in PM; molecular studies have also shown oligoclonality of endomysial infiltrating CD8[+] cells, and analysis of T-cell receptor rearrangements suggest an antigen-driven selection of cytotoxic T lymphocytes.[40] On the contrary, cells infiltrating muscle tissue in DM are predominantly B lymphocytes, although T lymphocytes can be found. The pathogenic mechanism in DM is mainly a humorally mediated process as demonstrated by the observation of immunoglobulin and complement fraction deposits occluding small vessels and capillaries. This is the basis for the microangiopathy that leads to the ischemic damage of muscle tissue. An antibody or a humoral factor–induced microangiopathy may be the cause of the diagnostic histologic finding of perifascicular atrophy typical of DM.[39] IBM is characterized by a T-cell infiltrate consisting mainly of CD8[+] T lymphocytes and macrophages as observed in PM. In addition to inflammation, the histologic hallmark of IBM is the presence of the typical rimmed vacuoles containing abnormal accumulation of β-amyloid, ubiquitin, and other proteins.[39] Whether this abnormal accumulation is a primary phenomenon or secondary to the inflammatory process is under investigation.

Different pathogenetic mechanisms underlying IM are likely to account for different responses to treatment.[41] Therapies for PM and DM are based on generalized immunosuppression with corticosteroids, immunosuppressive drugs, or a combination of the two, none of which has been investigated in a controlled fashion. On the contrary, IBM is resistant to immunosuppression. Despite the lack of controlled studies, prednisone is the drug of choice in PM and DM. Corticosteroid treatment should be started at full every-day dosage, then tapered to an alternate-day regimen and slowly tapered according to the clinical response. Combination with immunosuppressive drugs is advisable in the case of poor response to prednisone or in the case of severe side effects from corticosteroids. Acting on T-cell function, azathioprine is the immunosuppressive drug most often combined with prednisone. Its slowness of action requires several months of treatment to ascertain its efficacy. An alternative to azathioprine is methotrexate, an antagonist of folate metabolism, which is indicated in patients refractory to prednisone; dosages are usually between 7.5 and 15–25 mg per week. Cyclophosphamide, acting preferentially on B cells, is indicated in steroid-resistant DM, but its side effects must be carefully monitored. Cyclosporine A, an inhibitor of T-cell activation, can be considered in PM-DM patients refractory to first-choice treatments; severe nephrotoxicity may arise with daily doses more than 6 mg/kg of body weight. Treatment of IBM remains disappointing because the disease typically shows no response to immunosuppression with corticosteroids, suggesting that IBM may represent a degenerative muscle disease despite the presence of inflammation.[42] In general, treatment of IM relies on the data from open series, and no controlled studies are available on the use of corticosteroids or immunosuppressive drugs in any IM. On the contrary, controlled studies have been reported on the use of plasma exchange and IVIG in the different forms of IM.

Single case reports or small open studies suggested a positive effect of plasma exchange in IM.[43,44] However, plasma exchange has been more recently investigated in a controlled fashion in patients with PM or DM assigned randomly to plasma exchange, leukopheresis, or sham apheresis in a double-blind study.[45] Patients were submitted to twelve treatments given over a 1-month period. No significant differences were found in the final muscle strength or functional capacity measurements in the three treatment groups. The authors concluded that plasma exchange or leukopheresis is no more effective than sham apheresis for corticosteroid-resistant PM or DM. Although the lack of clinical benefit was clearly demonstrated in this controlled study, a required inclusion criteria for eligible patients was an incomplete response to high-dose prednisone therapy. The efficacy of apheresis should be further investigated, particularly in DM, in cases with a shorter disease duration than those enrolled in the study reported by Miller and coworkers.[45]

High-dose IVIGs has been extensively investigated in IM in open[46,47] and controlled fashion. A double-blind controlled study has been performed in 15 patients with treatment-resistant DM. Included patients were still on prednisone treatment and were assigned to receive one infusion of IVIG or placebo per month for 3 months. Patients were also allowed to cross over to the alternative treatment after 1 month of washout.[48] The authors reported that patients given IVIG had a significant improvement in muscle strength scores and neuromuscular symptoms. Improvement of muscle strength and skin findings were more evident after the second infusion. Muscle biopsies performed after treatment in five patients with a positive outcome showed a reduction of complement deposition in capillaries and a reduced expression of intercellular adhesion molecule 1. These results justify the use of IVIG in cases of poor response to, or treatment failure with, corticosteroid and immunosuppressive drug therapy. However, it must be remembered that improvement with IVIG, as in other immune-mediated disorders, is rather short-lived, usually no more than 8 weeks; this suggests the need for repeated courses in responding patients.[49] IVIG should be considered particularly for juvenile DM, due to the harmful side effects of corticosteroids in growing children.

Data on the use of IVIG in PM rely on small, open observations that suggest a positive effect, but results from controlled studies are awaited.[49]

The effect of IVIG is under investigation in IBM patients, as well. Open studies have provided conflicting results, indicating improvement in some patients and no benefit in others.[50,51] A double-blind, placebo-controlled study in 19 patients has been published.[52] The differences observed in muscle strength in IVIG-treated patients were not significantly different from placebo-treated patients. Despite the lack of effect on limb muscles, the authors report a significant difference in the effect on swallowing muscles assessed by ultrasound. A second double-blind, placebo-controlled study, in which patients were randomized to IVIG plus high-dose steroids or placebo plus steroids, has been undertaken, but results did not show a clear benefit from the combined therapy.[49] Apart from the reduction of inflammatory cells ascribed to corticosteroids, no major

318 *Clinical Trials in Neurologic Practice*

modifications of vacuoles, amyloid deposition, or expression of adhesion molecules was noted in treated patients. These findings give further indirect support to the degenerative features of IBM and leave the therapeutic decisions to be made on a patient-by-patient basis. A considerable amount of attention should be given to the histologic features of these patients at the time of diagnosis because several features are shared by PM and IBM; careful examination of muscle specimens is mandatory before starting any immunosuppressive treatment, because IBM is the most common IM in patients older than 50 years of age. The negative results obtained thus far also emphasize the need for better tools to evaluate muscle strength and function in patients eligible for controlled clinical trials in the field of IM.

A great body of data on the pathogenesis of IM has been reported, but the initiating factors, target antigens, precise function of inflammatory cells, and factors leading to chronic inflammation are largely unknown. Moreover, compared to other autoimmune disorders, no animal model of chronic muscle inflammation comparable to that observed in humans is available. New data have been reported on the role of cytokines and chemokines in IM. Although differences in inflammatory cells have been reported in IM, there are considerable similarities in the expression of such molecules in muscle tissue from IM patients. Cytokines and chemokines are involved in attracting leukocytes from blood vessels to the site of inflammation, and they may have a role in the genesis of muscle weakness and other associated clinical findings that are not directly correlated to the degree of infiltration of muscle tissue by mononuclear cells. A detailed description of chemokine expression in IM muscle is beyond the scope of this review. However, it is worth mentioning that considerable evidence has been produced on the predominant expression of cytokines such as interleukin-1α and -1β and transforming growth factor-β (TGF-β) in muscle from patients with PM, DM, and IBM. Moreover, macrophage inflammatory protein–1α has been reported to be upregulated among chemokines in IM muscle, and evidence exists on the possible pathogenetic contribution of tumor necrosis factor-α in these diseases. The increased expression of interleukin-1 in endothelial cells of capillaries and venules strengthens the pathogenetic role of blood vessels in IM. On the basis of these findings, speculations can be made on the future application of anticytokine therapies to the treatment of IM.[53]

## PRIMARY HEREDITARY MYOPATHIES

Several disorders mentioned in this chapter may be subdivided into the following categories: (1) muscular dystrophies, (2) congenital myopathies, and (3) myotonic syndromes. Because a treatise on the genetics and pathogenetic mechanisms of these diseases is beyond the scope of this review, we focus on the main diseases for which a major effort has been expended to perform clinical trials: the Xp21-linked muscular dystrophies (DMD or Becker muscular dystrophies [BMD]), facioscapulohumeral muscular dystrophy (FSHD), and myotonic dystrophy (MD).

DMD and BMD are X-linked recessive diseases that are characterized by progressive muscular weakness and wasting; DMD confines patients to a wheelchair before the age of 15 years, and the disease terminates fatally near the end of the second decade.[54,55] The severe DMD phenotype is caused by mutations in the dystrophin gene,[56] which lead to the absence of the cytoskeletal protein dystrophin, normally localized at the cytoplasmic face of the sarcolemma of skeletal muscle fibers.[57] In BMD, the benign phenotype is associated with a shorter dystrophin or with its patchy distribution on the sarcolemma. Characteristic histologic findings in DMD and BMD are the degeneration of fibers due to segmental necrosis, regeneration, and excessive connective tissue proliferation.[58] A portion of samples from DMD muscles shows a mononuclear cell infiltrate consisting of macrophages, T lymphocytes, and natural killer cells.[59,60] Large numbers of mast cells at the endomysium of dystrophic muscle were reported in the same area as focal necrosis, suggesting that mast cell degranulation plays a role in inducing myofiber death.[61,62] Moreover, we have demonstrated that fibrosis was significantly more prominent in DMD than BMD, spinal muscular atrophy, or controls. The proportion of connective tissue in muscle biopsies increased progressively with age in DMD, whereas levels of TGF-β1, a potent fibrogenic cytokine, peaked at 2 and 6 years of age. Our findings suggest that TGF-β1 stimulates fibrosis in DMD and that its expression in the early stages of DMD may be critical in initiating muscle fibrosis.[63] On the basis of these specific pathologic muscle alterations, and on the genetic alterations in Xp21-linked muscular dystrophies, the following two modes of treatment that culminated in clinical trials were developed: steroid usage as anti-inflammatory treatment and myoblast transfer.

Starting in 1974, a series of trials were performed using corticosteroids as a treatment for DMD and BMD[64–72]; most of them used prednisone at a dosage ranging from 0.3 to 1.5 mg per kg of body weight per day, but deflazacort and prednisolone were also used. Follow-up ranged from 6 to 36 months; apart from the first report, which determined that prednisone treatment is not effective ("transient and minimal slowing of the disease process in several patients"),[64] most of the other reports defined the results as effective.[65–72] As a whole, corticosteroid treatment can improve muscle force and function or diminish deterioration of muscle function in DMD and BMD. However, a significant problem in the evaluation of these clinical trials, as well as in other muscular dystrophies, is the end points used to evaluate treatment efficacy because the natural history of the disease should be clearly modified. The evaluation of the end points must rely on objective parameters such as manual muscle testing, maximal voluntary isometric contraction testing using a myometer, hand-grip strength by means of a strain gauge, functional tests, lean body mass assessed by dual energy x-ray absorptiometry, and laboratory tests.

Since the identification of the genetic defect of DMD and BMD, the idea of replacing dystrophin has been extensively explored in the animal model (*mdx* mouse) and in a few controlled trials in dystrophic children.[73–79] The rationale behind myoblast transfer relies on the possibility that dystrophin-positive myoblasts injected into muscles of affected patients can fuse with host muscle fibers to form multinucleated cells that are capable of replacing deficient gene products (i.e., a somatic gene therapy). Although this therapy has been proven effective in *mdx* mice, controlled trials involving a single transfer of myoblasts in humans were unsuccessful. Fifty to sixty $\times 10^6$ donor myoblasts were injected in multiple sites in one biceps muscle, the other biceps was injected with placebo. Patients, parents, and investigators were blinded to myoblast transfer procedure; patients received immunosuppression to avoid rejection reactions. Sixty DMD children worldwide were treated by myoblast transfer. Because single transfer was ineffec-

320    *Clinical Trials in Neurologic Practice*

tive for dystrophin replacement, an attempt was made using repetitive monthly cell transfer ($110 \times 10^6$) in 12 DMD boys over a 6-month period.[79] Patients were randomly assigned to receive immunosuppression, and a sham injection was performed in the contralateral arm. No significant difference in muscle strength was noticed in myoblast- and sham-injected arms. Four patients showed dystrophin expression in the injected muscle, although one showed only approximately 10% expression. A pilot study of myoblast transfer was performed in 1998 on three BMD patients who were injected with $60 \times 10^6$ cells into the tibialis anterior muscle while receiving cyclosporine for a period of 1 year; in this study, myoblast transfer did not improve strength of the implanted muscles.[80]

The reasons for the unsatisfactory results with myoblast transfer were as follows: (1) there was limited migration (a few millimeters) of injected myoblasts from local graft sites through the mass of skeletal muscles; (2) the compartmental structure of skeletal muscles further reduced the possibility of myoblast movement within injected muscles; (3) there was generation of an insufficient number of cells to obtain a successful engraftment; because of the aging of the cells generated by successive and continuous passages; (4) injected cells were unable to proceed normally to a myogenic differentiation; and (5) a rejection process was directed against donor myoblasts that may have been mediated by the generation of antidystrophin antibodies[81] or by the partial HLA matching of donor cells. Muscle biopsies from DMD patients involved in myoblast transfer were re-evaluated for dystrophin expression using a fluorescence in situ hybridization: 50% of donor nuclei were found fused into host myofibers, and half of these produced dystrophin. In three patients, more than 10% of the original number of donor cells were still present 6 months after injection. The authors concluded that, although donor myoblasts persisted for several months, their microenvironment influenced whether they fused and expressed dystrophin,[82] which suggests that an appropriate milieu is necessary for successful gene therapy. It should be emphasized that a solution to the processes of engraftment, survival, and proliferation of donor myoblasts into host muscles is of great importance, not only for therapeutic attempts in muscular dystrophy, but also to correct myopathies with metabolic defects.

FSHD is an autosomal-dominant disease in which the genetic defect seems to be associated with a deletion at 4q35. Neither the gene nor the gene product has been identified. Characteristically, facial or shoulder girdle muscles are affected at onset, and sparing of extraocular, pharyngeal, and lingual muscles is observed. Asymmetric involvement of shoulder girdle muscles is the rule, and facial weakness is detectable in 50% of affected family members. The pathologic features of FSHD include myopathic changes; and small angular fibers and moth-eaten fibers may be seen. FSHD is untreatable, and few therapeutic trials have been conducted in this disease. Inflammatory infiltrates can be a pathologic feature frequently observed (in up to 40% of the muscle biopsies) in FSHD, which can give rise to difficulties in making a distinction between an inflammatory myopathy.[83,84] There have been reports of FSHD patients treated with corticosteroids who showed improvement or failure to respond. Because of this, and because in DMD an improvement could be observed after corticosteroid treatment, a pilot open-label trial of prednisone was performed in eight FSHD patients. Prednisone was used at a dosage of 1.5 mg/kg per day and administered for 12 weeks. In this trial, manual muscle testing, maximum voluntary isometric contraction testing, muscle mass examination, and urinary creatinine excretion were assessed. No significant changes in muscle strength or mass could be observed. The study did not have sufficient power or length of follow-up to evaluate whether prednisone might arrest or slow disease progression.[85] Because it has been demonstrated that β2-adrenergic agonists can induce muscle hypertrophy or prevent atrophy in animals after physical or biochemical insults and can improve muscle strength in healthy volunteers, β2-adrenergic agonists have been proposed as a potential treatment in FSHD. An open-label trial of albuterol was conducted in 15 FSHD patients at a dosage of 16 mg per day for 3 months. The primary outcome was lean body mass and muscle strength as evaluated by maximal voluntary isometric contraction testing and manual muscle testing. Albuterol increased lean body mass ($p = .001$) and muscle strength ($p = .05$) with an overall 12% improvement in strength.[86] Albuterol efficacy is being investigated through a larger, randomized, double-blind, placebo-controlled trial.

MD is the most common inherited neuromuscular disease in adults, with an incidence of 1 in 8,000. MD is an autosomal-dominant multisystemic disorder that is characterized mainly by myotonia and progressive muscle weakness.[87] The disorder has been shown to be caused by an increased number of cytosine-thymine-guanine (CTG) repeats in the 3' untranslated region of the myotonic dystrophy protein kinase gene, which codes for the protein myotonin, a member of the protein kinase family. MD protein kinase maps to chromosome 19 (19q13.3).[88–93] Healthy individuals have 5–50 CTG repeats; mildly affected or asymptomatic MD patients have 50–180 repeats, whereas fully affected patients have 200–2,000 CTG repeats.[88,90–92,94] No effective treatment has been established for this disease, although many attempts have been made with diphenylhydantoin, procainamide, taurine, or mexiletine.[95–97]

It has been hypothesized that muscle weakness and wasting in MD are due to a decrease in muscle protein synthesis secondary to insulin resistance.[98,99] On the basis of this hypothesis, a 4-month, randomized, double-blind placebo-controlled study was undertaken to assess whether recombinant human insulin-like growth factor I (rhIGF-I) may overcome the insulin resistance.[100] MD patients were evaluated for glucose tolerance, leucine turnover, body composition, manual muscle strength, and neuromuscular function. Among the treated group, the insulin sensitivity index, insulin action, and glucose increased significantly. Leucine metabolism analysis was indicative of increased protein synthesis. Body weight and lean body mass increased, whereas body fat decreased. Muscle strength and neuromuscular function improved in patients who received more than 70 μg/kg of rhIGF-I. Long-term rhIGF-I treatment seems to induce metabolic and muscle improvement in MD patients when optimally treated. However, symptoms reverted to pretherapy levels as early as 1 month after discontinuation of treatment with rhIGF-I.

It has been reported that, in MD patients, a marked reduction of serum adrenal androgen can be observed when compared to age-matched healthy controls.[101] A 12-month randomized double-blind therapeutic trial of testosterone enanthate (3 mg/kg per week) was performed in 40 MD-affected men. In this study, the muscle mass was increased, but no muscle strength improvement was noted.[102] Because a direct effect of dehydroepiandrosterone sulfate (DHEAS) on smooth muscle cell lines has been observed, a pilot study with DHEAS in MD patients was undertaken; 200 mg per day by IV administration was given for 8 weeks in

322   *Clinical Trials in Neurologic Practice*

11 patients.[103] The following end points were evaluated: activities of daily living score, muscular strength, percussion and grip myotonia, and cardiac arrhythmia. The mean activities of daily living, manual muscle testing, and grasping power scores were significantly improved after 8 weeks of DHEAS treatment in all patients. Improvement of myotonia was seen in eight patients 2–4 weeks after DHEAS treatment. After 8 weeks, four patients exhibited no myotonia, and myotonia was markedly decreased in the other four patients. In the four patients with cardiac involvement, conduction block and premature beats improved. It should be emphasized that clinical improvement persisted long after discontinuation of the 8 weeks of DHEAS treatment. To assess its efficacy properly this study suggests the need for a controlled trial with DHEAS in patients with MD.

## REFERENCES

1. Marx A, Wilisch A, Schultz A, et al. Pathogenesis of myasthenia gravis. Virchows Arch 1997;430:355–364.
2. Engel AG. Myasthenic Syndromes. In AG Engel, C Franzini-Armstrong (eds), Myology (2nd ed). New York: McGraw-Hill, 1994;1798–1835.
3. Sinha SJ, Newsom-Davis J, Mills K, et al. Autoimmune etiology of acquired neuromyotonia (Isaac's syndrome). Lancet 1991;338:75–77.
4. Shillito P, Molenaar PC, Vincent A, et al. Acquired neuromyotonia: evidence for autoantibodies directed against K+ channels of peripheral nerves. Ann Neurol 1995;38:714–722.
5. Grob D, Arsura E, Brunner N, Namba T. The course of myasthenia gravis and therapies affecting outcome. Ann N Y Acad Sci 1987;505:472–499.
6. Drachman DB. Immunotherapy in neuromuscular disorders: current and future strategies. Muscle Nerve 1996;19:1239–1251.
7. Cornelio F, Antozzi C, Mantegazza R, et al. Immunosuppressive treatments: their efficacy on myasthenia gravis patients' outcome and on the natural course of the disease. Ann N Y Acad Sci 1993;681:594–602.
8. Jaretski A III. Thymectomy for myasthenia gravis. Analysis of the controversies regarding technique and results. Neurology 1997;48(Suppl 5):S52–S63.
9. Sghirlanzoni A, Peluchetti D, Mantegazza R, et al. Myasthenia gravis: prolonged treatment with steroids. Neurology 1984;34:170–174.
10. Mantegazza R, Antozzi C, Peluchetti D, et al. Azathioprine as a single drug or in combination with steroids in the treatment of myasthenia gravis. J Neurol 1988;235:449–453.
11. Hohlfeld R, Toyka K, Besinger UA, et al. Myasthenia gravis: reactivation of clinical disease and of autoimmune factors after discontinuation of long-term azathioprine. Ann Neurol 1985;17:238–242.
12. Palace J, Newsom-Davis J, Lecky B, the Myasthenia Gravis Study Group. A randomized double-blind trial of prednisolone alone or with azathioprine in myasthenia gravis. Neurology 1998;50:1778–1783.
13. Niakan E, Harati Y, Rolak LA. Immunosuppressive drug therapy in myasthenia gravis. Arch Neurol 1986;43:155–156.
14. Tindall RSA, Rollins JA, Phillips JT, et al. Preliminary results of a double-blind, randomized, placebo-controlled trial of cyclosporine in myasthenia gravis. N Engl J Med 1987;316:719–724.
15. Mantegazza R, Confalonieri P, Antozzi C. Video-assisted thoracoscopic extended thymectomy (VATET) in myasthenia gravis. Two-year follow-up in 101 patients and comparison with the transsternal approach. Ann N Y Acad Sci 1998;841:749–752.
16. Pinching AJ, Peters DK, Newsom-Davis J. Remission of myasthenia gravis following plasma exchange. Lancet 1976;1373–1376.
17. Dau PC, Lindstrom JM, Cassel CK, et al. Plasmapheresis and immunosuppressive drug therapy in myasthenia gravis. N Engl J Med 1977;297:1134–1140.
18. Antozzi C, Gemma M, Regi B, et al. A short plasma exchange protocol is effective in severe myasthenia gravis. J Neurol 1991;238:103–107.
19. Antozzi C, Berta E, Confalonieri P, et al. Protein-A immunoadsorption in immunosuppression-resistant myasthenia gravis. Lancet 1994:383:124.

## Clinical Trials in Muscle Disorders 323

20. Berta E, Confalonieri P, Simoncini O, et al. Removal of antiacetylcholine receptor antibodies by protein A immunoadsorption in myasthenia gravis. Int J Artif Organs 1994;11:603–608.

21. Howard JF. Intravenous immunoglobulins for the treatment of acquired myasthenia gravis. Neurology 1998;51(Suppl 5):S30–S36.

22. Gajdos P, Chevret S, Clair B, et al. for the Myasthenia Gravis Clinical Study Group. Clinical trial of plasma exchange and high-dose intravenous immunoglobulin in myasthenia gravis. Ann Neurol 1997;41:789–796.

23. Stricker RB, Kwiatkowska BJ, Habis JA, Kiprov DD. Myasthenia gravis: response to plasmapheresis following failure of intravenous immunoglobulins. Arch Neurol 1993;50:837–840.

24. Dau PC, Denys EH. Plasmapheresis and immunosuppressive drug therapy in the Eaton-Lambert syndrome. Ann Neurol 1982;11:570–575.

25. Newsom-Davis J, Murray NMF. Plasma exchange and immunosuppressive drug treatment in the Lambert-Eaton myasthenic syndrome. Neurology 1984;34:480–485.

26. Bain PG, Motomura M, Newsom-Davis J, et al. Effects of intravenous immunoglobulin on muscle weakness and calcium-channel autoantibodies in the Lambert-Eaton myasthenic syndrome. Neurology 1996;47:678–683.

27. Cornelio F, Antozzi C, Confalonieri P, et al. Plasma treatment in disorders of the neuromuscular junction. Ann N Y Acad Sci 1998;841:803–810.

28. Browne DL, Gancher ST, Nutt JG, et al. Episodic ataxia-myokymia syndrome is associated with point mutations in the human potassium channel gene KCNA1. Nat Genet 1994;8:136–140.

29. Newsom-Davis J, Mills KR. Immunological associations of acquired neuromyotonia (Isaacs' syndrome). Report of five cases and literary review. Brain 1993;116:453–469.

30. Hohlfeld H. Immunotherapeutic Strategies. In J Zhang, D Hafler, R Hohlfeld, A Miller (eds), Immunotherapy in Neuroimmunologic Diseases. London: Martin Dunitz, 1998;197–213.

31. Wang ZY, Qiao J, Link H. Suppression of experimental autoimmune myasthenia gravis by oral administration of acetylcholine receptor. J Neuroimmunol 1993;44:209–214.

32. Okumura S, McIntosh K, Drachman DB. Oral administration of acetylcholine receptor: effects on experimental autoimmune myasthenia gravis. Ann Neurol 1994;36:704–713.

33. Ma CG, Zhang GX, Xiao BG, et al. Suppression of experimental autoimmune myasthenia gravis by nasal administration of acetylcholine receptor. J Neuroimmunol 1995;58:51–60.

34. Shi FD, Bai XF, Huang YM, et al. Nasal tolerance in experimental autoimmune myasthenia gravis (EAMG): induction of protective tolerance in primed animals. Clin Exp Immunol 1998;111:506–512.

35. Wu B, Deng C, Goluszko E, Christadoss P. Tolerance to a dominant T cell epitope in the acetylcholine receptor molecule induces epitope spread and suppresses murine myasthenia gravis. J Immunol 1997:159:3016–3023.

36. Karachunski PI, Ostlie NS, Okita DK, Conti-Fine BM. Prevention of experimental myasthenia gravis by nasal administration of synthetic acetylcholine receptor T epitope sequences. J Clin Invest 1997; 100:3027–3035.

37. Antozzi C, Baggi F, Andreetta F, et al. Oral administration of an immunodominant TAChR epitope modulates antigen-specific T cell responses in mice. Ann N Y Acad Sci 1998;841:568–571.

38. Barchan D, Asher O, Tzartos S, et al. Modulation of the anti-acetylcholine receptor response and experimental autoimmune myasthenia gravis by recombinant fragments of the acetylcholine receptor. Eur J Immunol 1998;28:616–624.

39. Mantegazza R, Bernasconi P, Confalonieri P, Cornelio F. Inflammatory myopathies and systemic disorders: a review of immunopathogenetic mechanisms and clinical features. J Neurol 1997;244:177–287.

40. Mantegazza R, Andreetta F, Bernasconi P, et al. Analysis of T cell receptor repertoire of muscle-infiltrating T lymphocytes in polymyositis. Restricted V alpha/beta rearrangements may indicate antigen-driven selection. J Clin Invest 1993;91:2880–2886.

41. Dalakas M. Current treatment of inflammatory myopathies. Curr Opin Rheumatol 1994;6:595–601.

42. Barohn RJ, Amato AA, Sahenk Z, et al. Inclusion body myositis: explanation for poor response to immunosuppressive therapies. Neurology 1995;45:1302–1304.

43. Bennington JL, Dau PC. Patients with polymyositis and dermatomyositis who undergo plasmapheresis therapy. Arch Neurol 1981;38:553–560.

44. Clarke CR, Dyall-Smith T, Mackay IR. Plasma exchange in dermatomyositis/polymyositis: beneficial effects in three cases. J Clin Lab Immunol 1988;27:149–152.

45. Miller FW, Leitman SF, Cronin ME, et al. Controlled trial of plasma exchange and leukapheresis in polymyositis and dermatomyositis. N Engl J Med 1992;326:1380–1384.

46. Sussman GL, Pruzanski W. Treatment of inflammatory myopathy with intravenous gamma globulin. Curr Opin Rheumatol 1995;7:510–515.

47. Mastaglia FL, Phillips BA, Zilko PJ. Immunoglobulin therapy in inflammatory myopathy. J Neurol Neurosurg Psychiatry 1998;65:107–110.

324   *Clinical Trials in Neurologic Practice*

48. Dalakas MC, Illa I, Dambrosia JM, et al. A controlled trial of high-dose intravenous immune glob-ulin infusions as treatment for dermatomyositis. N Engl J Med 1993;329;1993–2000.
49. Dalakas MC. Controlled studies with high-dose intravenous immunoglobulin in the treatment of der-matomyositis, inclusion body myositis and polymyositis. Neurology 1998;51(Suppl 5):S37–S45.
50. Soueidan SA, Dalakas MC. Treatment of inclusion-body myositis with high-dose intravenous immunoglobulin. Neurology 1993;43:876–879.
51. Amato AA, Barohn RJ, Jackson CE, et al. Inclusion body myositis: treatment with intravenous immunoglobulins. Neurology 1994;43:876–879.
52. Dalakas MC, Sonies B, Dambrosia J, et al. Treatment of inclusion body myositis with IVIG: a dou-ble-blind, placebo-controlled study. Neurology 1997;48:712–716.
53. Lundberg IE, Nyberg P. New developments in the role of cytokines and chemokines in inflamma-tory myopathies. Curr Opin Rheumatol 1998;10:521–529.
54. Emery AEH. Duchenne Muscular Dystrophy. In P Harper, M Bobrow (eds), Oxford Monographs on Medical Genetics. Oxford, UK: Oxford University Press, 1987;71–91.
55. Engel AG, Yamamoto M, Fischbeck KH. Dystrophinopathies. In AG Engel, C Franzini-Armstrong (eds), Myology. New York: McGraw-Hill, 1994;1133–1187.
56. Koenig M, Beggs AH, Moyer M, et al. The molecular basis for Duchenne versus Becker muscular dystrophy: correlation of severity with type of deletion. Am J Hum Genet 1989;45:498–506.
57. Hoffman EP, Brown RH, Kunkel LM. Dystrophin: the protein product of the Duchenne muscular dystrophy locus. Cell 1987;51:919–928.
58. Dubowitz V. The Muscular Dystrophy. Muscle Biopsy: A Practical Approach. East Sussex, UK: Baillière Tindall, 1985;l289–1404.
59. McDouall RM, Dunn MJ, Dubowitz V. Nature of the mononuclear infiltrate and the mechanism of muscle damage in juvenile dermatomyositis and Duchenne muscular dystrophy. J Neurol Sci 1990;99:199–217.
60. Arahata K, Engel AG. Monoclonal antibody analysis of mononuclear cells in myopathies. I: Quan-titation of subsets according to diagnosis and sites of accumulation and demonstration and counts of muscle fibers invaded by T cells. Ann Neurol 1984;16:193–208.
61. Gorospe JRM, Tharp MD, Hinckley J, et al. A role for mast cells in the progression of Duchenne muscular dystrophy? Correlations in dystrophin-deficient humans, dogs and mice. J Neurol Sci 1994;122:44–56.
62. Gorospe JRM, Tharp MD, Demitsu T, Hoffman EP. Dystrophin-deficient myofibers are vulnerable to mast cell granule-induced necrosis. Neuromusc Disord 1994;4:325–333.
63. Bernasconi P, Torchiana E, Confalonieri P, et al. Expression of transforming growth factor-β1 in dystrophic patient muscles correlates with fibrosis: pathogenetic role of a fibrogenic cytokine. J Clin Invest 1995;96:1137–1144.
64. Siegel IM, Miller JE, Ray RD. Failure of corticosteroid in the treatment of Duchenne (pseudohy-pertrophic) muscular dystrophy: report on a clinically matched three year double-blind study. Ill Med J 1974;145:32–33.
65. Griggs RC, Moxley RT III, Mendell JR, et al. Prednisone in Duchenne dystrophy. A randomized, controlled study defining the time course and dose response. Arch Neurol 1991;84:383–388.
66. Griggs RC, Moxley RT III, Mendell JR, et al. Duchenne dystrophy: randomized, controlled trial of prednisone (18 months) and azathioprine (12 months). Neurology 1993;43:520–527.
67. Sansome A, Royston P, Dubowitz V. Steroids in Duchenne muscular dystrophy: pilot study of a new low-dosage schedule. Neuromusc Disord 1993;3:567–569.
68. Mesa LE, Dubrovski AL, Corderi J, et al. Steroids in Duchenne muscular dystrophy—Deflazacort trial. Neuromusc Disord 1991;1:261–266.
69. Mendel JR, Moxley RT, Griggs RC, et al. Randomized, double-blind six-month trial of prednisone in Duchenne's muscular dystrophy. N Engl J Med 1989;320:1592–1597.
70. Fenichel GM, Florence J, Pestronk A, et al. Prednisone slows strength decline in Duchenne muscu-lar dystrophy: two-year observation. Neurology 1991;41:166.
71. Backman E, Henriksson KG. Low dose prednisolone treatment in Duchenne and Becker muscular dystrophy. Neuromusc Disord 1995;5:233–241.
72. Angelini C, Pegoraro E, Turella E, et al. Deflazacort in Duchenne dystrophy: study of long-term effect. Muscle Nerve 1994;17:386–391.
73. Gussoni E, Pavlath G, Lanctot AM, et al. Normal dystrophin transcripts detected in Duchenne muscular dystrophy patients after myoblast transplantation. Nature 1992;356:435–438.
74. Karpati G, Ajdukovich D, Arnold D, et al. Myoblast transfer in Duchenne muscular dystrophy. Ann Neurol 1993;34:8–17.
75. Huard J, Bouchard JP, Roy R, et al. Human myoblast transplantation: preliminary results of 4 cases. Muscle Nerve 1992;15:550–560.

## Clinical Trials in Muscle Disorders    325

76. Tremblay JP, Malouin F, Roy R, et al. Results of a triple blind clinical study of myoblast transplantations without immunosuppressive treatment in young boys with Duchenne muscular dystrophy. Cell Transplant 1993;2:99–112.

77. Law PK, Goodwin TG, Fang Q, et al. Feasibility, safety and efficacy of myoblast transfer therapy on Duchenne muscular dystrophy boys. Cell Transplant 1992;1:235–244.

78. Morandi L, Bernasconi P, Gebbia M, et al. Lack of mRNA and dystrophin expression in DMD patients three months after myoblast transfer. Neuromusc Disord 1995,5:291–295.

79. Mendell JR, Kissel JT, Amato AA, et al. Myoblast transfer in the treatment of Duchenne's muscular dystrophy. N Engl J Med 1995;333:832–838.

80. Neumeyer AM, Cros D, McKenna-Yasek D, et al. Pilot study of myoblast transfer in the treatment of Becker muscular dystrophy. Neurology 1998;51:589–592.

81. Huard J, Roy R, Bouchard JP, et al. Human myoblast transplantation between immunohistocompatible donor and recipients produces immune reactions. Transplant Proc 1992;24:3049–3051.

82. Gussoni E, Blau HM, Kunkel LM. The fate of individual myoblasts after transplantation into muscles of DMD patients. Nature Med 1997;3:970–977.

83. Bates D, Stevens JC, Hodgson P. "Polymyositis" with involvement of facial and distal musculature. One form of the facioscapulohumeral syndrome? J Neurol Sci 1973;19:105–108.

84. Munsat TL, Piper D, Cancilla P, et al. Inflammatory myopathy with facioscapulohumeral distribution. Neurology 1972;22:335–347.

85. Tawil R, McDermott MP, Pandya S, et al. A pilot trial of prednisone in facioscapulohumeral muscular dystrophy. Neurology 1997;48:46–49.

86. Kissel JT, McDermott MP, Natarajan R, et al. Pilot trial of albuterol in facioscapulohumeral muscular dystrophy. Neurology 1998;50:1402–1406.

87. Harper PS, Rudel R. Myotonic Dystrophy. In AG Engel, C Franzini-Armstrong (eds), Myology. New York: McGraw-Hill 1994;1192–1219.

88. Aslanidis C, Jansen G, Amemiya C, et al. Cloning of the essential myotonic dystrophy region and mapping of the putative defect. Nature 1992;355:548–551.

89. Brook JD, McCurrach ME, Harley HG, et al. Molecular basis of myotonic dystrophy: expansion of a trinucleotide (CTG) repeat at the 3' end of a transcript encoding a protein kinase family member. Cell 1992;68:799–808.

90. Buxton J, Shelbourne P, Davies J, et al. Detection of an unstable fragment of DNA specific to individuals with myotonic dystrophy. Nature 1992;355:547–548.

91. Harley HG, Brook JD, Rundle SA, et al. Expansion of an unstable DNA region and phenotypic variation in myotonic dystrophy. Nature 1992;355:545–546.

92. Imbert G, Kretz C, Johnson K, Mandel JL. Origin of the expansion mutation in myotonic dystrophy. Nat Genet 1993;4:72–76.

93. Mahadevan M, Tsilfidis C, Sabourin L, et al. Myotonic dystrophy mutation: An unstable CTG repeat in the 3' untranslated region of the gene. Science 1992;255:1253–1255.

94. Fu YH, Pizzuti A, Fenwick RG, et al. An unstable triplet repeat in a gene related to myotonic muscular dystrophy, myotonin protein kinase. Science 1992;255:1256–1258.

95. Munsat TL. Therapy of myotonia. A double-blind evaluation of diphenylhydantoin, procainamide, and placebo. Neurology 1967;17:359–367.

96. Durelli L, Mutani R, Fassio F. The treatment of myotonia: evaluation of chronic oral taurine therapy. Neurology 1983;33:599–603.

97. Pouget J, Serratrice G. Myotonie avec faiblesse musculaire corrigée par l'exercice. Effet thérapeutique de la mexilétine. Rev Neurol 1983;139:665–672.

98. Rennie MJ. Muscle protein turnover and wasting due to injury and disease. Br Med Bull 1985;41:257–264.

99. Griggs RC, Jorefowicz R, Kingstone W, et al. Mechanism of muscle wasting in myotonic dystrophy. Ann Neurol 1990;27:505–512.

100. Vlachopapadopoulou E, Zachwieja JJ, Gertner JM, et al. Metabolic and clinical response to recombinant human insulin-like growth factor I in myotonic dystrophy—A clinical research center study. J Clin Endocrinol Metab 1995;80:3715–3723.

101. Carter JN, Steinbeck KS. Reduced adrenal androgens in patients with myotonic dystrophy. J Clin Endocrinol Metab 1985;60:611–614.

102. Griggs RC, Pandya S, Florence JM, et al. Randomized controlled trial of testosterone in myotonic dystrophy. Neurology 1989;39:219–222.

103. Sugino M, Ohsawa N, Ito T, et al. A pilot study of dehydroepiandrosterone sulfate in myotonic dystrophy. Neurology 1998;51:586–589.

# INDEX

Note: Numbers followed by *f* indicate figures; numbers followed by *t* indicate tables.

Absolute risk reduction, 22
Accidental bias, 10
Acetylcholine, in Alzheimer's disease, 155–156
Activities of daily living, in Alzheimer's disease, 152
Acyclovir
    for herpes simplex virus encephalitis, 245
    for varicella-zoster virus, 245–246
Adenosine antagonists, for tremor, 205
Beta-adrenergic receptor antagonists, for tremor, 203–204
Adrenocorticotropic hormone, for multiple sclerosis, 222–223
Adverse events, in randomized clinical trials, monitoring of, 14
AIDS Clinical Trials Group, 250
Akathisia, 214–215
Albuterol, for facioscapulohumeral muscular dystrophy, 321
Aldose reductase inhibitors, for diabetic neuropathy, 280–282, 281t
α Variable, in sample size calculation, 7–9, 7t
Alprazolam, for tremor, 205
Alzheimer's disease. *See also* Dementia
    behavioral interventions in, 164–165
    behavioral symptoms in, 162–163
    diagnostic criteria for, 148–149
    prevention in, primary and secondary, 164–165
    psychosocial interventions in, 163
    rehabilitation in, 163
    study goals in, 157–158, 158f

therapeutic efficacy in, assessment of, 150–164
    anti-inflammatory agents, 157
    antioxidants, 156
    attenuating potentiation of glutamate toxicity, 156
    cholinergic treatment, 155–156
    crossover design in, 160
    donepezil, 159
    enrichment design in, 160
    estrogens, 157
    free-radical scavengers, 156
    guidelines for, 161–162
    neuroprotective agents, 156
    neurotrophic agents, 156
    parallel group design in, 161
    randomized withdrawal design in, 161
    rivastigmine, 159
    run-in-period in, 161–162
    studies testing slowing of decline, 160
    tetrahydroaminoacridine, 158
    variables and outcome measures in, 150–154
        activities of daily living, 152
        behavioral rating scales, 152–153
        caregiver burden, 153
        clinical global outcome measure, 151–152
        cognitive measures, 150–151
        quality of life, 153–154
        rate of progression to end point, 154
        staging measures, 150
        treatment of, goals of, 150
    variants of, 163–164

327

**328** *Clinical Trials in Neurologic Practice*

Alzheimer's Disease Assessment Scale, 151
American Academy of Neurology, diagnostic criteria for HIV-dementia, 246
American Association of Neurological Surgeons, 77
American Heart Association, Stroke Council of, 63
American Spinal Injury Association, 104
4-Aminopyridine, for spinal cord injury, 113
Amphotericin B, intravenous, vs. fluconazole, for cryptococcal meningitis, 250–251
Ampicillin, for bacterial meningitis, 238–239
Amyotrophy, diabetic, 284
Aneurysm(s)
  rupture of, subarachnoid hemorrhage due to, 63–75. *See also* Subarachnoid hemorrhage, aneurysmal
  ruptured, treatment of, 64
Angioplasty, transluminal balloon, for vasospasm after subarachnoid hemorrhage, 69
Antibiotic(s), prophylactic, for head injury, 92
Anticoagulant(s)
  for acute stroke, 43
  in stroke prevention, 37–38, 39f
Anticonvulsant(s), for head injury, 84–85
Antiepileptic drugs, 121–145. *See also specific drug*
Antifibrinolytic agents, for aneurysmal subarachnoid hemorrhage, 64–65
Anti-inflammatory drugs
  adjuvant, for bacterial meningitis, 241–243
  in Alzheimer's disease, 157
Antimicrobial therapy, empiric, for bacterial meningitis, 238–239
Antimyelin-associated glycoprotein, treatment of, 273t, 274–275
Antimyelin-associated glycoprotein neuropathy, 273–275
Antioxidant(s)
  in Alzheimer's disease, 156
  for head injury, 87–88
Apomorphine, for chorea, 209–210
Asilomar Working Group on Recommendations for Reporting of Clinical Trials in the Biomedical Literature, 21

Aspirin
  dipyridamole with, in stroke prevention, 35–37
  in stroke prevention, 30–32, 31t
  vs. clopidogrel, in stroke prevention, 34–35, 36t
  vs. ticlopidine, in stroke prevention, 32–34
  vs. warfarin, in stroke prevention, 37–38, 39f
Aspirin Myocardial Infarction Study, 20
Asymptomatic Carotic Atherosclerosis Study, 20, 46t–47t
Asymptomatic Carotid Atherosclerosis Study, 41–42
Athetosis, 214–215
Atovaquone, for toxoplasma encephalitis, 254
Autoimmune neuromuscular ion channel disorders, 312–315
Azathioprine
  for chronic inflammatory demyelinating neuropathy, 270, 271t
  for inflammatory myopathies, 316
  for multiple sclerosis, 231
  for myasthenia gravis, 299, 312–313
  vs. corticosteroid, for myasthenia gravis, 299

Bacterial meningitis, 238–243
  anti-inflammatory therapy for, adjuvant, 241–243
  cefepime for, 241
  corticosteroids for, 242–243
  dexamethasone for, 239–240, 242–243
  empiric antimicrobial therapy for, 238–239
  meropenem for, 240–241
  vancomycin for, 239–240
Balloon angioplasty, transluminal, for vasospasm after subarachnoid hemorrhage. *See* Vasospasm, after aneurysmal subarachnoid hemorrhage, prevention and treatment of, transluminal balloon angioplasty in
Barbiturate(s)
  for head injury, 85–86
  for intracerebral hemorrhage, 53
Becker muscular dystrophy, 318–320
Behavioral rating scales, in Alzheimer's disease, 152–153
Benserazide, for Parkinson's disease, 175–176

Benzodiazepine(s), for tremor, 205
β Variable, in sample size calculation, 7–9, 7t
Betaferon, for multiple sclerosis, 224–225, 226–227
Bias
  accidental, 10
  in randomized clinical trials, 19
  selection, 10
Biopsy, brain, for herpes simplex virus encephalitis, 244–245
Blinding, in randomized clinical trials, 11–13
Blocked randomization, 11
Botulinum toxin type A, for tremor, 205
Brain biopsy, for herpes simplex virus encephalitis, 244–245
Brain Trauma Foundation, 77
Bromocriptine, for Parkinson's disease, 180

Cabergoline, for Parkinson's disease, 182–183
Calcium antagonists, for vasospasm after subarachnoid hemorrhage, 65–66
Calcium channel blockers
  for head injury, 86–87
  for tremor, 205
California Collaborative Treatment Group, 250
Canadian Aspirin Sulfinpyrazone Transient Ischemic Attack trial, 5
Canadian Cooperative Study Group Randomized Trial of Aspirin and Sulfinpyrazone in Threatened Stroke, 30–32, 31t, 46t–47t
Cannabidiol, for chorea, 211
CAPRIE trial (Clopidogrel versus Aspirin in Patients at Risk of Ischemic Events Trial), 22, 34–35, 36t, 46t–47t
Carbamazepine
  for epilepsy, 124–125
  for head injury, 84–85
  vs. gabapentin, for epilepsy, 129
  vs. lamotrigine, for epilepsy, 131
  vs. oxcarbazepine, for epilepsy, 133
  vs. phenobarbital, for epilepsy, 122–123
  vs. valproate, for epilepsy, 126
  vs. zonisamide, for epilepsy, 140
Carbidopa, for Parkinson's disease, 175–176
Cardiac Arrhythmia Suppression Trial, 16

Caregiver burden, in Alzheimer's disease, 153
Carotid endarterectomy, in stroke prevention, 40–42
Catechol-O-methyltransferase inhibitors, in Parkinson's disease, 184–187. See also specific inhibitor
Cefepime, for bacterial meningitis, 241
Cefotaxime
  for bacterial meningitis, 238–239
  vs. meropenem, for bacterial meningitis, 240–241
Ceftriaxone
  for bacterial meningitis, 238–239
  for chemoprophylaxis, 244
  vs. meropenem, for bacterial meningitis, 240–241
Cefuroxime, for head injury, 92
Central nervous system (CNS)
  infections of, 237–259. See also specific infection
    bacterial meningitis, 238–243
    chemoprophylaxis for, 243–244
    herpes simplex virus encephalitis, 244–246
    HIV, 246–255. See also Human immunodeficiency virus (HIV)
    varicella-zoster virus, 244–246
  lymphoma of, primary, 252–255
    treatment of, 254–255
Cephalosporin(s)
  for bacterial meningitis, 238–239
  vs. meropenem, for bacterial meningitis, 241
Chemoprophylaxis, 243–244
Chemotherapy, for primary CNS lymphoma, 254
Chlorambucil
  for antimyelin-associated glycoprotein neuropathy, 273t, 274
  for neuropathies with monoclonal gammopathy of uncertain significance, 276
Chloramphenicol, for bacterial meningitis, 238–239
Cholinergic hypothesis, in Alzheimer's disease, 155–156
Cholinesterase inhibitors, for myasthenia gravis, 297
Chorea, 207–211. See also Huntington's chorea
  diagnosis of, 208–209
  receptor types in, 209
  treatment of, 209–211

## 330   *Clinical Trials in Neurologic Practice*

Chronic inflammatory demyelinating neur-
    opathy, 267–270
  treatment of
    azathioprine, 270, 271t
    corticosteroids, 267, 268t
    cyclophosphamide, 270
    intravenous immunoglobulin,
        268–270, 270t
    plasma exchange, 267–268, 269t
Cilostazol, for diabetic neuropathy, 284
Cladribine, for multiple sclerosis, 231–232
Clindamycin, for toxoplasma encephalitis,
    254
Clinician's Interview-Based Impression of
    Change (CIBIC), in Alzhei-
    mer's disease, 151–152
Clinician's Interview-Based Impression of
    Change-Plus (CIBIC-Plus),
    in Alzheimer's disease, 152
Clonazepam
  for chorea, 210
  tremor and, 207
  vs. carbamazepine, for epilepsy, 125
Clonidine
  for tics, 212
  tremor and, 207
Clopidogrel, in stroke prevention, 34–35,
    36t
Clopidogrel versus Aspirin in Patients at
    Risk of Ischemic Events Trial,
    22, 34–35, 36t, 46t–47t
Close contacts, defined, 244
Clozapine
  for chorea, 208, 209
  for tremor, 204–205
CNS. *See* Central nervous system (CNS)
Coenzyme Q$_{10}$, for chorea, 210–211
Cognitive measures, in Alzheimer's disease,
    150–151
Coiling, for aneurysmal subarachnoid hem-
    orrhage, 64
Compliance, in randomized clinical trials,
    monitoring of, 15
Computed tomography (CT)
  for intracerebral hemorrhage, 55–57,
    56t
  in primary CNS lymphoma vs. toxo-
    plasma encephalitis, 252–253
Consent, informed, in dementia, 166
Consolidated Standards of Reporting Trials,
    21
CONSORT statement, 21
Construct validity, 17–18
Content validity, 17

Control groups, types of, in randomized
    clinical trials, 28, 28t
Copolymer 1, for multiple sclerosis,
    229–230
Coronary Drug Project, 19–20
Corticosteroid(s)
  for bacterial meningitis, 242–243
  for chronic inflammatory demyelinating
    neuropathy, 267, 268t
  for facioscapulohumeral muscular dys-
    trophy, 320–321
  for Guillain-Barré syndrome, 266–267,
    266t
  for head injury, 87
  for intracerebral hemorrhage, 50–51
  for multifocal motor neuropathy, 271
  for myasthenia gravis, 298, 312
  for Xp21-linked muscular dystrophies,
    319
  vs. azathioprine, for myasthenia gravis,
    299
Corticosteroid Randomization After Signifi-
    cant Head Injury Trial, 87
Craniotomy, for intracerebral hemorrhage,
    54–57
Criterion-related validity, 17
Cronbach's alpha, 17
Crossover design, 5–6, 6f
  in Alzheimer's disease, 160
Cryptococcal meningitis, 250–251
Cyclophosphamide
  for antimyelin-associated glycoprotein
    neuropathy, 273t, 274
  for chronic inflammatory demyelinating
    neuropathy, 270
  for inflammatory myopathies, 316
  for multifocal motor neuropathy,
    271–272
  for multiple sclerosis, 231
Cyclosporine, for myasthenia gravis, 300,
    313
Cytarabine, for progressive multifocal leu-
    koencephalopathy, 249
Cytomegalovirus encephalitis, 251–252

Danaparoid, for acute stroke, 43
Data, missing, in randomized clinical trials,
    14
Data analysis, in randomized clinical trials.
    *See* Randomized clinical trials,
    data analysis in
Data collection, in randomized clinical tri-
    als, 13–14
Deanol, for chorea, 211

*Index* 331

Deep brain stimulation
of globus pallidus interna, for Parkinson's
disease, 190
of subthalamic nucleus, for Parkinson's
disease, 191
thalamic, for Parkinson's disease, 188
Dehydroepiandrosterone sulfate, for myotonic dystrophy, 321–322
δ Variable, in sample size calculation, 7–9,
7t
Dementia, 147–172. *See also* Alzheimer's
disease
defined, 148
diagnostic criteria for, 148–149
ethical issues in, 165–166
frontotemporal, 164
history of clinical trials in, 149
incidence of, 147
informed consent in, 166
with Lewy bodies, 147, 163
origins of, 147
prevalence of, 147
vascular, 164
diagnostic criteria for, 149
Deprenyl, for Parkinson's disease,
177–179
Deprenyl and Tocopherol Antioxidative
Therapy of Parkinsonism,
177–178
Dermatomyositis, 315–318. *See also* Inclusion body myositis; Myopa-
thy(ies), inflammatory;
Polymyositis
Dexamethasone
for bacterial meningitis, 242–243
for intracerebral hemorrhage, 49–51, 50t
vancomycin with, for bacterial meningitis, 239–240
Diabetes Control and Complications Trial
Research Group, 277
Diabetic amyotrophy, 284
Diabetic lumbosacral radiculoplexus neuropathy, 284, 285t
Diabetic neuropathy, 276–284
aldose reductase inhibitors for, 280–282,
281t
diabetic lumbosacral radiculoplexus neuropathy in, 284, 285t
glycemic control in, 277–280, 277t
investigational therapies for, 283–284
myoinositol for, 282
pancreatic transplantation in, 278–280,
279t
pathogenesis of, 276–277

trophic factors for, 282, 283t
types of, 276
Didanosine, for HIV-dementia, 247–248
Dipyridamole, aspirin with, in stroke pre-
vention, 35–37
Diuretic(s), osmotic, for intracerebral hem-
orrhage, 53
Donepezil, for Alzheimer's disease, 159
Dopa-decarboxylase inhibitors, peripheral,
for Parkinson's disease,
175–176
Dopamine agonists, for Parkinson's disease,
179–184. *See also specific drug*
Double-blind study, 12
Drug holiday, levodopa and, 175
Dystonia, 214–215
Dystrophy(ies). *See specific type*

EC/IC Bypass Study Group, 38–40, 40t,
46t–47t
Effect size, calculation of, responsiveness
and, 18, 18t
Encephalitis
cytomegalovirus, 251–252
herpes simplex virus, 244–246
toxoplasma, 252–255
Endarterectomy, carotid, in stroke preven-
tion, 40–42
Endothelin receptor antagonists, for vaso-
spasm after subarachnoid hem-
orrhage, 71–72
Enrichment design, in Alzheimer's disease,
160
Entacapone, for Parkinson's disease,
186–187
Epilepsy, drugs for. *See* Antiepileptic drugs
Equivalency studies, 2
Estrogen, in Alzheimer's disease, 157
Ethanol, for tremor, 204
Ethical issues, in dementia, 165–166
Ethosuximide, vs. valproate, for epilepsy,
126
European Medical Evaluating Agency, 150
European Stroke Prevention Study 2, 12,
46t–47t
European Stroke Prevention Study Group,
35–37
Extracranial-intracranial (EC/IC) arterial
bypass, in stroke prevention.
*See* Stroke prevention, surgery
in, extracranial-intracranial
(EC/IC) arterial bypass

Face validity, 17

Facioscapulohumeral muscular dystrophy,
320–321
Factorial design, 5
Famciclovir, for varicella-zoster virus,
246
Felbamate, for epilepsy,
127–128
Fetal nigral grafts, for Parkinson's disease,
191–192
Fibrinolytic therapy, intracisternal, for
vasospasm after subarachnoid
hemorrhage, 70–71
Fluconazole, vs. intravenous amphotericin
B, for cryptococcal meningitis,
250–251
Flucytosine, for cryptococcal meningitis,
250–251
Fludarabine, for antimyelin-associated glycoprotein neuropathy, 273t,
274
Flunarizine
for tics, 213
for tremor, 205
Flutamide, for tics, 213
Folinic acid, for toxoplasma encephalitis,
253–254
Foscarnet, for cytomegalovirus encephalitis,
252
Free-radical scavengers
for head injury, 87–88
in Alzheimer's disease, 156
Frontotemporal dementia, 164

Gabapentin
for epilepsy, 128–130
tremor and, 206–207
Gacyclidine, for spinal cord injury,
108t–109t, 110
Gammopathy, monoclonal, neuropathies
with, of uncertain significance,
275–276
Ganciclovir, intravenous, for cytomegalovirus encephalitis, 252
Ganglioside(s), GM-1, for spinal cord
injury, 108t–109t, 110
Gilles de la Tourette, 212–214. See also
Pimozide; Tic(s)
Glasgow Coma Scale, 81
Glasgow Outcome Scale, 83
Glatiramer acetate, for multiple sclerosis,
229–230
Globus pallidus interna
stimulation of
for Parkinson's disease, 190

vs. subthalamic nucleus deep brain
stimulation, for Parkinson's
disease, 191
surgery on, for Parkinson's disease,
189–190
Glutamate, toxicity of, attenuating potentiation of, in Alzheimer's disease,
156
Glycemic control, in diabetic neuropathy,
277–280, 277t
Glycerol, for intracerebral hemorrhage, 49,
50t, 51
Glycoprotein, antimyelin-associated, treatment of, 273t, 274–275
Glycoprotein neuropathy, antimyelin-associated, 273–275
GM-1 ganglioside, for spinal cord injury,
108t–109t, 110
Graft(s), tissue, for Parkinson's disease,
191–192
Guillain-Barré syndrome, 263–267
Hughes' six-grade disability scale for,
263, 263t
treatment of
corticosteroids, 266–267, 266t
intravenous immunoglobulin vs.
plasma exchange, 265–266,
265t
overview of, 264
plasma exchange, 264–265, 264t

*Haemophilus influenzae* type B. *See* Bacterial meningitis
Haloperidol
for tics, 213
vs. pimozide, for tics, 212
Head injury, 77–98. *See also* Traumatic
brain injury
anticonvulsants for, 84–85
antioxidants for, 87–88
barbiturates for, 85–86
calcium channel blockers for, 86–87
corticosteroids for, 87
critical assessment of clinical trials of,
80–84
data collection sources for clinical trials
of, 78–79, 78t, 79f
free radical scavengers for, 87–88
gastric protection in, 92–93
hypertonic saline for, 90–91
hyperventilation for, 88–89
hypothermia for, 89–90
immune response in, 92–93
infection control in, 92–93

mannitol for, 90–91
mortality of, 77
neuropsychologic therapy for, 93–94
nutrition in, 91–92
prevention of, 93
sedation in, 93
standards of clinical care in, 77
Head Injury Trials, 86–87
Head position, in intracerebral hemorrhage, 52
Health-related quality of life, assessment of, in randomized clinical trials, 16–18
Helmet(s), in head injury prevention, 93
Hemodilution
for intracerebral hemorrhage, 51–52
for vasospasm after subarachnoid hemorrhage, 66–68
Hemorrhage
intracerebral. *See* Intracerebral hemorrhage
subarachnoid, aneurysmal. *See* Subarachnoid hemorrhage, aneurysmal
Heparin, for acute stroke, 43
Herpes simplex virus encephalitis, 244–246
acyclovir for, 245
HIV. *See* Human immunodeficiency virus (HIV)
HIV-dementia, 246–249
American Academy of Neurology's diagnostic criteria for, 246
treatment of, 247–248
Hughes' six-grade disability scale. *See* Guillain-Barré syndrome
Human immunodeficiency virus (HIV), 246–255. *See also* Central nervous system (CNS), HIV
combination drug therapy for, 248
cryptococcal meningitis in, 250–251
cytomegalovirus encephalitis in, 251–252
dementia in, 246–249
American Academy of Neurology's diagnostic criteria for, 246
treatment of, 247–248
primary CNS lymphoma in, 252–255
progressive multifocal leukoencephalopathy in, 249–250
toxoplasma encephalitis in, 252–255
treatment of, 247–248
Huntingtin, 211
Huntingtin-associated protein, 211
Huntington's chorea, 207–211. *See also* Chorea
Hyperexplexia, 214–215

Hyperglycemia, in head injury, 92
Hyperkinetic movement disorders, 201–219. *See also specific disorder*
Hypertension
in intracerebral hemorrhage, 52
in vasospasm after subarachnoid hemorrhage, 66–68
Hyperthermia, in intracerebral hemorrhage, 52
Hypertonic saline, for head injury, 90–91
Hyperventilation
in head injury, 88–89
in intracerebral hemorrhage, 53
Hypervolemia, in vasospasm after subarachnoid hemorrhage, 66–68
Hypotension, in spinal cord injury, 102–103
Hypothermia
in head injury, 89–90
in intracerebral hemorrhage, 52
Hypothesis, in randomized clinical trials, 2
Hypoxia, in intracerebral hemorrhage, 52

Immune system, response of, head injury and, 92–93
Immunoglobulin, intravenous
for antimyelin-associated glycoprotein neuropathy, 273–274, 273t
for inflammatory myopathies, 317–318
for Lambert-Eaton myasthenic syndrome (LEMS), 314–315
for multifocal motor neuropathy, 271, 272t
for multiple sclerosis, 230–231
for myasthenia gravis, 314
vs. plasma exchange
for chronic inflammatory demyelinating neuropathy, 268–270, 270t
in Guillain-Barré syndrome, 265–266, 265t
for myasthenia gravis, 300–301
Immunosuppressive drugs, for multiple sclerosis, 231–232. *See also specific drug*
Inclusion body myositis, 315–318. *See also* Dermatomyositis; Myopathy(ies), inflammatory; Polymyositis
Indinavir, lamivudine and zidovudine with, for HIV, 248
Infection(s), head injury and, 92–93
Informed consent, in dementia, 166
Injury(ies). *See specific type*

## 334　Clinical Trials in Neurologic Practice

Insulin-like growth factor 1, for head injury, 92

Intention to treat, 33

Interferon-γ, for multiple sclerosis, 223–228, 224t
　therapeutic approaches with, 228–229

Interleukin-1, for bacterial meningitis, 241–242

International Cooperative Study on Timing of Aneurysm Surgery, 64

International League Against Epilepsy, 121

International Medical Society of Paraplegia, 104

International normalized ratio (INR), 37–38

International Subarachnoid Aneurysm Trial, 64

International Working Group on Harmonization of Dementia Drug Guidelines, 165, 166

Intracerebral hemorrhage, 49–62
　increased intracranial pressure in, 49–53, 50t
　management of
　　barbiturates, 53
　　continuous intracranial pressure monitoring in, 53
　　corticosteroids in, 50–51
　　glycerol, 51
　　hemodilution in, 51–52
　　osmotic diuretics, 53
　　surgical
　　　novel techniques in, 59–61
　　　vs. nonsurgical, 54–59
　　　　nonrandomized clinical trials, 54–57, 54t, 56t
　　　　randomized clinical trials, 57–59, 58t

Intracranial pressure
　continuous monitoring of, in intracerebral hemorrhage, 53
　increased, prevention and treatment of, in intracerebral hemorrhage, 49–53, 50t

Isoniazid, for tremor, 205

Italian Haemodilution Trial, 52

Itraconazole, for cryptococcal meningitis, 250

Joint Study of Extracranial Arterial Occlusion, 19

Kaplan-Meier graphs, in stroke clinical trials, 27

Lambert-Eaton myasthenic syndrome, 314–315

Lamivudine, indinavir and zidovudine with, for HIV, 248

Lamotrigine, for epilepsy, 130–132

Leg(s), painful, 214–215

Lennox-Gastaut syndrome, 127–128, 132, 137, 140

Leukoencephalopathy, progressive multifocal, 249–250

Levodopa
　for Parkinson's disease, 174–177
　　controlled release vs. immediate release preparations of, 176–177
　　mortality associated with, 174–175
　　peripheral dopa-decarboxylase inhibitors and, 175–176
　　toxic effect of, 174–175
　　vs. deprenyl, for Parkinson's disease, 178–179
　　vs. dopamine agonists, for Parkinson's disease, 179–184
　　vs. entacapone, for Parkinson's disease, 186–187
　　vs. tolcapone, for Parkinson's disease, 184–186

Lewy bodies, dementia with. *See* Dementia, with Lewy bodies

γ-Linolenic acid, for diabetic neuropathy, 283

Linomide, for multiple sclerosis, 232

α-Lipoic, for diabetic neuropathy, 283–284

Lithium, for chorea, 211

Lymphoma, of primary CNS, 252–255
　treatment of, 254–255

Magnetic resonance imaging (MRI)
　in multiple sclerosis, 221
　in primary CNS lymphoma vs. toxoplasma encephalitis, 252–253

Mannitol
　for head injury, 85–86, 90–91
　for intracerebral hemorrhage, 53

Meningitis
　bacterial. *See* Bacterial meningitis
　cryptococcal, 250–251

Meropenem, for bacterial meningitis, 240–241

Methazolamide, tremor and, 206

Methotrexate
　for inflammatory myopathies, 316
　for multiple sclerosis, 231

Methylphenidate, for head injury, 93–94

Methylprednisolone
  for multiple sclerosis, 222–223
  for spinal cord injury, 107–110,
        108t–109t
Michigan Diabetic Neuropathy Score,
        262–263
Milacemide, for chorea, 210
Minimally important difference, calculation
        of, responsiveness and,
        18, 18t
Mitoxantrone, for multiple sclerosis, 231
Model Spinal Cord Injury System Program,
        103
Monoclonal anti-TNF-$\alpha$ antibody, for multiple
        sclerosis, 232
Monoclonal gammopathy, neuropathies
        with, of uncertain significance,
        275–276
Morphine sulfate, in head injury, 93
Movement disorders, hyperkinetic,
        201–219. *See also specific disorder*
Moving toes, 214–215
MRI. *See* Magnetic resonance imaging
        (MRI)
Multicenter AIDS Cohort Study, 246–247
Multifocal motor neuropathy, 270–272
  treatment of, 271–272, 272t
Multiple comparisons, in randomized clinical
        trials, 20
Multiple sclerosis, 221–236
  acute relapse in, management of,
        222–229
    adrenocorticotropic hormone for,
        222–223
    interferon-$\gamma$ for, 223–228, 224t
      therapeutic approaches with,
        228–229
    methylprednisolone for, 222–223
  glatiramer acetate for, 229–230
  immunosuppressive treatments for,
        231–232
  intravenous immunoglobulin for,
        230–231
  methodology of clinical trials in, limitations
        of, 232–233
  MRI in, 221
Muscle disorders, 311–325. *See also specific disorder*
  autoimmune neuromuscular ion channel
        disorders, 312–315
  inflammatory myopathies, 315–318
  primary hereditary myopathies,
        318–322

Muscular dystrophy(ies)
  Becker, 318–320
  facioscapulohumeral, 320–321
  Xp21-linked, 318–320
Myasthenia gravis, 293–310, 312–314
  clinical manifestations of, 293–294
  diseases associated with, 293
  future of clinical trials in, 303–306
  Myasthenia Gravis Foundation of America
        clinical classification of,
        303, 304t
  Myasthenia Gravis Foundation of America
        postintervention status of,
        305, 307t
  Myasthenia Gravis Foundation of America
        therapy status of, 305, 306t
  myasthenic crisis in, 300–303
  natural course of, 294–295
  prevalence of, 293
  quantitative score for disease severity,
        304–305, 305t
  severe, 300–303
  thymectomy for, classification of, 306,
        308t
  treatment of, 295–300, 312–314
    azathioprine, 298
    cholinesterase inhibitors, 297
    corticosteroids, 297
      vs. azathioprine, 299
    cyclosporine, 299–300
    intravenous immunoglobulin vs.
        plasma exchange, 300–301
    thymectomy, 295–297
Myasthenia Gravis Foundation of America
  in clinical classification of myasthenia
        gravis, 303, 304t
  in postintervention status, 305, 307t
  in therapy status, 305, 306t
Myasthenic crisis, 300–303
Mycosis Study Group, 250
Myoblast transfer, for Xp21–linked muscular
        dystrophies, 319–320
Myoclonus, 214–215
Myoinositol, for diabetic neuropathy, 282
Myopathy(ies)
  inflammatory, 315–318. *See also* Dermatomyositis; Inclusion body
        myositis; Polymyositis
    characteristics of, 316
    pathogenesis of, 318
    treatment of, 316–318
  primary hereditary, 318–322. *See also specific type*
Myotonic dystrophy, 321–322

336    *Clinical Trials in Neurologic Practice*

National Acute Spinal Cord Injury Studies, 107–111, 108t–109t
National Institute of Allergy and Infectious Diseases Collaborative Antiviral Study Group, 245
National Institute of Neurologic and Communicative Disorders and Stroke–Alzheimer's Disease and Related Disorders Association, 148–149
National Institute of Neurological and Communicative Disorders and Stroke—Association Internationale pour le Recherché et l'Enseignement en Neurosciences, 149
National Institute of Neurological Disorders and Stroke, 41, 44–45, 46t–47t
National Spinal Cord Injury Database, 103
Neurologic recovery, after spinal cord injury, natural history of, 103–104
Neuromyotonia, 315
Neuropathy(ies)
    antimyelin-associated glycoprotein, 273–275
    chronic inflammatory demyelinating. *See* Chronic inflammatory demyelinating neuropathy
    diabetic. *See* Diabetic neuropathy
    diabetic lumbosacral radiculoplexus, 284, 285t
    glycoprotein, antimyelin-associated, 273–275
    with monoclonal gammopathy of uncertain significance, 275–276
    multifocal motor, 270–272
    peripheral. *See* Peripheral neuropathy
Nicardipine, for head injury, 86
Nifedipine, for tics, 213
Nigral grafts, fetal, for Parkinson's disease, 191–192
Nimodipine
    for head injury, 86–87
    for spinal cord injury, 108t–109t, 110–111
    for tremor, 205
    for vasospasm after subarachnoid hemorrhage, 65–66
Nitrogen wasting, in head injury, 91–92
North American Symptomatic Carotid Endarterectomy Trial, 32, 41–42, 46t–47t
Nutrition, in head injury, 91–92

OKY-046, for vasospasm after subarachnoid hemorrhage, 71
Osmotic diuretics, for intracerebral hemorrhage, 53
Outcome(s)
    patient-centered, in randomized clinical trials, 16–18
    primary, assessment of, in randomized clinical trials, 15
    secondary, assessment of, in randomized clinical trials, 15
Oxcarbazepine, for epilepsy, 132–134

Painful legs, 214–215
Pallidotomy, for Parkinson's disease, 189–190
Pancreatic transplantation, in diabetic neuropathy, 278–280, 279t
Parallel design, 5
Parallel group design, in Alzheimer's disease, 161
Parkinson's disease, 173–199
    catechol-O-methyltransferase inhibition in, 184–187
        entacapone, 186–187
        tolcapone, 184–186
    dopamine agonists for, 179–184
        bromocriptine, 180
        cabergoline, 182–183
        pergolide, 180
        pramipexole, 181
        ropinirole, 181–182
    levodopa for. *See* Levodopa, for Parkinson's disease
    prevalence of, 173
    selegiline for, 177–179
    surgical treatment of, 187–192
        globus pallidus interna stimulation, 190
        history of, 187
        pallidotomy, 189–190
        subthalamic nucleus deep brain stimulation, 191
        thalamic deep brain stimulation, 188
        thalamotomy, 187–188
        tissue graft therapies, 191–192
    tremor and. *See* Tremor
Pegorgotein, for head injury, 87–88
Pentobarbital, for head injury, 85–86
Pergolide, for Parkinson's disease, 180
Peripheral neuropathy. *See also specific disorder*
    immune-mediated, 263–276
        antimyelin-associated glycoprotein neuropathy, 273–275

chronic inflammatory demyelinating neuropathy, 267–270
diabetic neuropathy, 276–284
Guillain-Barré syndrome, 263–267
multifocal motor neuropathy, 270–272
neuropathies with monoclonal gammopathy of uncertain significance, 275–276
treatment of, 261–291
Phase I trials, 2–3
Phase II trials, 3
Phase III trials, 3
Phase IV trials, 3
Phenobarbital
for epilepsy, 122–123
for head injury, 85
vs. carbamazepine, for epilepsy, 124–125
vs. primidone, for tremor, 204
Phenytoin
for epilepsy, 123
for head injury, 85
vs. carbamazepine, for epilepsy, 124–125
vs. lamotrigine, for epilepsy, 131
vs. oxcarbazepine, for epilepsy, 133
vs. phenobarbital, for epilepsy, 122–123
Pimozide. See also Gilles de la Tourette; Tic(s)
for tics, 213
vs. haloperidol, for tics, 212
Piracetam, for chorea, 210
Placebo effect, 12–13
Plasma exchange
for antimyelin-associated glycoprotein neuropathy, 273t, 274
for chronic inflammatory demyelinating neuropathy, 267–268, 269t
for Guillain-Barré syndrome, 264–265, 264t
for inflammatory myopathies, 317
for multifocal motor neuropathy, 271
for myasthenia gravis, 313–314
for neuropathies with monoclonal gammopathy of uncertain significance, 275–276, 275t
vs. intravenous immunoglobulin
for chronic inflammatory demyelinating neuropathy, 268–270, 270t
in Guillain-Barré syndrome, 265–266, 265t
for myasthenia gravis, 300–301
Platelet antiaggregants, in stroke prevention, 30–37

Polyethylene glycol conjugated superoxide dismutase, for head injury, 87–88
Polymerase chain reaction technique, for herpes simplex virus encephalitis, 244–245
Polymyositis, 315–318. See also Dermatomyositis; Inclusion body myositis; Myopathy(ies), inflammatory
Ponalrestat, for diabetic neuropathy, 281
Population, of randomized clinical trials, 3–5, 4f
Positron emission tomography (PET), in primary CNS lymphoma vs. toxoplasma encephalitis, 253
Postmarketing study, 3
Power, of randomized clinical trials, 7
Pramipexole, for Parkinson's disease, 181
sleep attacks with, 183
Preclinical studies, 2
Prednisolone
for chronic inflammatory demyelinating neuropathy, 267, 268t
for Guillain-Barré syndrome, 266–267, 266t
vs. azathioprine, for myasthenia gravis, 299
Prednisone
for facioscapulohumeral muscular dystrophy, 320–321
for inflammatory myopathies, 316
for multifocal motor neuropathy, 271
for myasthenia gravis, 298, 312
for Xp21-linked muscular dystrophies, 319
Primary central nervous system (CNS) lymphoma. See Central nervous system (CNS), lymphoma of, primary
Primidone
for tremor, 204
vs. carbamazepine, for epilepsy, 124–125
vs. phenobarbital, for epilepsy, 122–123
Progabide, tremor and, 206–207
Progressive multifocal leukoencephalopathy, 249–250
Propentofylline, in Alzheimer's disease, 156
Propofol, in head injury, 93
Propranolol, for tremor, 203–204
Prostaglandin $E_1$, for diabetic neuropathy, 284
Protein(s), huntingtin-associated. See Huntingtin-associated protein

Pyridostigmine, for myasthenic crisis, 302–303
Pyrimethamine, for toxoplasma encephalitis, 253–254

Quality of life, assessment of, in Alzheimer's disease, 153–154

Radiation therapy, for primary CNS lymphoma, 254
Randomization
blocked, 11
in randomized clinical trials, 10–11
simple, 10–11
Randomized clinical trials, 1–26
blinding in, 11–13
components of, 1–2
control groups in, types of, 28, 28t
data analysis in, 19–22
bias in, 19
interpreting results, 21–22
multiple comparisons in, 20
reporting results, 21
data collection in, 13–14
defined, 1
design of, 5–9, 6f
sample size calculation in, 7–9, 7t, 9t
trial power in, 7–9
historical background of, 1
hypothesis in, 2
outcomes of
assessment of, 13–16
patient-centered, 16–18
phases of, 2–3
randomization in, 10–11
safety in, 33
study population in, 3–5, 4f
Randomized withdrawal design, in Alzheimer's disease, 161
Ranitidine, for head injury, 93
Rebleeding, after aneurysmal subarachnoid hemorrhage, 64–65
Recombinant human insulin-like growth factor I, for myotonic dystrophy, 321
Recombinant human nerve growth factor, for diabetic neuropathy, 282, 283t
Recombinant tissue plasminogen activator, for vasospasm after subarachnoid hemorrhage, 70–71
Reflex(es), loss of, in spinal cord injury, 103
Rehabilitation, in Alzheimer's disease, 163

Relative risk reduction, 22
Reliability, 17
Remacemide, for chorea, 210
Responsiveness, of scale, 18, 18t
Restless legs syndrome, 214–215
Rifampin, for chemoprophylaxis, 244
Ritanserin, for tremor, 206
Rituximab, for antimyelin-associated glycoprotein neuropathy, 273t, 275
Rivastigmine, for Alzheimer's disease, 159
Ropinirole, for Parkinson's disease, 181–182
sleep attacks with, 183

Safety, in randomized clinical trial, 33
Saline, hypertonic, for head injury, 90–91
Sample size calculation, in randomized clinical trials, 7–9, 7t, 9t
Second International Study of Infarct Survival, 20
Sedation, in head injury, 93
Seizure(s), in intracerebral hemorrhage, 52
Selection bias, 10
Selegiline
in Alzheimer's disease, 156
in Parkinson's disease, 177–179
Shock, in spinal cord injury, 103
Sickness Impact Profile, 18
Significance level, in sample size calculation, 7–9
Simple randomization. See Randomization, simple
Single-blind study, 12
Sleep, attacks of, with dopamine agonists, 183
Sodium nitroprusside, for vasospasm after subarachnoid hemorrhage, 71–72
Sorbinil, for diabetic neuropathy, 280, 281t
Sorbinil Retinopathy Trial, 280
Spinal cord injury, 99–120
acute
mechanisms of injury in, primary and secondary, 100, 100t
neurologic recovery after, natural history of, 103–104
nonrandomized studies in, 111–112, 114t–115t
randomized prospective control trials in, 107–111, 108t–109t
surgical decompression for, 108t–109t, 111–112, 114t–115t
treatment of

early, biologic rationale for, 100–101, 100t
optimal, 102–103, 102t
chronic, 113, 116t
importance of, 99–100
incidence of, 99
outcome studies and measures used in methodology of clinical trials, 104–107, 105t
Staging measures, in Alzheimer's disease, 150
Standardized effect size, calculation of, responsiveness and, 18, 18t
Standardized response mean, calculation of, responsiveness and, 18, 18t
Standards of Reporting Trials, 21
State of California Alzheimer's Disease Diagnostic and Treatment Centers, 149
Stroke, 27–48
Kaplan-Meier graphs in, 27
overview of, 27–30
prevention of. *See* Stroke prevention
treatment of, 43–45
Stroke Council of the American Heart Association, 63
Stroke prevention, 30–42
anticoagulants in, 37–38, 39f
warfarin, 37–38, 39f
platelet antiaggregants in, 30–37
aspirin, 30–32, 31t
clopidogrel, 34–35, 36t
dipyridamole with aspirin, 35–37
ticlopidine, 32–34
surgery in, 38–42
carotid endarterectomy, 40–42
extracranial-intracranial (EC/IC) arterial bypass, 38–40, 40t
Stroke Prevention in Atrial Fibrillation, 37–38, 39f, 46t–47t
Study population, of randomized clinical trials, 3–5, 4f
Subarachnoid hemorrhage, aneurysmal, 63–75. *See also* Aneurysm(s), rupture of, subarachnoid hemmorhage due to
coiling for, 64
morbidity of, 63
mortality of, 63
rebleeding in, 64–65
vasospasm after, prevention and treatment of. *See* Vasospasm, after aneurysmal subarachnoid hem-

orrhage, prevention and treatment of
Subgroup analysis, 20–21
Subthalamic nucleus deep brain stimulation, for Parkinson's disease, 191
Sulfadiazine, for toxoplasma encephalitis, 253–254
Sulfinpyrazone, in stroke prevention, 30–32, 31t
Superoxide dismutase, for head injury, 87–88
Surgical decompression, for spinal cord injury
acute, 108t–109t, 111–112, 114t–115t
chronic, 113, 116t
Surrogate outcome variables, 15–16
Swedish Aspirin Low-Dose Trial, 7–8, 9

Tacrine, for Alzheimer's disease, 158
Tardive dyskinesia. *See* Chorea
Testosterone enanthate, for myotonic dystrophy, 321–322
Tetrabenazine, for chorea, 210
Tetrahydroaminoacridine, for Alzheimer's disease, 158
Thalamic deep brain stimulation, for Parkinson's disease, 188
Thalamotomy
for Parkinson's disease, 187–188
for tremor, 206
vs. thalamic deep brain stimulation, for Parkinson's disease, 188
Thalamus, surgery on, for Parkinson's disease, 187–188
Theophylline, for tremor, 205
Thiopental, for intracerebral hemorrhage, 53
Thromboxane synthetase inhibitor, intravenous, for vasospasm after subarachnoid hemorrhage, 71
Thymectomy, for myasthenia gravis, 295–297, 313
classification of, 306, 308t
Thyrotropin-releasing hormone, for spinal cord injury, 108t–109t, 110
Tiagabine, for epilepsy, 134–136
Tic(s), 212–214. *See also* Gilles de la Tourette; Pimozide
assessment of, 212
treatment of, 212–214
Ticlopidine, in stroke prevention, 32–34
Ticlopidine Aspirin Stroke Study Group, 32–34, 46t–47t

## 340 Clinical Trials in Neurologic Practice

Tirilazad mesylate
for head injury, 81, 87–88
for vasospasm after subarachnoid hemorrhage, 68–69
Tissue grafts, for Parkinson's disease. See Parkinson's disease, surgical treatment of, tissue graft therapies
Tissue plasminogen activator, for acute stroke, 44–45
α-Tocopherol, in Alzheimer's disease, 156
Tocopherol, vs. deprenyl, for Parkinson's disease, 177–179
Toe(s), moving, 214–215
Tolcapone, for Parkinson's disease, 184–186
Tolrestat, for diabetic neuropathy, 280–281, 281t
Topiramate, for epilepsy, 136–137
Total neuropathy score, 262–263, 262t
Total parenteral nutrition, in head injury, 91
Tourette Syndrome Classification Study Group, 212
Toxoplasma encephalitis, 252–255
treatment of, 253–254
Transient ischemic attack. See Stroke
Transluminal balloon angioplasty, for vasospasm after subarachnoid hemorrhage, 69
Transplantation, pancreatic, in diabetic neuropathy, 278–280, 279t
Traumatic brain injury, 77–98. See also Head injury
Tremor, 201–207
adenosine antagonists for, 205
benzodiazepines for, 205
beta-adrenergic receptor antagonists for, 203–204
botulinum toxin type A for, 205
calcium channel blockers for, 205
clozapine for, 204–205
duration of, 202
ethanol for, 204
inclusion criteria for, 202
isoniazid for, 205
primidone for, 204
recording of, 203
ritanserin for, 206
surgical treatment of, 206
test conditions in, 202
Trial(s), randomized clinical. See Randomized clinical trials

Trial of Organon 10172 in Acute Stroke Treatment, 43, 46t–47t
Triamcinolone, for head injury, 87
Triple-H therapy, for vasospasm after subarachnoid hemorrhage, 66–68
Tromethamine, for head injury, 89
Tumor necrosis factor, for bacterial meningitis, 241–242
Type I error, 7
Type II error, 7

Ubiquinone, for chorea, 211
Unblinded study, 11–12
Unified Parkinson's Disease Rating Scale, 174
Unified Huntington's Disease Rating Scale, 208–209
United Parkinson's Disease Rating Scale, 203
University of Toronto Head Injury Treatment Study, 90–91
Urokinase, for vasospasm after subarachnoid hemorrhage, 71

Valacyclovir, for varicella-zoster virus, 245–246
Validity, 17–18
Valproate
for epilepsy, 125–127
for head injury, 85
vs. felbamate, for epilepsy, 127–128
vs. lamotrigine, for epilepsy, 131
vs. zonisamide, for epilepsy, 140
Vancomycin
dexamethasone with, for bacterial meningitis, 239–240
for bacterial meningitis, 239–240
Varicella-zoster virus, 244–246
treatment of, 245–246
Vascular dementia, 164
diagnostic criteria for, 149
Vasospasm, after aneurysmal subarachnoid hemorrhage, prevention and treatment of, 65–69
calcium antagonists in, 65–66
endothelin receptor antagonists in, 71–72
intracisternal fibrinolytic treatment in, 70–71
intravenous thromboxane synthetase inhibitor in, 71
natrium nitroprusside in, 71–72
tirilazad mesylate in, 68–69
transluminal balloon angioplasty in, 69
triple-H therapy in, 66–68

Vigabatrin
   for epilepsy, 137–139
   vs. lamotrigine, for epilepsy, 132

Warfarin, in stroke prevention, 37–38,
         39f

Zidovudine
   for HIV-dementia, 247
   indinavir and lamivudine with, for HIV,
         248
Zonisamide, for epilepsy. *See* Antiepileptic
         drugs